Stem Cell and Bone Marrow Transplantation

Stem Cell and Bone Marrow Transplantation

Editor: Williams Douglas

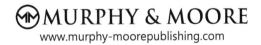

MURPHY & MOORE

www.murphy-moorepublishing.com

www.murphy-moorepublishing.com

ⓂMURPHY & MOORE

Cataloging-in-Publication Data

Stem cell and bone marrow transplantation / edited by Williams Douglas.
　　p. cm.
Includes bibliographical references and index.
ISBN 978-1-63987-507-8
1. Bone marrow--Transplantation. 2. Hematopoietic stem cells--Transplantation.
3. Transplantation of organs, tissues, etc. I. Douglas, Williams.
RD123.5 .S74 2022
61744--dc23

Murphy & Moore Publishing,
1 Rockefeller Plaza,
New York City, NY 10020, USA

ISBN 978-1-63987-507-8 (Hardback)

Contents

Permissions

List of Contributors

Index

Preface

Bone marrow transplantation involves introducing healthy blood-forming cells in order to supplant diseased or impaired bone marrow. It is also known as a stem cell transplant. It is used to treat numerous medical conditions such as acute leukemia, adrenoleukodystrophy, aplastic anemia and chronic leukemia. The procedure involves pretransplant procedures and examinations wherein the health of the patient is monitored. There are two major types of cell transplant procedures, namely, autologous stem cell transplant and allogeneic stem cell transplant. Autologous stem cell transplant makes use of healthy stem cells from a person's own body to replace damaged bone marrow. Allogeneic stem cell transplants take cells from another donor for the treatment of the bone marrow. This book discusses the fundamentals as well as modern approaches of stem cell and bone marrow transplantation. It will also provide interesting topics for research which interested readers can take up. The book is appropriate for medical students seeking detailed information in this area as well as for experts.

Various studies have approached the subject by analyzing it with a single perspective, but the present book provides diverse methodologies and techniques to address this field. This book contains theories and applications needed for understanding the subject from different perspectives. The aim is to keep the readers informed about the progresses in the field; therefore, the contributions were carefully examined to compile novel researches by specialists from across the globe.

Indeed, the job of the editor is the most crucial and challenging in compiling all chapters into a single book. In the end, I would extend my sincere thanks to the chapter authors for their profound work. I am also thankful for the support provided by my family and colleagues during the compilation of this book.

Editor

Part I
Introduction

Topic leaders: Mohamad Mohty and Jane Apperley

HSCT: Historical Perspective

Rainer Storb

1.1 Introduction

HSCT has evolved from a field that was declared dead in the 1960s to the amazing clinical results obtained today in the treatment of otherwise fatal blood disorders. This chapter will reflect upon how HSCT has progressed from the laboratory to clinical reality.

1.2 Early Enthusiasm and Disappointment

Research efforts on how to repair radiation effects resulted from observations on radiation damage among survivors of the atomic bomb explosions in Japan (reviewed in van Bekkum and de Vries 1967). In 1949, Jacobson and colleagues discovered protection of mice from TBI by shielding their spleens with lead. Two years later, Lorenz and colleagues reported radiation protection of mice and guinea pigs by infusing marrow cells. Initially many investigators, including Jacobson, thought that the radiation protection was from some humoral factor(s) in spleen or marrow. However, by the mid-1950s, this "humoral

R. Storb (✉)
Clinical Research Division,
Fred Hutchinson Cancer Research Center and
University of Washington, School of Medicine,
Seattle, WA, USA
e-mail: rstorb@fredhutch.org

hypothesis" was firmly rejected, and several laboratories convincingly demonstrated that the radiation protection was due to seeding of the marrow by donor cells.

This discovery was greeted with enthusiasm because of the implications for cell biology and for therapy of patients with life-threatening blood disorders. The principle of HSCT was simple: high-dose radiation/chemotherapy would both destroy the diseased marrow and suppress the patient's immune cells for a donor graft to be accepted. Within 1 year of the pivotal rodent studies, Thomas and colleagues showed that marrow could safely be infused into leukemia patients and engraft, even though, in the end, the leukemia relapsed. In 1958, Mathé's group attempted the rescue, by marrow transplantation, of six nuclear reactor workers accidentally exposed to TBI. Four of the six survived, although donor cells persisted only transiently. In 1965, Mathé and colleagues treated a leukemia patient with TBI and then marrows from six relatives, absent any knowledge of histocompatibility (Mathe et al. 1965). A brother's marrow engrafted. The patient went into remission but eventually succumbed to a complication, GVHD. Following up on early observations by Barnes and Loutit in mice, Mathé coined the term "graft-vs.-leukemia effect." In 1970, Bortin summarized results of 200 human marrow grafts reported between 1957 and 1967 (Bortin 1970). All 200 patients died of either graft failure, GVHD, infections, or recurrence of leukemia.

These transplants were performed before a clear understanding of conditioning regimens, histocompatibility matching, and control of GVHD. They were based directly on work in inbred mice, for which histocompatibility matching is not absolutely required. In 1967, van Bekkum and de Vries stated, "These failures have occurred mainly because the clinical applications were undertaken too soon, most of them before even the minimum basic knowledge required to bridge the gap between mouse and patient had been obtained." Clinical HSCT was declared a total failure and prominent immunologists pronounced that the barrier between individuals could never be crossed.

1.3 Back to the Laboratory: Focus on Animal Studies

Most investigators left the field, pronouncing it a dead end. However, a few laboratories continued animal studies aimed at understanding and eventually overcoming the obstacles encountered in human allogeneic HSCT. Van Bekkum's group in Holland used primates, George Santos at Johns Hopkins chose rats, and the Seattle group chose outbred dogs as experimental models. One reason behind using dogs was that, besides humans, only dogs combine unusual genetic diversity with a widespread, well-mixed gene pool. Also, dogs share spontaneous diseases with humans, such as non-Hodgkin lymphoma and X-linked SCID. In addition to determining the best ways to administer TBI, new drugs with myeloablative or immunosuppressive qualities were introduced, including cyclophosphamide, ATG, and BU (Santos 1995). These agents improved engraftment and provided for tumor cell killing similar to TBI. Based on the mouse histocompatibility system defined 10 years earlier, in vitro histocompatibility typing for dogs was developed. Studies from 1968 showed that dogs given grafts from dog leukocyte antigen (DLA)-matched littermates or unrelated donors survived significantly longer than their DLA-mismatched counterparts, even though typing techniques were very primitive and the complexity of the genetic region coding for major antigens

was far from understood (Epstein et al. 1968). Serious GVHD was first described in H-2 mismatched mice and in randomly selected monkeys. However, the canine studies first drew attention to fatal GVHD across minor histocompatibility barriers.

These pivotal observations drove the search for Post transplant drug regimens to control GVHD. The most promising drug was the folic acid antagonist, MTX (Storb et al. 1970). Further work in canines showed that transfusion-induced sensitization to minor antigens caused rejection of DLA-identical grafts (reviewed in Georges and Storb 2016). Subsequent canine studies eventually led to ways of understanding, preventing, and overcoming transfusion-induced sensitization. Next, mechanisms of graft-host tolerance were investigated. It turned out that IS could often be discontinued after 3–6 months, and donor-derived T lymphocytes were identified that downregulated immune reactions of other donor T cells against GVHD targets. Immune reconstitution was found to be complete in long-term canine chimeras, enabling them to live in an unprotected environment. Techniques for isolating transplantable stem cells from peripheral blood were refined in dogs and primates. Importantly, studies in pet dogs with non-Hodgkin lymphoma showed cures, in part due to graft-vs.-tumor effects.

1.4 Resuming Clinical Transplantation: 1968–1980s

The second half of the 1960s saw the refinement of high-intensity conditioning regimens, including fractionated TBI and maximally tolerated doses of CY or BU (Santos 1995). Histocompatibility matching was confirmed to be of utmost importance for reducing both graft rejection and GVHD (Thomas et al. 1975). However, even when donor and recipient were well matched, GVHD was a problem unless postgrafting MTX was given, which slowed donor lymphocyte replication. Rapid progress in understanding the molecular nature of the major human histocompatibility complex—HLA—improved matching of donor recipient pairs.

By 1968, the stage was set to resume clinical trials. The first successful transplants were for patients with primary immune deficiency disorders. A 5-month-old boy with "thymic alymphoplasia and agammaglobulinemia" was not perfectly matched with his sister (Gatti et al. 1968). Marrow and peripheral blood cells were infused intraperitoneally without conditioning. After a booster infusion several months later, the patient fully recovered with donor hematopoiesis and is well. A patient with Wiskott-Aldrich syndrome received a first unsuccessful marrow infusion from an HLA-identical sister without conditioning (Bach et al. 1968). A second transplant following CY conditioning resulted in full T- and B-cell recovery, but thrombocytopenia persisted.

During the first 7 or 8 years, most clinical studies were for patients with advanced hematological malignancies and SAA, who were in poor condition and presented tremendous challenges in supportive care (Thomas et al. 1975). They required transfusions and prophylaxis or treatment of bacterial, fungal, and viral infections. Therefore, in addition to discoveries made in marrow transplantation, these early trials stimulated advances in infectious diseases and transfusions (reviewed in Forman et al. 2016). The longest survivors from that era are patients with aplastic anemia who are approaching their 47th anniversary from HSCT with fully recovered donor-derived hematopoiesis and leading normal lives. Chronic GVHD emerged as a new problem among long-term survivors.

The initial studies saw GVHD among approximately half of the patients, despite HLA matching and despite receiving methotrexate. This stimulated further research in the canine system. Major improvements in GVHD control and patient survival were made when combining MTX with CNI inhibitors such as CSA or TAC (Storb et al. 1986). Combinations of drugs have remained a mainstay in GVHD prevention. GVHD treatment with PRD was introduced.

Early results with marrow grafts from HLA-identical siblings after CY for SAA showed 45% long-term survival (reviewed in Georges and Storb 2016). The major cause of failure was graft rejection as expected from canine studies on transfusion-induced sensitization to minor antigens. Canine studies identified dendritic cells in transfusions to be the key element in sensitization. Depleting transfusions of white cells, therefore, reduced the rejection risk. Further canine studies generated a clinical conditioning regimen that alternated CY and ATG, which greatly reduced the rates of both graft rejection and chronic GVHD (Storb et al. 1994). Finally, irradiation of blood products with 2000 cGy in vitro almost completely averted sensitization to minor antigens. Consequently, graft rejection in transplantation for AA has become the exception, and current survivals with HLA-identical sibling and HLA-matched unrelated grafts range from 90% to 100%. First successful grafts for thalassemia (Thomas et al. 1982) and sickle cell disease were reported.

For patients with leukemia and other malignant blood diseases, disease relapse after HSCT has remained a major problem. Attempts to reduce relapse by increasing the intensity of systemic conditioning regimens have met with success, but this benefit was offset by higher non-relapse mortality. Reports by Weiden and the Seattle group in 1979/1981 firmly established the existence of graft-vs.-leukemia (GvL) effects in humans (Weiden et al. 1979). DLI to combat relapse were introduced by Kolb and colleagues in 1990 (Kolb et al. 1990) (see Chap. 59).

Some investigators have removed T cells from the marrow as a means of preventing GVHD (reviewed in Soiffer 2016). Early studies showed high incidences of graft rejection, relapse of underlying malignancies, and infections. More recent studies showed that relapse seemed a lesser problem in patients with acute leukemia. Others have used T-cell depletion with close disease monitoring and treating recurrence with DLI in hopes of initiating GvL responses without causing GVHD. Most recently, younger patients have been given high-intensity conditioning for grafts which were depleted of naïve T cells with a resulting decrease in GVHD (Bleakley et al. 2015).

The late 1980s saw the introduction of G-CSF-mobilized PBSC (reviewed in Schmitz and

Dreger 2016). These were equivalent to marrow as far as engraftment and survival were concerned; however, they seemed to increase the risk of chronic GVHD. For patients with nonmalignant diseases, marrow has therefore remained the preferred source of stem cells in order to keep the rate of chronic GVHD low.

Only approximately 35% of patients have HLA-identical siblings. Therefore, alternative donors have been explored, predominantly HLA-matched unrelated volunteers. The first successful unrelated transplant for leukemia was reported in 1980. In order to expand the donor pool, national registries were established, with currently more than 30 million HLA-typed unrelated volunteers (reviewed in Confer et al. 2016). The likelihood of finding suitable unrelated donors is approximately 80% for Caucasians, although this percentage declines dramatically for patients from minority groups. A second, important alternative stem cell source has been unrelated cord blood (Gluckman et al. 1989), not requiring complete HLA matching and resulting in encouraging outcomes among patients with malignant blood diseases. First attempts with yet another donor source have included TCD megadose CD34+ cell grafts from related HLA-haploidentical donors to treat acute leukemia (Aversa et al. 1998).

1.5 Moving Ahead: The 1990s and Beyond

Conventional HSCT following high-intensity conditioning is risky and requires specialized intensive care wards. The associated toxicities restrict the therapy to younger, medically fit patients. To allow the inclusion of older (highest prevalence of hematological malignancies), medically infirm or very young immunodeficiency patients, less intensive conditioning programs have been developed. In patients with malignancies, these rely less on high-dose chemoradiation therapy and more on graft-vs.-tumor effects.

One outpatient transplant strategy combines FLU and 2–3 Gy TBI conditioning with Post transplant IS using an inhibitor of purine synthesis MMF and CSA or TAC. Figure 1.1 illustrates the spectrum of current conditioning regimens (reviewed in Storb and Sandmaier 2016).

A transplant regimen combining fludarabine and 2 Gy TBI conditioning with additional cyclophosphamide before and after HSCT has encouraged widespread use of unmodified HLA-haploidentical grafts (Luznik et al. 2008). It is well tolerated with low incidences of graft rejection and of acute and chronic GVHD, but relapse remains a problem. Strategies addressing relapse have included infusion of donor lymphocytes or NK cells. Retrospective multicenter analyses show comparable outcomes after HLA-matched vs. HLA-haploidentical HSCT.

While reduced-intensity regimens have been well tolerated, relapse and GVHD need improving. Adding targeted radioimmunotherapy against host hematopoietic cells, using anti-CD45 antibody coupled to beta and alpha emitting radionuclides to standard conditioning, has the potential to decrease the pre-transplant tumor burden, thereby lessening the relapse risk (Chen et al. 2012; Pagel et al. 2009). As for GVHD, a recent phase III randomized trial convincingly demonstrated that a triple combination of MMF/cyclosporine/sirolimus significantly reduced both acute GVHD and non-relapse mortality and improved survival (Sandmaier et al. 2016).

Survival of patients with primary immune deficiency diseases given NMA conditioning before HLA-matched and HLA-mismatched grafts between 1998 and 2006 has stabilized at 82% (Moratto et al. 2011).

In the future, better understanding of hematopoietic cell-specific polymorphic minor histocompatibility antigens might result in ways of directing donor immune cells toward hematopoietic targets, thereby controlling relapse without inducing GVHD. Another major research target is containment of chronic GVHD.

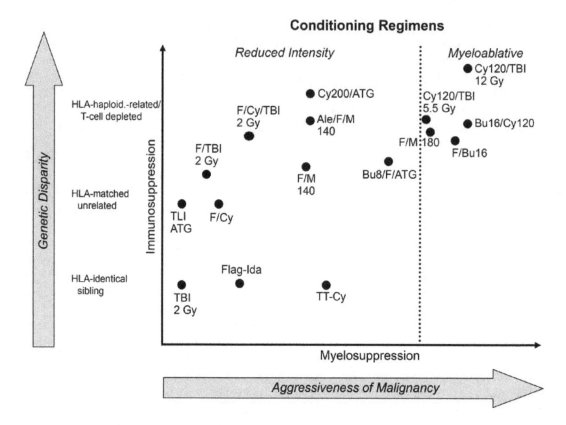

Fig. 1.1 Spectrum of current conditioning regimens. Reproduced with permission from Sandmaier, B.M. and Storb, R. Reduced-intensity allogeneic transplantation regimens (Ch. 21). In Thomas' Hematopoietic Cell Transplantation, fifth edition (ed. by Forman SJ, Negrin RS, Antin JH, & Appelbaum FR) 2016, pp. 232–243. John Wiley & Sons, Ltd., Chichester, UK

Key Points
- Radiation protection of rodents by shielding the spleen or marrow infusion
- First human transplants all failed
- Allogeneic HSCT called a total failure
- HSCT studies in large animals: Histocompatibility matching; MTX for GVHD prevention; CY, ATG, and BU; rejection from transfusion-induced sensitization; PBSC; graft-versus-lymphoma effect
- Fractionated TBI
- HSCT for patients with immunodeficiency diseases, aplastic anemia, leukemia, hemoglobinopathies

- Advances in infection prophylaxis and treatment
- Graft-versus-leukemia effects
- Donor lymphocyte infusions
- ATG conditioning
- Unrelated donors
- Cord blood transplants
- Mega CD34+ HLA-haploidentical grafts
- MTX/CNI GVHD prophylaxis
- Reduced and minimal intensity conditioning
- Outpatient transplantation
- PT-CY GVHD prophylaxis
- Targeted radioimmunotherapy

References

Aversa F, Tabilio A, Velardi A, et al. Treatment of high-risk acute leukemia with T-cell-depleted stem cells from related donors with one fully mismatched HLA haplotype. N Engl J Med. 1998;339:1186–93.

Bach FH, Albertini RJ, Joo P, et al. Bone-marrow transplantation in a patient with the Wiskott-Aldrich syndrome. Lancet. 1968;2:1364–6.

van Bekkum DW, de Vries MJ. Radiation chimaeras. London: Logos Press; 1967.

Bleakley M, Heimfeld S, Loeb KR, et al. Outcomes of acute leukemia patients transplanted with naive T cell-depleted stem cell grafts. J Clin Invest. 2015;125:2677–89.

Bortin MM. A compendium of reported human bone marrow transplants. Transplantation. 1970;9:571–87.

Chen Y, Kornblit B, Hamlin DK, et al. Durable donor engraftment after radioimmunotherapy using alpha-emitter astatine-211-labeled anti-CD45 antibody for conditioning in allogeneic hematopoietic cell transplantation. Blood. 2012;119:1130–8.

Confer DL, Miller JP, Chell JW. Bone marrow and peripheral blood cell donors and donor registries. In: Forman SJ, Negrin RS, Antin JH, Appelbaum FR, editors. Thomas' hematopoietic cell transplantation. 5th ed. Chichester: Wiley; 2016. p. 423–30.

Epstein RB, Storb R, Ragde H, Thomas ED. Cytotoxic typing antisera for marrow grafting in littermate dogs. Transplantation. 1968;6:45–58.

Forman SJ, Negrin RS, Antin JH. F.R.A. complications of hematopoietic cell transplantation. (Ch. Part 7). In: Thomas' hematopoietic cell transplantation. 5th ed. Chichester: Wiley; 2016. p. 944–1306.

Gatti RA, Meuwissen HJ, Allen HD, et al. Immunological reconstitution of sex-linked lymphopenic immunological deficiency. Lancet. 1968;2:1366–9.

Georges GE, Storb R. Hematopoietic cell transplantation for aplastic anemia. In: Forman SJ, Negrin RS, Antin JH, Appelbaum FR, editors. Thomas' hematopoietic cell transplantation. 5th ed. Chichester: Wiley; 2016. p. 517–36.

Gluckman E, Broxmeyer HE, Auerbach AD, et al. Hematopoietic reconstitution in a patient with Fanconi's anemia by means of umbilical-cord blood from an HLA-identical sibling. N Engl J Med. 1989;321:1174–8.

Kolb HJ, Mittermüller J, Clemm C, et al. Donor leukocyte transfusions for treatment of recurrent chronic myelogenous leukemia in marrow transplant patients. Blood. 1990;76:2462–5.

Luznik L, O'Donnell PV, Symons HJ, et al. HLA-haploidentical bone marrow transplantation for hematologic malignancies using nonmyeloablative conditioning and high-dose, post-transplantation cyclophosphamide. Biol Blood Marrow Transplant. 2008;14:641–50.

Mathe G, Amiel JL, Schwarzenberg L, Cattan A, Schneider M. Adoptive immunotherapy of acute leukemia: experimental and clinical results. Cancer Res. 1965;25:1525–31.

Moratto D, Giliani S, Bonfim C, et al. Long-term outcome and lineage-specific chimerism in 194 patients with Wiskott-Aldrich syndrome treated by hematopoietic cell transplantation in the period 1980-2009: an international collaborative study. Blood. 2011;118:1675–84.

Pagel JM, Gooley TA, Rajendran J, et al. Allogeneic hematopoietic cell transplantation after conditioning with 131 I-anti-CD45 antibody plus fludarabine and low-dose total body irradiation for elderly patients with advanced acute myeloid leukemia or high-risk myelodysplastic syndrome. Blood. 2009;114:5444–53.

Sandmaier BM, Maloney DG, Storer BE, et al. Sirolimus combined with mycophenolate mofetil (MMF) and cyclosporine (CSP) significantly improves prevention of acute graft-versus-host-disease (GVHD) after unrelated hematopoietic cell transplantation (HCT): results from a phase III randomized multi-center trial. Blood. 2016;128:#506. (abstract); http://www.bloodjournal.org/content/128/522/506

Santos GW. Preparative regimens: chemotherapy versus chemoradiotherapy. A historical perspective. (review). Ann N Y Acad Sci. 1995;770:1–7.

Schmitz N, Dreger P. Peripheral blood hematopoietic cells for allogeneic transplantation. (Ch. 41). In: Forman SJ, Negrin RS, Antin JH, Appelbaum FR, editors. Thomas' hematopoietic cell transplantation. 5th ed. Chichester: Wiley; 2016. p. 460–8.

Soiffer RJ. T-cell depletion to prevent graft-versus-host disease. (Ch. 82). In: Forman SJ, Negrin RS, Antin JH, Appelbaum FR, editors. Thomas' hematopoietic cell transplantation. 5th ed. Chichester: Wiley; 2016. p. 965–72.

Storb R, Deeg HJ, Whitehead J, et al. Methotrexate and cyclosporine compared with cyclosporine alone for prophylaxis of acute graft versus host disease after marrow transplantation for leukemia. N Engl J Med. 1986;314:729–35.

Storb R, Epstein RB, Graham TC, Thomas ED. Methotrexate regimens for control of graft-versus-host disease in dogs with allogeneic marrow grafts. Transplantation. 1970;9:240–6.

Storb R, Etzioni R, Anasetti C, et al. Cyclophosphamide combined with antithymocyte globulin in preparation for allogeneic marrow transplants in patients with aplastic anemia. Blood. 1994;84:941–9.

Storb R, Sandmaier BM. Nonmyeloablative allogeneic hematopoietic cell transplantation. Haematologica. 2016;101:521–30.

Thomas ED, Buckner CD, Sanders JE, et al. Marrow transplantation for thalassaemia. Lancet. 1982;2:227–9.

Thomas ED, Storb R, Clift RA, et al. Bone-marrow transplantation. N Engl J Med. 1975;292:832–43. 895–902.

Weiden PL, Flournoy N, Thomas ED, et al. Antileukemic effect of graft-versus-host disease in human recipients of allogeneic-marrow grafts. N Engl J Med. 1979;300:1068–73.

The EBMT: History, Present, and Future

Alois Gratwohl, Mohamad Mohty,
and Jane Apperley

2.1 Introduction

"Only he/she who knows the past has a future" is a proverb attributed to Wilhelm von Humboldt (1767–1835), a great historian, scientist, and philosopher (Spier 2015). It appears as an ideal introduction to a chapter on the history of EBMT. The context by which HSCT evolved in the middle of last century fits with modern views on history. The novel "big history" concept attempts to integrate major events in the past, beginning with the "big bang" up to today's industrial revolution number IV (Spier 2015). According to this model, nothing "just happens." Progress occurs when the conditions fit, at the right time and at the right place. Such circumstances are called "Goldilocks conditions," according to the novel by Robert Southey (https://en.wikipedia.org/wiki/Goldilocks_and_the_Three_Bears. accessed November 6, 2018). They hold true for the formation of galaxies, suns, and planets, for the appearance of life on earth, or for

A. Gratwohl (✉)
Hematology, Medical Faculty, University of Basel, Basel, Switzerland
e-mail: alois.gratwohl@unibas.ch

M. Mohty
Hematology, Hôpital St. Antoine, Sorbonne University, Paris, France

J. Apperley
Centre for Haematology, Hammersmith Hospital, Imperial College London, London, UK

the evolution of mankind. They apply specifically to the latter: as the one and only species, *Homo sapiens* managed to create "Goldilocks conditions" by him or herself. They allowed man to fit religion, art, or beliefs in such ways to master society. In our perspective, big history thinking helps to understand the development of HSCT and EBMT and to view it in a broader framework. It provides as well a caveat for the future.

2.2 The Past: Development of HSCT and EBMT

The use of bone marrow (BM) for healing purposes dates back long in history, and BM from hunted animals might have contributed as rich nourishment to the evolution of *Homo sapiens* (McCann 2016). Its recognition as primary hematopoietic organ in adult life with a hematopoietic stem cell as source of the circulating blood cells began in the middle of the nineteenth century (Schinck 1920). It did result in some early recommendations on the potential therapeutic use of bone marrow (JAMA 1997; Osgood et al. 1939), but with no broader application. All changed after the explosions of atomic bombs in Hiroshima and Nagasaki in World War II, when survivors of the immediate exposure died from BM failure (Van Bekkum and De Vries 1967). Research was directed to find ways to treat this lethal complication. It led to the discovery that bone marrow-derived stem cells from a healthy donor could replace hematopoiesis after total body irradiation (TBI); it provided at the same time, a tool, TBI, to eradicate aberrant hematopoiesis (Van Bekkum and De Vries 1967; Jacobson et al. 1949; Lorenz et al. 1951; Ford et al. 1956). The concept of HSCT was born, and "the conditions were right." It is to no surprise that the first clinical BMT centers in Europe started in hospitals with close links to radiobiology research institutes in the UK, the Netherlands, France, and Germany. Funding of radiobiology fostered basic research and stimulated clinical application. In the first series of patients reported in the NEJM in 1957 by the late Nobel Prize winner ED Thomas, all six patients died but two of them with clear signs of donor chimerism (Thomas et al. 1957). And, BMT "saved" accidentally irradiated workers of a radiation facility in Vinca, a town in former Jugoslawia (Mathé et al. 1959). Hence, the clinical results confirmed the "proof of principle" obtained in mice: TBI could eradicate normal and malignant bone marrow cells, and the infusion of healthy donor bone marrow cells could restore the recipient's depleted hematopoiesis with functioning donor cells. In reality, of more than 200 patients reported by M. Bortin for the IBMTR, all patients with leukemia had died, many of them free of their disease. Three patients survived, all with congenital immune deficiency and transplanted from HLA-identical sibling donors (Bortin 1970). Despite the dismal results, Goldilocks conditions prevailed. Armed forces were convinced of the need for a rescue tool in the event of a nuclear war, physicians viewed BMT as an instrument to treat hitherto incurable blood disorders, and patients envisioned a cure of their lethal disease.

In order to improve outcome, the "believers" joined forces. They met each other, openly reviewed their cases and charts one by one, exchanged views on hurdles and opportunities, spent time together on the slopes in the Alps, and became friendly rivals: EBMT was born. Goldilocks conditions still prevailed. Leukemia could be eradicated. BMT with haploidentical donor bone marrow for SAA after conditioning with ATG yielded spectacular results (Speck et al. 1977). Today, we know that ATG, rather than the cells, was responsible for the outcome.

The introduction of intensive induction regimens for AML enabled stable phases of complete first remission (CR1) (Crowther et al. 1970). The discovery of CSA, as the first of its kind of novel IS agents, opened new dimensions in BMT and other organ transplantation (Kay et al. 1980). It became acceptable to transplant patients in early phase of their disease, e.g., CR1 or first chronic phase (CP1) (Thomas et al. 1975). The boom of BMT began (Thomas 2007; Gratwohl et al. 2015a). The first patient in the EBMT database dates back to 1965. In 1973, at the first informal gathering in St. Moritz, the database comprised 13 patients; 4 transplanted in that year. In 1980, a total of 285 HSCT were performed, increasing to 4025 10 years later.

HSCT rapidly diversified in terms of donor type, by including autologous and allogeneic stem cells from related and unrelated donors, and of stem cell source, from bone marrow and peripheral blood to cord blood. Indications expanded from the early congenital immunodeficiency, leukemia, and aplastic anemia to a full variety of severe congenital disorders of the hematopoietic system, to other hematological malignancies such as myeloma and lymphoma, and to non-hematological malignancies, e.g., germ cell tumors. The HSCT technology improved to encompass a variety of in vivo and ex vivo GvHD prevention methods and conditioning regimens of varying intensities with or without TBI. HSCT became open to centers with no links to radiobiology institutes and was no longer bound to "sterile units" and to selected countries (Gratwohl et al. 2015a; Copelan, 2006).

The previously informal gatherings and the database no longer sufficed to share the urgently needed information exchange. EBMT became a formal structure, with elections for presidents and working party chairs. It was listed in PubMed for the first time in 1985 (EBMT 1985). The meetings were no longer confined to ski resorts and became open to all involved in patient care and scientific analyses (Table 2.1). Obviously, organization of the annual meeting is today a major undertaking and only possible with the support of corporate sponsors. Still, the initial spirit remains.

Table 2.1 List of EBMT meetings and presidents

Year	Location annual meeting	Participating groups	EBMT president
1974			Informal gathering
1975	St. Moritz, Switzerland	1st P	
1976	St. Moritz, Switzerland	2nd P	B. Speck[a]
1977	Courchevel, France	3rd P	B. Speck[a]
1978	Courchevel, France	4th P	B. Speck[a]
1979	St. Moritz, Switzerland	5th P	E. Gluckman
1980	Sils-Maria, Switzerland	6th P	E. Gluckman
1981	Courchevel, France	7th P	E. Kubanek
1982	Courmayeur, Italy	8th P	E. Gordon-Smith
1983	Oberstdorf, Germany	9th P	E. Gordon-Smith
1984	Granada, Spain	10th P	J. Barrett
1985	Bad Hofgastein, Austria	11th P, 1st N	J. Barrett
1986	Courmayeur, Italy	12th P, 2nd N	A. Marmont[a]
1987	Interlaken, Switzerland	13th P, 3rd N	A. Marmont[a]
1988	Chamonix, France	14th P, 4th N	G. Gharton
1989	Bad Hofgastein, Austria	15th P, 5th N	G. Gharton
1990	The Hague, Netherlands	16th P, 6th N	J. Goldman[a]
1991	Cortina d'Ampezzo, Italy	17th P, 7th N	J. Goldman[a]
1992	Stockholm, Sweden	18th P, 8th N	J. Goldman[a]
1993	Garmisch-Partenkirchen, Germany	19th P, 9th N	J. Goldman[a]
1994	Harrogate, UK	20th P, 10th N	A. Gratwohl
1995	Davos, Switzerland	21st P, 11th N	A. Gratwohl
1996	Vienna, Austria	22nd P, 12th N	A. Gratwohl
1997	Aix-les-bains, France	23rd P, 13th N	A. Gratwohl
1998	Courmayeur, Italy	24th P, 14th N	A. Bacigalupo
1999	Hamburg, Germany	25th P, 15th N	A. Bacigalupo
2000	Innsbruck, Germany	26th P, 16th N	A. Bacigalupo
2001	Maastricht, Netherlands	27th P, 17th N	A. Bacigalupo
2002	Montreux, Switzerland	28th P, 18th N, 1st DM	J. Apperley
2003	Istanbul, Turkey	29th P, 19th N, 2nd DM	J. Apperley
2004	Barcelona, Spain	30th P, 20th N, 3d DM	J. Apperley
2005	Prague, Czech Republic	31st P, 21st N, 4th DM	J. Apperley
2006	Hamburg, Germany	32nd P, 22nd N, 5th DM	D. Niederwieser
2007	Lyon, France	33rd P, 23d N, 6th DM, 1st P&F	D. Niederwieser
2008	Florence, Italy	34th P, 24th N, 7th DM, 2nd P&F	D. Niederwieser
2009	Goteborg, Sweden	35th P, 25th N, 8th DM, 3rd P&F	D. Niederwieser
2010	Vienna, Austria	36th P, 26th N, 9th DM, 4th P&F	A. Madrigal
2011	Paris, France	37th P, 27th N, 10th DM, 5th P&F	A. Madrigal
2012	Geneva, Switzerland	38th P, 28th N, 11th DM, 6th P&F, 1st QM, 1st Ped	A. Madrigal
2013	London, UK	39th P, 29th N, 12th DM, 7th P&F, 2nd QM, 2nd Ped	A. Madrigal
2014	Milan, Italy	40th P, 30th N, 13th DM, 8th P&F, 3d QM, 3d Ped	A. Madrigal
2015	Istanbul, Turkey	41st P, 31st N, 14th DM, 9th P&F, 4th QM, 4th Ped	M. Mohty
2016	Valencia, Spain	42nd P, 32nd N, 15th DM, 10th P&F, 5th QM, 5thPed, 1stPha	M. Mohty
2017	Marseille, France	43rd P, 33rd N, 16th DM, 11th P&F, 6th QM, 6thPed, 2nd Pha	M. Mohty
2018	Lisbon, Portugal	44th P, 34th N, 17th DM, 12th P&F, 7th QM, 7thPed, 3d Pha	M. Mohty
2019	Frankfurt, Germany	45th P, 35th N, 18th DM, 13th P&F, 8th QM, 8th Ped, 4th Pha	N. Kröger

Participating groups: *P* physicians, *N* nurses, *DM* data manager, *P&F* patient and family day, *QM* quality manager, *Ped* pediatricians, *Pha* pharmacists
[a]deceased

2.3 The Present

Today, EBMT (www.ebmt.org) is a nonprofit organization with a clear mission statement: "To save the lives of patients with blood cancers and other life-threatening diseases by advancing the fields of blood and marrow transplantation and cell therapy worldwide through science, education and advocacy" (https://portal.ebmt.org/Contents/About-EBMT/ Mission-Vision/Pages/Mission%2D%2DVision. aspx. Accessed 26 Feb 2018). It is formally a professional society with legal residence in the Netherlands and an administrative office in Barcelona, Spain. EBMT is chaired by the president, who is elected by the members for 2 years and for a maximum of two terms. He/she is supported by the board of association as the executive committee and the board of counselors as external advisors. The scientific council which represents the 11 working parties, the seven committees, and the groups guides the scientific work with the help of the seven offices (Table 2.2). The main task of the organizational body of EBMT is to collect, analyze, and disseminate scientific data; to conduct clinical trials; to improve quality through the close cooperation with JACIE and FACT; to plan the annual meeting, the educational events, and training courses, including the EBMT Handbook; and to provide assistance to patients, donors, physicians, and competent authorities.

Members of the EBMT are mainly centers active in transplantation of hematopoietic stem cells (HSC) or any other organization involved in the care of donors and recipients of HSC. Currently (January 1, 2018), EBMT holds 509 full center members and 55 associate center members, 122 individual, and 35 honorary members, from 65 different countries. EBMT is supported in its activities through the membership fees and the revenue of the annual meetings and by its corporate sponsors (https://www2.ebmt. org/Contents/Members-Sponsors/Sponsors/ Listofcorporatesponsors/Pages/List-of-corporate-sponsors.aspx. Accessed 26 Feb 2018). EBMT is part of the global network of organizations involved in HSCT, the Worldwide Network for Blood and Marrow Transplantation (WBMT), and in close link with national and other

international professional organizations involved in HSCT, such as AFBMT, APBMT, CIBMTR, EMBMT, LABMT, or WMDA. The EBMT database now holds information on more than 500,000 transplants. Over 35,000 new patients were treated annually over the last 5 years and more than 40,000 HSCT performed (Fig. 2.1). An estimated number of more than 400,000 patients are currently alive after HSCT in Europe; they reflect the EBMT achievements and the challenges ahead.

Table 2.2 EBMT working parties, committees, groups and offices

Working parties	
ADWP	Autoimmune Diseases Working Party
ALWP	Acute Leukemia Working Party
CMWP	Chronic Malignancies Working Party
CTIWP	Cellular Therapy & Immunobiology Working Party
IDWP	Infectious Diseases Working Party
IEWP	Inborn Errors Working Party
LWP	Lymphoma Working Party
PDWP	Paediatric Diseases Working Party
SAAWP	Severe Aplastic Anaemia Working Party
STWP	Solid Tumors Working Party
TCWP	Transplant Complications Working Party
Committees	
	Nuclear Accident Committee
	Donor Outcomes Committee
	Statistical Committee
	Registry Committee
	JACIE Committee
	Global Committee
	Legal & Regulatory Affairs Committee
Groups	
	EBMT nurses' group with its own president
	Data managers' group
	Statisticians' group
EBMT units	
	EBMT Executive Office, Barcelona, Spain
	JACIE Accreditation Office, Barcelona, Spain
	EBMT Central Registry Office, London, UK
	EBMT Data Office, Leiden, The Netherlands
	EBMT Clinical Trials Office, Leiden, The Netherlands
	EBMT Data Office/CEREST-TC, Paris, France
	EBMT Activity Survey Office, Basel, Switzerland

Courtesy: EBMT office Barcelona, Marta Herrero Hoces

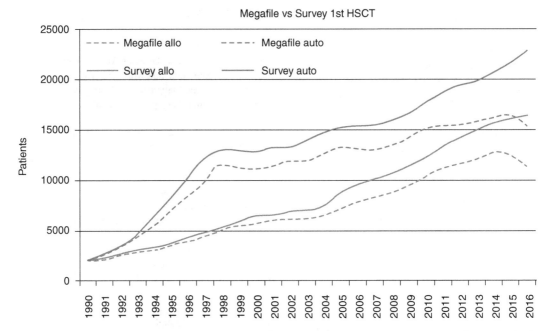

Fig. 2.1 Numbers of patients with a first HSCT by main donor type and year of transplant. The lines reflect the difference in patient numbers with and without information in the database (megafile). Courtesy: Carmen Ruiz de Elvira, EBMT megafile office, London; Helen Baldomero, EBMT activity survey office, Basel

2.4 The Future

Again, according to the Big History concept, predicting the future is a difficult task: "There are no data about the future; from an empirical scientific point of view, it is impossible to say what lies ahead of us." (Spier 2015). But we can project scenarios; we know the past, and we see the today. We live in the rapidly evolving world of the industrial revolution IV, dominated by globalization, digitization, and personalized medicine. Targeted therapies promise cures; gene-modified cells destroy hitherto untreatable cancers; immunomodulation with checkpoint inhibitors has become a reality (Hochhaus et al. 2017; Tran et al. 2017; Le et al. 2015). If HSCT is to remain a valuable treatment, mentalities and methods of the past no longer suffice. The idea of beliefs, hence physicians creating their own Goldilocks conditions, will lead to the end of HSCT. It has to be replaced by a stringent scientific approach. The sad story of HSCT for breast cancer, with more than 40,000 transplants but no clear answer, must not to be repeated (Gratwohl et al. 2010).

Hence, prediction number one: The idea of "a donor for everybody" will be abandoned. HSCT has to provide for the individual patient the best outcome regarding overall survival, quality of life and costs. The outcome after HSCT must be superior, in these three aspects, to any of the modern drugs or treatments, including "watch and wait" strategies or palliation. Assessment of risks needs to integrate risk factors relating to the patient, his or her disease, the donor, the stem cell source, the transplant technology, as well as micro- and macroeconomic risk factors (Gratwohl et al. 2015b; Gratwohl et al. 2017). For some patients, early transplant will be the optimal approach; for others, HSCT may need to be delayed. For others, HSCT will never be the preferred option. Obviously, the transplant physician is no longer in a position to adequately assess risk in comparison to the multiple alternative strategies, as it was possible in the old times of the simple EBMT risk score. Machine-learning algorithms will replace risk assessment; the competent physician will still be needed to discuss the results with his or her patients and their families and to conduct the transplant (Verghese et al. 2018).

Hence, prediction number two: The WHO guiding principles for cell, organ, and tissue transplants, "data collection and data analysis are integral parts of the therapy", need to become a mandatory reality for all transplant teams (WHO 2010). The gap between transplant numbers and reports (Fig. 2.1) has to be closed. Reporting has to become real-time and life-long. The EBMT and transplant centers have to adapt. Data and quality management will become a "condition sine qua non" for all, with close interactions between local, national, and international organizations. Machine learning will end the individualistic center unique transplant techniques. It will no longer be possible to apply hundreds of different GvHD prevention methods and a multitude of conditioning regimens, just by the argument "I have good experience with my method." Standardization will permit correct personalized medicine, as outlined above. Obviously, assessment of outcome can no longer be restricted to transplanted patients; it will need the correct comparison with non-transplant strategies on a routine basis.

Hence, prediction number three: HSCT centers and the EBMT will no longer be isolated in the treatment landscape. HSCT will need to be integrated into the treatment chain, from diagnosis to early treatment, transplant decisions, and secondary treatment, up to life-long follow-up. Not all of these steps have to occur at the transplant center, but they need to be coordinated by the expert team. Data have clearly shown that transplant experience, as measured in patient numbers and years, is associated with outcome (Gratwohl et al. 2015b). No center will have sufficient expertise for all diseases amenable to HSCT or for all transplant techniques, e.g., bone marrow harvest. HSCT centers will have to decide on their priorities, jointly with their referral and their after-care chain, within their city, their country, or with neighboring countries for coordination.

Hence, final prediction: EBMT can take the science-based lead for coordination and standardization, guide in reorganization of networks with non-transplant treatment chains, and prioritize comparative studies, independent of pressure groups. Then, history will tell, whether the proverb from a contemporary of von Humboldt, Georg Wilhelm Friedrich Hegel (1770–1831) "History teaches us that man learns nothing from history." (Spier 2015), can be overcome. The potential is here.

References

11th annual meeting of the EBMT (European Cooperative Group for Bone Marrow Transplantation). Bad Hofgastein (Salzburg). Austria, January 28–30, 1985. Exp Hematol. 1985;13(Suppl 17):1–154.

Bortin MM. A compendium of reported human bone marrow transplants. Transplantation. 1970;9:571–87.

Copelan EA. Hematopoietic stem cell transplantation. N Engl J Med. 2006;354:1813–26.

Crowther D, Bateman CJ, Vartan CP, et al. Combination chemotherapy using L-asparaginase, daunorubicin, and cytosine arabinoside in adults with acute myelogenous leukaemia. Br Med J. 1970;4(5734):513–7.

Ford CE, Hamerton JL, Barnes DW, Loutit JF. Cytological identification of radiation-chimaeras. Nature. 1956;177:452–4.

Gratwohl A, Pasquini MC, Aljurf M, Worldwide Network for Blood and Marrow Transplantation (WBMT), et al. One million haemopoietic stem-cell transplants: a retrospective observational study. Lancet Haematol. 2015a;2:e91–100.

Gratwohl A, Schwendener A, Baldomero H, et al. Changes in the use of hematopoietic stem cell transplantation: a model for diffusion of medical technology. Haematologica. 2010;95:637–43.

Gratwohl A, Sureda A, Baldomero H, Joint Accreditation Committee (JACIE) of the International Society for Cellular Therapy (ISCT), the European Society for Blood and Marrow Transplantation (EBMT), the European Leukemia Net (ELN), et al. Economics and outcome after hematopoietic stem cell transplantation: a retrospective cohort study. EBioMedicine. 2015b;2:2101–9.

Gratwohl A, Sureda A, Cornelissen J, et al. Alloreactivity: the Janus-face of hematopoietic stem cell transplantation. Leukemia. 2017;31:1752–9.

Hochhaus A, Larson RA, Guilhot F, et al. IRIS investigators. Long-term outcomes of Imatinib treatment for chronic myeloid leukemia. N Engl J Med. 2017;376:917–27.

Jacobson LO, Marks EK, Gaston EO, Robson M, Zirkle RE. The role of the spleen in radiation injury. Proc Soc Exp Biol Med. 1949;70:740–2.

Kay HE, Powles RL, Sloane JP, Farthing MG. Cyclosporin A in human bone marrow grafts. Haematol Blood Transfus. 1980;25:255–60.

Le DT, Uram JN, Wang H, et al. PD-1 blockade in tumors with mismatch-repair deficiency. N Engl J Med. 2015;372:2509–20.

Lorenz E, Uphoff D, Reid TR, Shelton E. Modification of irradiation injury in mice and Guinea pigs by bone marrow injections. J Natl Cancer Inst. 1951;12:197–201.

Mathé G, Jammet H, Pendic B, et al. Transfusions and grafts of homologous bone marrow in humans after accidental high dosage irradiation. Rev Fr Etud Clin Biol. 1959;4:226–38.

McCann SR. A history of haematology. From herodotus to HIV. Oxford medical histories. London: Oxford University Press; 2016.

Osgood EE, Riddle MC, Mathews TJ. Aplastic anemia treated with daily transfusions and intravenous marrow; a case report. Ann Intern Med. 1939;13:357–67.

Schinck P. Ernst Neumann als Begründer der Hämatologie. Dissertation Königsberg; 1920.

Speck B, Gluckman E, Haak HL, van Rood JJ. Treatment of aplastic anaemia by antilymphocyte globulin with and without allogeneic bone-marrow infusions. Lancet. 1977;2(8049):1145–8.

Spier F, editor. Big history and the future of humanity. Chichester: Wiley; 2015.

The bone-marrow. JAMA. 1908;LI(23):1997. https://doi.org/10.1001/jama.1908.02540230083025.

Thomas ED. A history of allogeneic hematopoietic cell transplantation. In: Appelbaum FR, Forman SJ, Negrin RS, Blume KG, editors. Thomas' hematopoietic cell transplantation. Chichester: Wiley; 2007. p. 3–7.

Thomas ED, Lochte HL Jr, Lu WC, Ferrebee JW. Intravenous infusion of bone marrow in patients receiving radiation and chemotherapy. N Engl J Med. 1957;257:491–6.

Thomas ED, Storb R, Clift RA, et al. Bone-marrow transplantation (second of two parts). N Engl J Med. 1975;292:895–902.

Tran E, Longo DL, Urba WJ. A milestone for CAR T cells. N Engl J Med. 2017;377:2593–6.

Van Bekkum DW, De Vries MJ. Radiation chimeras. New York: Academic Press; 1967.

Verghese A, Shah NH, Harrington RA. What this computer needs is a physician humanism and artificial intelligence. JAMA. 2018;319:19–20.

World Health Organization. WHO guiding principles on human cell, tissue and organ transplantation. Transplantation. 2010;90:229–33.

The Role of Unrelated Donor Registries in HSCT

Irina Evseeva, Lydia Foeken, and Alejandro Madrigal

3.1 Introduction

3.1.1 From Anthony Nolan to 32 Million Volunteer Donors Worldwide

Bone marrow donor registries (hereinafter referred to as registries) have been playing an important role in developing the treatment of HSCT for more than four decades. In 1974, the world's first registry was founded by Shirley Nolan in London. Shirley's son, a 3-year-old, Anthony, had been diagnosed with Wiskott-Aldrich syndrome and needed a transplant. Following the example of Anthony Nolan, a large number of registries have been established around the world, mainly in the late 1980s to early 1990s and have increased over the years. The growing pool of donors has contributed to the development of stem cell transplantation as a treatment method and a field of science (Fig. 3.1).

I. Evseeva
Anthony Nolan, London, UK

L. Foeken
Word Marrow Donor Association (WMDA),
Leiden, The Netherlands

A. Madrigal (✉)
Anthony Nolan, London, UK

UCL Cancer Institute, Royal Free Campus,
London, UK
e-mail: a.madrigal@ucl.ac.uk

3.1.2 Registry: Structure and Duties

A registry is "an organisation responsible for coordination of the search for haematopoietic progenitor cells from donors (including cord blood) unrelated to the potential recipient" (WMDA International Standards 2017).

Registries play the main role in communication between the physician in the transplant centre and the healthcare professional contacting the donor at national and international level. Search requests for adult unrelated donors (AUDs) and cord blood units (CBUs) are usually sent to the national registry, which facilitates all stages of search and provision of the graft for a patient.

A typical registry performs different interrelated functions, including donor recruitment and management and search and interact with HLA-typing laboratories, apheresis and marrow collection centres, cord blood banks (CBBs), stem cell couriers and transplant centres.

Some registries recruit donors themselves, while others have an agreement with blood banks, donor centres or donor recruitment groups. The donor's or cord blood information is provided by the donor centre or CBB to a registry. The registry is responsible for listing the donors on the global database and handling communication with national and international transplant centres (through their national registries) if a potential match for a patient has been found.

The search for a suitable stem cell source is based on the HLA-type of the patient.

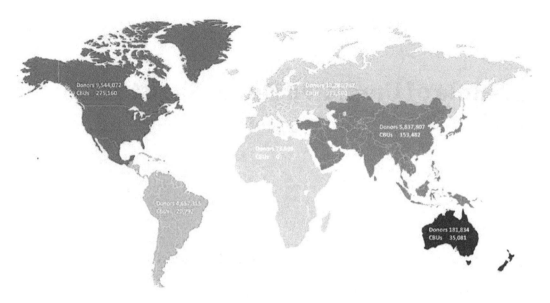

Fig. 3.1 Volunteer donors and cord blood units recruited around the wold (data from WMDA web page)

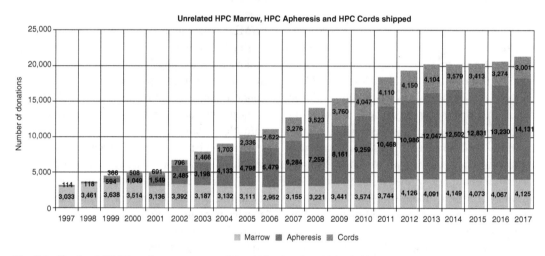

Fig. 3.2 Unrelated HSC from bone marrow, peripheral blood and cord blood shipped annually (data from WMDA)

Transplant centres and search coordinators within donor registries have access to the Search & Match Service of WMDA (https://search.wmda. info/login), where they can register patient data and get a match list to see if there is a potential stem cell source in the global database.

When the transplant centre identifies a potentially matched stem cell source, the national registry will contact the relevant organisation and facilitate the delivery of stem cells for the patient. Annually, more than 20,000 stem cell products of different sources are shipped within and across borders to patients in need of a HSCT (see Fig. 3.2).

3.2   Current Landscape

3.2.1   Ethnic Diversity and Chance to Find a Donor

As of January 2018, more than 32 million potential AUDs and CBUs are listed in the global Search & Match Service of WMDA. Almost 95%

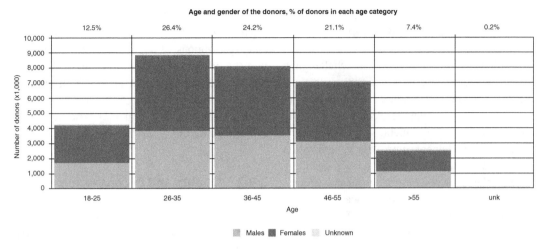

Fig. 3.3 Age and gender of unrelated donors and percentage of donors in each category

of these donors have DNA-based HLA-A, HLA-B and HLA-DRB1 phenotype presented, and more than half are listed with additional information on HLA-C, HLA-DQB1 and HLA-DPB1. Every year, registries across the world add approximately two million new volunteer donors to the worldwide pool, with the vast majority being HLA-typed at high and allelic level resolution.

The chance of finding a well-matched donor varies for patients belonging to different ethnic groups. In 2014, the National Marrow Donor Program (NMDP) study demonstrated that whereas approximately 75% of Caucasian patients are likely to identify an 8/8 HLA-matched AUD, the rate is much lower for ethnic minority and mixed-race patients. This is due to the higher genetic diversity of HLA haplotypes in African and Asian populations compared to Europeans and the lower representation and poorer availability of ethnic minority donors in the worldwide pool (Gragert et al. 2014).

3.2.2 Donor Profile

WMDA defines an unrelated donor as "a person who is the source of cells or tissue for cellular therapy product. Donors are unrelated to the patient seeking a transplant".

Donor centres recruit volunteer donors from 16 to 55 years of age with variations in individual policies. Although donors can remain on the database until they are 60, donor centres try to recruit more young volunteers, as donor age has been proven to be linked to better HSCT outcomes (Kollman et al. 2016). According to the World Marrow Donor Association (WMDA) data, approximately 50% of donors listed globally are younger than 35 (see Fig. 3.3).

Medical suitability for donation, gender diversity, behaviour and psychological risks are constantly changing factors in donor recruitment and management. Donor centres align their policies with national and international standards and recommendations, including donor suitability guidelines produced by the WMDA on https://share.wmda.info/x/FABtEQ and published in 2014 (Lown et al. 2014).

Unrelated donors are acting voluntarily and altruistically and have a right to withdraw from the process at any stage. To avoid such cases, donor centres focus on informing volunteers about all aspects of donation, including risks, at the very early stage of recruitment. When a donor is identified as a potential match for a patient and is asked to provide a blood sample for verification or extended testing, healthcare professionals will have further detailed conversations with the donor addressing any possible questions and concerns. Full informed consent is usually given at the donor's medical, prior to the conditioning of the patient for transplant.

3.2.3 Recruitment, Retention and Data Confidentiality

Recruiting volunteer donors is challenging. Registries and donor centres must ensure they are recruiting the preferred donors (usually younger donors) who are appropriately counselled to fully understand their commitment.

Registries and donor centres use a combination of methods to recruit potential donors including patient-related drives, targeting special groups, e.g. universities, uniformed services, engaging blood donors or online recruitment. The approach depends on the laws of the country and takes traditions, religion and habits into account. The same factors influence donor retention. Considering several options and alternative donors in urgent cases is a recommended practice.

By signing to a donor centre or registry, a potential donor agrees that his/her data are registered in the global database. The donor also provides biological material (blood sample, saliva or buccal swab) for tests, such as HLA typing and infectious disease markers, along with their personal details, in order to be searched as a match for a patient. The registry or donor centre has an obligation to adhere to national and international data protection laws and to keep donor personal and medical information confidentially and use it strictly in line with the donor's informed consent.

While social media helps enormously with donor recruitment and retention, it can present a challenge for confidentiality of both the donor and the recipient. Registries and donor centres in different countries have different policies on donor/patient post-donation contact and on the level of information provided to each other. These should be respected by all sides involved.

3.3 Connections and Worldwide Collaboration

3.3.1 WMDA

In 1988, three pioneers in the field of transplantation, Professors John M. Goldman (United Kingdom), E. Donnell Thomas (United States) and Jon J. van Rood (the Netherlands), informally initiated the WMDA, which became a formal organization in 1994. It is made up of individuals and organizations who promote global collaboration and best practices for the benefit of stem cell donors and patients requiring HSCT. It aims to give all patients worldwide equal access to high-quality stem cells from donors, whose rights and safety are carefully protected.

3.3.2 Quality and Accreditation

In 2017, WMDA took the lead role in the merging of three key organizations: WMDA, BMDW and the NetCord Foundation. This allowed WMDA to streamline resources to provide a global platform for facilitating international search, to support members to develop and grow and to promote safety, quality and global collaboration through accreditation and standardisation. Eighty-four percent of AUDs available for search are provided by WMDA qualified/accredited registries (WMDA Annual Report 2017). WMDA accreditation of the registries along with FACT-NetCord accreditation of the CBBs reassures recipients in the quality of product and services provided. A complete list of the accreditation status of organisations can be found on WMDA Share: https://share.wmda.info/x/4gdcAQ.

3.3.3 Network Formalities

All registries, donor centres and CBBs providing stem cells for HSCT nationally and internationally have legal agreements and contracts with each other within the network. The contracts cover legal, financial and ethical questions of collaboration in respect of obtaining, testing and shipment of stem cells.

3.4 Challenges and Opportunities

3.4.1 Donor Attrition

Time to transplant is reported to be a factor of overall survival (Craddock et al. 2011). Formal search for an unrelated donor on average takes about 2 months. However, more and more urgent search requests are made to the registries, where transplant centres are hoping to get a donor work-up in weeks rather than months.

Not all potential donors listed on the database will be available for donation due to different reasons, including medical or personal circumstances or loss of contact with the registry. It varies in different countries. According to WMDA annual questionnaire, in 2017, the recommended target for donor availability at verification typing stage was 80% and at work-up stage 95%. Registries and donor centres are working hard to keep in contact with their donors to have updated information to help reach the donor without delays. Some donor centres use private healthcare providers to speed-up blood sample collection and increase the number of apheresis centres in order to meet desirable turnaround times.

3.4.2 Ethical Challenges

HSCT is an evolving field of medical science. Volunteer donors can be asked to be a subject of research and clinical trials as part of their stem cell donation for a particular patient or not. In the majority of cases, this is covered by the informed consent given at the recruitment and donor medical stages, but in some cases, additional consent is required. It is the obligation of registries and donor centres to make sure that donors are well informed and free to withdraw.

3.4.3 Donor Pool HLA Diversity

Current trends in HSCT (with high requirements for patient/donor matching, complexity of standard and research protocols and a growing index of indications) present challenges for registries, donor centres and CBBs. Different strategies need to be applied to recruit not only a larger number of potential donors but also increase HLA diversity of the pool. As HLA allele and haplotype frequencies have population-specific patterns, there are limitations to how many different phenotypes can be obtained by adding new donors. In 2016, the WMDA reported no more than 50 different phenotypes per thousand new AUDs and CBUs submitted to the global database. This can be addressed by recruiting among ethnic minority groups or in parts of the world with a wider genetic diversity, e.g. Africa (see Fig. 3.4).

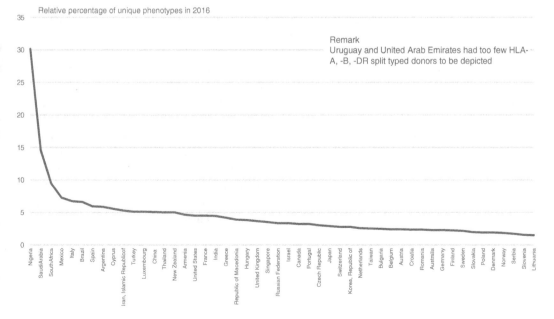

Fig. 3.4 Relative percentage of unique HLA-A, HLA-B and HLA-DR split phenotypes of stem cell donors per country contributed to the entire database of BMDW

Although the majority of stem cell provisions worldwide are currently coming from Northern America and Europe, a few large registries arose in South America and Asia over recent years. WMDA is encouraging and supporting new and growing registries. The WMDA handbook: "A gift for life: the essential WMDA handbook for stem cell donor registries & cord blood banks" (2016) provides all necessary information and advice for starting a registry in your country.

3.5   Future Developments

3.5.1   New Level of HLA Matching

As of January 2018, classic criterion for HLA matching with a patient is 10/10 at HLA-A, HLA-B, HLA-C, HLA-DRB1 and HLA-DQB1 for AUDs and 8/8 on HLA-A, HLA-B, HLA-C and HLA-DRB1 for CBUs, all at high-resolution level, with mismatches associated with inferior patient outcome (Shaw et al. 2017, Eapen et al. 2017). Many transplant centres are now considering HLA-DPB1 allele or epitope matching (Fleischhauer et al. 2012). There are also trends to include other genes like MICA and MICB in donor selection (Fuerst et al. 2016; Carapito et al. 2016; Kitcharoen et al. 2006).

The resolution of HLA matching is important. The advantage of allelic/ultrahigh-resolution HLA matching on OS and NRM compared to high-resolution level was presented by Anthony Nolan at the 2018 BMT Tandem meetings (Mayor et al. 2018). Full/extended gene sequencing results in fully phased phenotypes, thus significantly reduced allelic ambiguity, and can reveal mismatches not otherwise identified by high-resolution typing.

Following these developments, some registries and donor centres have already implemented HLA allelic level typing for their donors and

make additional non-HLA genetic information available for transplant centres at the search stage. It is expected that transplant centres will also be able to type patients at this level of resolution to achieve better matching and additional survival advantages.

3.5.2   Related Donors Provision and Follow–Up

Historically, registries have not been closely involved with the provision of related donors. However, in recent years, many registries have begun to support related donors internationally (i.e. where the patient is living in one country and their related donor is living in another) and domestically (e.g. where the patient and donor live far apart or the transplant centre cannot facilitate a collection). Some registries also provide support in following-up related donors post-collection and in providing information and support for related donors.

3.5.3   Advisory Services Provided by Registries

Nowadays, many registries are taking additional advisory roles in supporting transplant centres in stem cell searches as they accumulate knowledge and expertise over an ever-growing number of stem cell provisions. Working closely with clinical teams, national registries may offer advice and consultancy in donor selection, product quality evaluation, education and training.

As part of research and business development strategy, registries are looking at other products and services to further support HSCT. A range of cell therapy products may be provided along with standard stem cell donation or under a separate service agreement.

Key Points

- International collaboration over the last four decades resulted in more than 32 million unrelated donors potentially available to donate stem cells for patients requiring HSCT.
- Donor search and provision are carried out via national registries to ensure quality and legal compliances.
- Unrelated donors act voluntarily and altruistically; their availability varies due to medical and personal reasons.
- Big efforts are made to increase HLA diversity of the donor pool to address the lower chance of finding a well-matched donor for ethnic minority and mixed-race patients.
- Registries continue to develop HSCT by contributing to research, enhancing services and extending the range of cell products provided.

Acknowledgements The authors are grateful to Ms. Ann O'Leary, Ms. Nicola Alderson, Dr. Neema Mayor and Mrs. Pauline Dodi at Anthony Nolan for providing information and advising on the content of this chapter.

References

Carapito R, Jung N, Kwemou M, et al. Matching for the nonconventional MHC-I MICA gene significantly reduces the incidence of acute and chronic GVHD. Blood. 2016;128:1979–86.

Craddock C, Labopin M, Pillai S, et al. Factors predicting outcome after unrelated donor stem cell transplantation in primary refractory acute myeloid leukaemia. Leukemia. 2011;25:808–13.

Eapen M, Wang T, Veys PA, et al. Allele-level HLA matching for umbilical cord blood transplantation for non-malignant diseases in children: a retrospective analysis. Lancet Haematol. 2017;4:325–33.

Fleischhauer K, Shaw BE, Gooley T, et al. Effect of T-cell-epitope matching at HLA-DPB1 in recipients of unrelated-donor haematopoietic-cell transplantation: a retrospective study. Lancet Oncol. 2012;13:366–74.

Fuerst D, Neuchel C, Niederwieser D, et al. Matching for the MICA-129 polymorphism is beneficial in unrelated hematopoietic stem cell transplantation. Blood. 2016;128:3169–76.

Gragert L, Eapen M, Williams E, et al. HLA match likelihoods for hematopoietic stem-cell grafts in the US registry. N Engl J Med. 2014;371:339–48.

Kitcharoen K, Witt C, Romphruk A, et al. MICA, MICB, and MHC beta block matching in bone marrow transplantation: relevance to transplantation outcome. Hum Immunol. 2006;67:238–46.

Kollman C, Spellman SR, Zhang MJ, et al. The effect of donor characteristics on survival after unrelated donor transplantation for hematologic malignancy. Blood. 2016;127:260–7.

Lown RN, Philippe J, Navarro W, et al. Unrelated adult stem cell donor medical suitability: recommendations from the World Marrow Donor Association Clinical Working Group Committee. Bone Marrow Transplant. 2014;49:880–6.

Mayor NP, Hayhurst JD, Turner TR, et al. Better HLA matching as revealed only by next generation sequencing technology results in superior overall survival post-allogeneic haematopoietic cell transplantation with unrelated donors. Biol Blood Marrow Transplant. 2018;24(3):63–4.

Shaw BE, Mayor NP, Szydlo RM, et al. Recipient/donor HLA and CMV matching in recipients of T-cell-depleted unrelated donor haematopoietic cell transplants. Bone Marrow Transplant. 2017;52:717–25.

WMDA Finance and Activities Report. WMDA, 2018. 2017. https://share.wmda.info

WMDA Handbook. A gift for life: the essential handbook for stem cell donor registries and cord blood banks (freely available for WMDA members); 2016.

WMDA International Standards for unrelated haematopoietic stem cell donor registries, January 2017. https://www.wmda.info/professionals/quality-and-accreditation/wmda-standards/.

The HSCT Unit

Walid Rasheed, Dietger W. Niederwieser, and Mahmoud Aljurf

4.1 Introduction

HSCT is an advanced therapeutic intervention that is required for a number of malignant and nonmalignant medical conditions, often for critically ill patients. The establishment of an HSCT program requires the efforts of experienced and appropriately trained personnel to lead the program. Clearly, this also requires financial, legal, ethical, and other institutional support. For newly starting programs, it would be essential to identify minimal requirements for establishing an HSCT unit in order to optimize resource utilization as well as maintain safe patient care. While these minimal requirements also apply to well-established units, its structure helps to understand and implement additional steps for larger units which plan to offer additional transplant services and have access to more resources.

Approximately 20 years ago, the EBMT and the ISCT (International Society for Cellular Therapy) formed the Joint Accreditation Committee— ISCT and EBMT (JACIE) based on the FACT (Foundation for the Accreditation of Cellular Therapy) program. Efforts of these bodies have cul-

minated in the establishment of standards related to HSCT and cellular therapies to assure quality and safety in the practice of HSCT. Although pro gram accreditation with JACIE is not mandatory worldwide, these standards are very helpful as guidelines to understand requirements to establish an HSCT unit. Table 4.1 summarizes basic mini mal requirements of an HSCT unit, which are dis_ cussed in more details in the following sections. _

4.2 Inpatient Unit

The inpatient HSCT unit should have a minimum number of single-bedded rooms with isolation capability. The number and space of rooms should be adequate for the type and volume of transplant activity performed at the transplant center. These rooms must adhere to the standards of safety and comfort of patients in a tertiary care hospital facility. Every location or room should have a sink and tap for hand washing.

There needs to be a working station or room for nurses involved in patient care. A similar working space for physicians is required. Medical and nurs ing staff coverage should be available 24 h a day, including public holidays. The ratio of nurses to patient beds depends on the type and intensity of transplants being performed, e.g., autologous versus allogeneic, but generally, a ratio one nurse to three patients is reasonable. Emergency cart with drugs for resuscitation should be available in the inpatient unit.

W. Rasheed (✉) · M. Aljurf
King Faisal Specialist Hospital and Research Centre, Riyadh, Saudi Arabia
e-mail: wrasheed@kfshrc.edu.sa

D. W. Niederwieser
University of Leipzig, Leipzig, Germany

Table 4.1 HSCT unit minimal requirements

Inpatient unit	– Clean single-bedded rooms with isolation capability
Ancillary medical services	– Intensive care unit – Emergency room service – Gastroenterology and pulmonary service[a]
Outpatient clinic	– Single patient examination rooms
Blood bank	– Twenty-four hour on-site blood bank service: ABO typing and cross match, RBC, and platelets for transfusion – Irradiation and leukocyte depletion of blood products
Laboratory	– Hematology cell count and chemistry lab – Serology for viral screen – Microbiology for basic bacterial and fungal cultures – CMV PCR or antigenemia[a] – Access to CSA/tacrolimus levels[a]
HLA typing lab[a]	– Access to ASHI or similarly accredited HLA typing lab
Stem cell collection	– PBSC apheresis capability – Bone marrow harvesting facility and expertise for matched sibling donor[a]
Stem cell processing facility	– FACS CD34 enumeration – Refrigerator for blood and bone marrow – Controlled cryopreservation capability for freezing of autologous stem cell product – Equipment and expertise to process ABO-mismatched cellular product[a]
Radiology	– Routine x-ray radiology, ultrasound, and CT scanner – Placement of central venous catheters
Pharmacy	– Availability of conditioning chemotherapy drugs – Availability of antimicrobial agents (broad-spectrum antibiotics, antiviral, and antifungal drugs) – Availability of immunosuppressive agents for GVHD prophylaxis and treatment[a]
Human resources	– Medical director: Licensed physician with adequate training and experience in HSCT – Nursing staff with training in chemotherapy administration, infection control, and handling of stem cell products – Clinical laboratory director: Clinical pathology trained. – Appropriately trained lab scientist and technicians – Multidisciplinary medical staff (radiology, pathology, ICU, surgery, gastroenterology[a], pulmonary[a])
Outcome database	– Monitor patient demographics, treatment, and outcomes (level I data reporting)
Quality management	– Written institutional protocols/guidelines – Regular audits of various HSCT procedures and patient treatment outcomes – System to detect errors or adverse events for corrective or preventative actions

[a]Requirements for allogeneic HSCT programs

Infections, including bacterial, viral, or fungal infections, are potential significant complications in transplant recipient and may lead to significant morbidity and mortality. Therefore, HSCT units should have established measures for infection control. Guidelines for infection prevention and prophylaxis in HSCT patients, endorsed by several scientific organizations, are available and highly recommended to follow. HSCT recipients should be placed in single-patient rooms. Furthermore, at a minimum, standard precautions should be followed in all patients including hand hygiene and wearing of appropriate protective equipment (gloves, surgical masks or eye/face protection, gowns) during procedures/activities that are likely to generate splashes or spray of blood, body fluids, or secretions. Hand hygiene is essential, using alcohol-based hand rubs or washing with soap and water. In patients with suspected or proven of having an infection, additional precautions are required accordingly, e.g., airborne, droplet, or contact isolation. HSCT units should be cleaned at least daily with special attention to dust control. During building construction, intensified mold control measures are required, and a multidisciplinary team should be involved.

Other important infection control measures include well-sealed rooms, positive pressure differential between patient rooms and the hall-way, self-closing doors, more than 12 air exchanges per hour, and continuous pressure monitoring. HEPA (high efficiency particulate air) filters have shown efficacy in providing protection against acquisition of fungal infections in immune-compromised hematology patients, including HSCT patients, and during hospital construction or renovation works. While HEPA filters are not absolutely required as a minimal requirement in newly established centers with less complicated transplant activities, they are certainly preferred and highly recommended as newly established centers expand their activities to include more complicated (especially allogeneic) transplant activities.

There is no agreed upon minimum number of transplants to be performed in a program. However, to ensure continuing proficiency in a transplant program, the ASBMT recommends for programs performing only one type of HSCT (autologous or allogeneic), at least ten transplants of that type are to be performed per annum; programs performing both allogeneic and autologous transplantations should perform a minimum of ten transplants of each kind per annum.

4.3   Ancillary Medical Services

HSCT patients often require other medical specialties involvement in their complicated care. This includes the risk of developing life-threatening infections or other post transplant complications, hence the importance of having access to emergency room as well as intensive care services at the same tertiary care hospital facility where transplant program is being established. Intensive care units should have the ability of providing inotropic support, respiratory support (including mechanical ventilation) as well as renal replacement (hemodialysis) if required.

Input from infectious disease physicians can be valuable in HSCT patients who are at risk of a multitude of opportunistic and potentially life-threatening infections; this is especially important for programs that perform allogeneic

transplants. Availability of gastroenterology specialist with endoscopy services is critical for allogeneic programs, as often diagnostic endoscopy is required to differentiate GVHD from other etiologies of gastrointestinal complications. Similarly, pulmonary medicine service with access to diagnostic bronchoscopies is required for such patients with pulmonary abnormalities.

HSCT programs that perform transplants using radiotherapy as part of conditioning regimen (total body irradiation) should have available radiation oncology service on site. The radiation oncology team, including the radiation oncologist and physicist, should have adequate training in the technique of total body irradiation and appropriate equipment, and procedures must be in place to deliver successful and safe radiation component of these conditioning regimen.

4.4   Outpatient Unit

HSCT patients attend to the outpatient unit, both for pretransplant assessment and work-up and post transplant follow-up and management. Single patient examination rooms are a minimal requirement for the outpatient service of the program. These rooms should be adequately equipped to allow clinical assessment of patients. It is important to implement infection control measures to minimize risk of transmitting infections, including hand hygiene measures and availability of appropriate room to isolate patients who are identified to be potentially infectious to others, e.g., due to herpes zoster infection. A dedicated infusion area would be ideal as transplant recipients often require IV fluid and electrolyte replacement or blood product administration.

4.5   Blood Bank

Availability of blood banking services is a critical component of a successful transplant program. A 24-h on-site blood banking service is required for ABO typing, cross match, and urgent supply of red blood cells and platelets for transfusion. Meeting minimal standard criteria according to recognized international blood bank societies such as the American Association of Blood Banks (AABB) or equivalent is important. Blood bank staff, including blood bank director, scientists, and technicians should be adequately qualified and trained in blood banking procedures.

Transplant recipients are severely immune-compromised and are at risk of transfusion-associated GVHD, caused by unrestricted proliferation of donor lymphocytes in the immune-compromised host. Hence, it is critical that transplant recipients receive irradiated blood products to prevent this complication. The use of leukocyte-depleted blood products is recommended to reduce the risk of HLA alloimmunization in the multiply transfused hematology patients, as well as to reduce the incidence of transfusion reactions. In allogeneic programs, clear documented pathways for transfusion support in cases of ABO mismatch should be available for both blood bank and clinical staff as guidance.

4.6 Laboratory

A 24-h on-site hematology cell count and basic chemistry lab are required. Furthermore, microbiology laboratory service is essential in the clinical management of transplant recipients, including routine bacterial and fungal cultures of various patient specimens. Serology screening for relevant viral and bacterial infections is also required for pretransplant work-up of recipients as well as donor screening. For allogeneic transplant recipients, monitoring for cytomegalovirus (CMV) reactivation is essential, and results must be available in a timely manner to allow therapeutic intervention; both molecular technique by quantitative PCR (preferable) and antigenemia method are acceptable. In the allogeneic setting, monitoring drug levels, e.g., cyclosporine or tacrolimus, is required, and same-day service is recommended to allow interventions aiming at keeping levels of these important drugs within the target therapeutic range.

4.7 HLA Typing Lab

Access to HLA typing laboratory is mandatory for allogeneic programs. Such service can be available on-site or alternatively provided in reference laboratory. JACIE standards state that clinical programs performing allogeneic transplantation shall use HLA testing laboratories that are capable of carrying out DNA-based intermediate and high-resolution HLA typing and are appropriately accredited by the American Society for Histocompatibility and Immunogenetics (ASHI), European Federation for Immunogenetics (EFI), or other accrediting organizations providing histocompatibility services appropriate for hematopoietic cellular therapy transplant patients.

4.8 Stem Cell Collection

Access to peripheral blood stem cell apheresis service on-site is a minimal requirement in each program. This is often part of the blood bank service or alternatively under the administration of the clinical program. Having at least two cell separators would be beneficial, as the second cell separator would be a backup in situations of unexpected machine faults and for routine servicing. Daily operation of apheresis facility requires appropriately trained and experienced nursing staff and a medical director with adequate qualification and experience in clinical and laboratory aspects of the apheresis procedure. Institutional written protocols and policies covering all aspects of apheresis procedure should be available for guidance. JACIE standards require a minimum average of ten cellular therapy products collected by apheresis per year for program accreditation.

A bone marrow stem cell source is sometimes recommended for better patient outcome, e.g., patients with bone marrow failure. Programs performing allogeneic transplants for such indication should have a bone marrow harvest facility on-site. This requires convenient and easy access to surgical operating room with anesthesia service. Appropriate equipment for the bone marrow harvest procedure are required. Physicians with adequate training and experience in bone marrow harvesting are crucial to perform the procedure successfully.

4.9   Stem Cell Processing Facility

The stem cell processing facility requires a designated area, usually within the laboratory. It should be appropriately equipped for the processing of various stem cell products depending on the types of transplants performed and the size of the program. Availability of flow cytometry for the enumeration of CD34 cell count is mandatory. Controlled cryopreservation capability, using liquid nitrogen, for freezing of autologous stem cell product is essential. This may also be used in allogeneic sibling products. Standard quality control measures, including systems to closely monitor and record the temperature in all freezes and refrigerators, are critical. Allogeneic programs should have appropriate equipment and expertise on-site for the timely and safe processing of ABO-mismatched stem cell products as required, including the need to perform red cell or plasma depletion procedures when indicated. The processing facility should be operated by adequately trained staff, including scientist, technicians, and a medical director. Written standard operating procedures explaining all aspects of stem cell processing performed at the facility are required.

4.10   Radiology

Standard routine (X-ray), ultrasound, and computed tomography (CT scan) imaging services are the minimal requirements and should be available on site for the routine diagnostic imaging. Availability of magnetic resonance imaging (MRI) is preferred, as it is often useful in the diagnosis of specific clinical conditions relevant to stem cell transplant recipients, such as iron overload, CNS infections, and posterior reversible encephalopathy syndrome (PRES) related to

calcineurin inhibitor toxicity. Placement of central venous catheters in transplant recipients is obviously required in each program. Depending on the institutional setting, this service may be provided by various hospital services; often this is done by the radiology service under ultrasound guidance. Having well trained and experienced interventional radiologist to perform this procedure is crucial for the safety of patients.

4.11   Pharmacy

Pharmacy services are essential in each HSCT program. Availability of conditioning chemotherapy agents is clearly required; specific drugs depend on the type and complexity of transplant procedures performed in each program. Commonly used agents in conditioning regimens include BU, CY, FLU, and MEL. ATG may also be required in the allogeneic setting (e.g., in aplastic anemia) and requires special attention and training by nursing, pharmaceutical, and medical staff in relation to its administration.

Broad-spectrum antibiotics should be available for urgent use as required in transplant recipient. Likewise, access to antiviral and antifungal agents is important for both prophylaxis and treatment. Allogeneic programs should also have access to immunosuppressive drugs used for GVHD prophylaxis such as CSA, MTX, and TAC.

A trained pharmacist is crucial for the HSCT program. The pharmacist should review all conditioning chemotherapy protocols and ensure appropriate dispensing and administration of cytotoxic agents.

4.12   Staffing and Human Resources

Appropriately trained and experienced medical and nursing staffs are crucial for the HSCT program. The clinical medical director of the program should be a licensed physician (specialty certification in hematology, oncology, or immunology) with adequate training at a BMT program. A minimal BMT training duration of 6–12 months is suggested. JAICIE standards indicate that the clinical program director shall have 2 years of experience as an attending physician responsible for the direct clinical management of HSCT patients in the inpatient and outpatient settings. A minimum of one (1) additional attending transplant physician is required in the program.

The success of a transplant program relies heavily on the presence of appropriately trained and experienced nursing staff. This includes training in chemotherapy administration, infection control, management of neutropenic patients, and handling of stem cell products.

Other important staff includes appropriately trained and experienced personnel in the laboratory (including laboratory director, scientist, and technicians), trained pharmacist, as well as medical professionals of ancillary medical services. Continuous education activities are required for all healthcare professionals involved in the management of HSCT patients.

4.13 Institutional Database and Data Manager

Monitoring patient demographics, treatment details, and outcomes is an essential minimal requirement. Each program should keep complete and accurate patient records, and a database containing relevant patient data should be established and regularly maintained. Appropriate patient consent needs to be obtained for such database. An example of the minimal data required to be obtained on each transplant patient is the information required in the CIBMTR or EBMT mid A forms. Having a data manager in a transplant program to initiate and maintain this institutional transplant database is highly recommended. Often data managers have nursing background with experience in stem cell transplantation. Attending training data management courses during international meetings or through links with other experienced and well-established programs would be valuable.

4.14 Quality Control

The JACIE standards require that all essential clinical collection and processing facilities in the transplant center evaluate and report patient outcomes. Regular audits of various HSCT procedures and patient treatment outcomes are required. Essentially, a system is required to be in place to detect errors/adverse events, so that these can be evaluated in order to implement preventative measures to minimize the risk of recurrence of these incidents. Furthermore, each program should have written institutional clinical protocols in relation to the various aspects of the transplant patient care to standardize practice. Likewise, stem cell collection and processing facilities should have standard operating procedures that serve as a guidance for all staff to follow to enhance patient's safety. Access to or relationship with experienced HSCT program is often very helpful and highly recommended via shared protocols/telemedicine and/or web-based conferencing.

4.15 Transplant Coordinator

HSCT is a complex therapeutic intervention, and coordination of the pretransplant, transplant, and post transplant patient care is important. A transplant coordinator can play pivotal role in this context, acting as a facilitator, educator, as well as a point of contact for the patient and their families. Transplant coordinators ensure the smooth and safe running of the HSCT service starting from scheduling and arranging pretransplant work-up of patient and planning the roadmap for the transplant recipient with continued involvement and education of the patients and their families until the time of admission. Furthermore, transplant coordinator would play a significant role in the coordination of post HSCT follow-up and care in clinics. For allo-HSCT, the transplant coordinator would be very valuable in arranging donor search starting from HLA typing of the recipient and his/her family members, in addition to initiating and following a search for unrelated donor in national or international registries.

The transplant coordinator involvement may extend to organizing the logistics of getting the stem cells from the donor from the donor center where the recipient may be in another health facility (national or international). Moreover, transplant coordinators will often lead the HSCT team weekly planning meetings and discussions with the arrangement of the HSCT waiting list. Typically, transplant coordinators have nursing background with significant experience in stem cell transplantation.

Key Points
- The inpatients unit should have single-bedded rooms with isolation capabilities. Single outpatient examination rooms are also required.
- Laboratory, blood bank, and pharmacy services are critical to the success of HSCT programs.
- Stem cell collection and processing capabilities are minimal requirements for any HSCT program; the level of such capabilities depends on the type and complexity of HSCT performed in each center.
- Ancillary medical services are essential components of successful HSCT programs, including intensive care and emergency and radiology services. Additional medical services are required in allogeneic programs.
- Appropriately trained and experienced staff (medical, nursing, laboratory, pharmacy) are crucial for the HSCT program.
- Monitoring patient characteristics and transplant outcomes is essential.
- A local quality control system is required in all aspects involved in the HSCT procedure.
- Having a data manager for the HSCT program, to initiate and maintain institutional minimal transplant data base is highly recommended.

- Transplant coordinators play pivotal role the management of HSCT patients, starting from pre SCT work up, right through post transplant care.

Recommended References

Booth GS, Gehrie EA, Bolan CD, Savani BN. Clinical guide to ABO-incompatible allogeneic stem cell transplantation. Biol Blood Marrow Transplant. 2013;19:1152–8.

Chang CC, Ananda-Rajah M, Belcastro A, et al. Consensus guidelines for implementation of quality processes to prevent invasive fungal disease and enhanced surveillance measures during hospital building works, 2014. Intern Med J. 2014;44:1389–97.

Crysandt M, Yakoub-Agha I, Reiß P, et al. How to build an allogeneic hematopoietic cell transplant unit in 2016: proposal for a practical framework. Curr Res Transl Med. 2017;65:149–54.

Daniele N, Scerpa MC, Rossi C, et al. The processing of stem cell concentrates from the bone marrow in ABO-incompatible transplants: how and when. Blood Transfus. 2014;12:150–8.

FACT/JACIE. FACT-JACIE 7th edition standards; 2018. http://www.jacie.org/.

Hahn T, Cummings KM, Michalek AM, et al. Efficacy of high-efficiency particulate air filtration in preventing aspergillosis in immunocompromised patients with hematologic malignancies. Infect Control Hosp Epidemiol. 2002;23:525–31.

Krüger WH, Zöllner B, Kaulfers PM, Zander AR. Effective protection of allogeneic stem cell recipients against Aspergillosis by HEPA air filtration during a period of construction--a prospective survey. J Hematother Stem Cell Res. 2003;12:301–7.

Leemhuis T, Padley D, Keever-Taylor C, et al. Essential requirements for setting up a stem cell processing laboratory. Bone Marrow Transplant. 2014;49:1098–105.

Napier A, Williamson LM. British Committee for Standards in Haematology, Blood Transfusion Task Force, et al. Guidelines on the clinical use of leucocyte – depleted blood components. Transfusion Med. 1998;81:59–71.

Phillip G, Armitage J, Bearman S. American Society for Blood and Marrow Transplantation guidelines for clinical centers. Biol Blood Marrow Transplant. 1995;1:54–5.

Tomblyn M, Chiller T, Einsele H, et al. Guidelines for preventing infectious complications among hematopoietic cell transplantation recipients: a global perspective. Biol Blood Marrow Transplant. 2009;15:1143–238.

Treleaven J, Gennery A, Marsh J, et al. Guidelines on the use of irradiated blood components prepared by the British committee for standards in haematology blood transfusion task force. Br J Haematol. 2011;152:35–51.

5

JACIE Accreditation of HSCT Programs

Riccardo Saccardi, Eoin McGrath,
and John A. Snowden

5.1 Introduction

The complexity of HSCT as a medical technology and the frequent need for close interaction and interdependence between different services, teams, and external providers (donor registries, typing laboratories, etc.) distinguish it from many other medical fields. Approximately 20 years ago, this complexity led to efforts by transplantation professionals to standardize processes based on consensus as a way to better manage inherent risks of this treatment. HSCT was, and continues to be, a pioneer in the area of quality and standards.

R. Saccardi (✉)
Department of Cellular Therapies and Transfusion Medicine, Careggi University Hospital, Florence, Italy
e-mail: riccardo.saccardi@unifi.it

E. McGrath
European Society for Blood and Marrow Transplantation (EBMT), Barcelona, Spain

J. A. Snowden
Department of Haematology, Sheffield Teaching Hospitals NHS Foundation Trust, University of Sheffield, Sheffield, UK

5.2 Background

In 1998, EBMT and the International Society for Cell & Gene Therapy (ISCT) established the Joint Accreditation Committee, ISCT and EBMT (JACIE), aimed to offer an inspection-based accreditation process in HSCT against established international standards. JACIE is a committee of the EBMT, its members are appointed by and are accountable to the EBMT Board, and ISCT is represented through two members of the Committee. JACIE collaborates with the US-based Foundation for the Accreditation of Cellular Therapy (FACT) to develop and maintain global standards for the provision of quality medical and laboratory practice in cellular therapy.

The JACIE and FACT accreditation systems stand out as examples of profession-driven initiatives to improve quality in transplantation and which have subsequently been incorporated by third parties, such as healthcare payers (health insurers, social security) and competent authorities (treatment authorization). The JACIE Accreditation Program was supported in 2004 by the European Commission under the public health program 2003–2008 and was acknowledged as an exemplary project in a 2011 review of spending under the public health program.

5.3   Impact of Accreditation in Clinical Practice

Much literature indicating a better clinical outcome in teaching hospitals and centers of excellence has been available since the 1990s (Hartz et al. 1989; Birkmeyer et al. 2005; Loberiza et al. 2005). Initial evidence of a positive relationship between the implementation of a quality management system and outcome of HSCT in Europe was published in 2011 (Gratwohl et al. 2011). In this paper, patients' outcome was systematically better when the transplantation center was at a more advanced phase of JACIE accreditation, independent of year of transplantation and other risk factors.

Another analysis (Gratwohl et al. 2014) was performed on a large cohort of patients who received either an allogeneic or an autologous transplantation between 1996 and 2006 and reported to the EBMT database. The authors showed that the decrease of overall mortality in allogeneic procedures over the 14-year observation period was significantly faster in JACIE-accredited centers, thus resulting in a higher relapse-free survival and overall survival at 72 months from transplant. Such improvement was not shown in autologous transplantation.

Similar results published by Marmor et al. (2015) in an American study showed that centers accredited by both FACT and Clinical Trial Network (CTN) demonstrated significantly better results for more complex HSCT such as HLA-mismatched transplants.

These data reinforce the concept that clinical improvement is driven by the implementation of a quality management system embedded in external accreditation standards, especially in the context of more complex procedures. This process also results in a wider standardization of procedures across different countries and geographic areas, therefore contributing to providing patients with similar treatment expectations even when accessing different health management systems. A comprehensive review of this was recently published (Snowden et al. 2017).

5.4   JACIE-FACT Accreditation System

JACIE and FACT accreditation systems are based on the development and continuous update of standards covering the entire transplantation process, from selection of the donor/patient to follow-up, including collection, characterization, processing, and storage of the graft. Considering the different competences included in the process, the standards are articulated in four parts:

- Clinical Program,
- Bone Marrow Collection,
- Apheresis Collection and
- Processing Facility.

A quality management (QM) section is embedded in each section, aimed at providing a tool for both the applicants to develop a comprehensive system of quality assessment and for the inspectors to check the compliance of the program to the standard. Stand-alone processing labs can apply; however, the target of the accreditation is the transplantation program, intended as a process in its entirety, thus requiring a full integration of units, laboratories, services, and professionals. Each section focusses on the competence of personnel, listing topics for which the evidence of a specific training is required which also includes the minimum experience requirements for positions of responsibility. Maintaining these competences is also required for all professionals.

The standards are revised on a 3-year basis by a commission formed of experts appointed by JACIE and FACT, including HSCT administration, cell processing and storage, blood apheresis, transplant registries, and QM specialists. The standards are based on published evidence and, when this is not available, on expert consensus. A legal review and comparison with current regulations are carried out for each version. When the developmental phase is finalized, the standards are published for public review and comment and finally approved by JACIE and FACT.

The standards incorporate sound principles of quality medical and laboratory practice in cellular therapy, but do not cover legal requirements of local competent authorities.

The compliance to the standards is ensured through an inspection system, carried out by voluntary inspectors, trained and coordinated by the JACIE office in Barcelona. The JACIE inspection is a multistep procedure: the applicant center is provided with all the application documents and is then required to submit a set of documentation to the JACIE accreditation coordinators. If the first review is positive, the on-site inspection is then planned in agreement with the applicant.

JACIE inspections are carried out in most cases in the language of the applicant. The inspectors' report is then assessed by the JACIE accreditation committee, which may request supplementary information, modifications, or another on-site visit. If all aspects are shown to be compliant, accreditation is awarded. An accreditation cycle is 4 years for JACIE, and facilities must complete an interim desk-based audit after 2 years post-accreditation. Accredited facilities must reapply for reaccreditation and may also be reinspected in response to complaints or information that a facility may be noncompliant with the standards, in response to significant changes in the program and/or facility or as determined by JACIE.

Many tools are made available to prepare the accreditation through the JACIE website, including a quality management guide, the welcome guide, and webinars. JACIE runs training courses throughout the year, and the Barcelona-based staff are available to support the applicants. An accreditation manual provides detailed explanations and examples for each single item of the standards. A special approach is under development for transplant programs in low- and middle-income countries (LMICs), where full accreditation might not be feasible due to resources and/or cultural issues. In this case, a stepped process toward accreditation is being developed, based on the selection of organizational items of the standard which may be ful-

filled by the implementation of a QM system, without requiring specific investments in infrastructures and/or equipment. This "stepwise" option will also encourage the programs to connect with an international network of professionals and may also stimulate local authorities to support further progress toward full accreditation in the interests of patients, donors, and the professional community.

The standards cover the use of different sources of hematopoietic stem cells and nucleated cells from any hematopoietic tissue source administered in the context of the transplant process, such as DLI. The term "hematopoietic" in the title is to define the scope of these standards, due to an increasing number of accredited facilities that also support non-hematopoietic cellular therapies. Starting with version 6.1, the standards include new items specifically developed for other cellular therapy products, with special reference to immune effector cells (IECs). This reflects the rapidly evolving field of cellular therapy through mainly, but not exclusively, genetically modified cells, such as CAR-T cells. The standards do not cover the manufacturing of such cells but include the chain of responsibilities where the product is provided by a third party and ensure the competence of the personnel in the management of adverse events related to the infusion.

Another recent development has been the introduction of "benchmarking" standards related to 1-year survival and other patient outcomes. If center performance is below the expected range, then a corrective action plan is mandated. The requirement for a risk-adapted "benchmarking" system is being addressed in the development of the new EBMT MACRO registry, which will enable centers to address these new JACIE standards within their own BMT community and across international boundaries.

JACIE is run on a non-profit basis, resourced almost entirely on application fees. Fees depend on the configuration of the program and its EBMT membership status. At the time of writing in February 2018, the application fee for a transplant program made up of collection, processing, and clinical units is €14,600 for EBMT members and €29,200 for non-EBMT members. Supplementary fees for additional sites and discounts for active inspectors in the team are applied (*see* JACIE website for details).

Overall, over 600 accreditation inspections have been carried out in 25 countries, representing over 40% transplant centers in Europe (Figs. 5.1 and 5.2), many of which have been through more than one accreditation cycle. JACIE accreditation is now mandatory in several European countries, to apply for reimbursement of the procedure and/or to be authorized to perform HSCT. JACIE also represents an opportunity for centers in LMICs to align their organizations with practice in the more advanced HSCT programs.

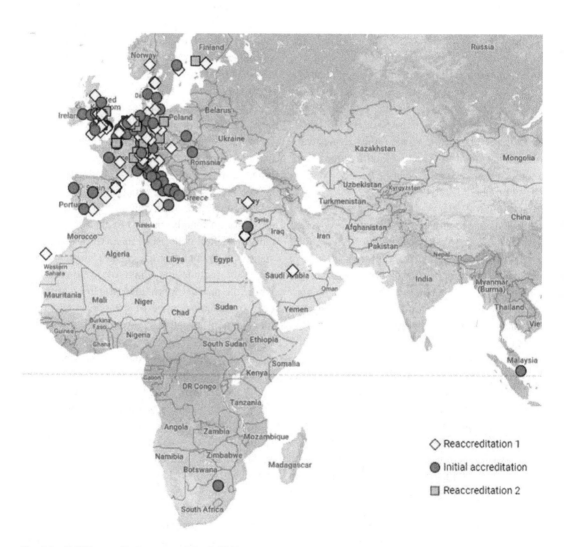

Fig. 5.1   JACIE-accredited programs March 2018

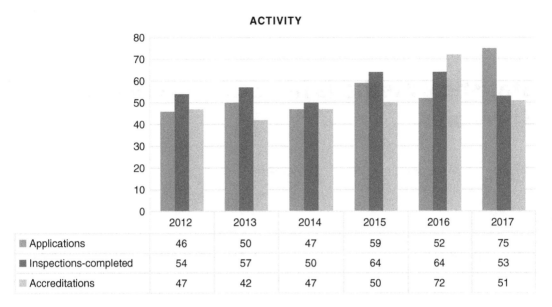

ACTIVITY

	2012	2013	2014	2015	2016	2017
■ Applications	46	50	47	59	52	75
■ Inspections-completed	54	57	50	64	64	53
▦ Accreditations	47	42	47	50	72	51

Fig. 5.2 JACIE activity 2012–2017

Key Points

- JACIE accreditation is based on an internationally agreed quality standard system led and delivered by HSCT and cell therapy professionals.
- The standards are regularly updated, incorporating advances in the evidence base while reflecting the practical view of experienced experts on clinical and laboratory practice of HSCT and cell therapy.
- Published data support a positive improvement in the clinical outcome related to the accreditation process, also promoting a progressive standardization of HSCT practice across different countries.
- Recent developments in the standards include development of standards for CAR-T and other immune effector cells (IEC), "benchmarking" of patient survival and access of centers in LMIC to the "stepwise" accreditation.

References

Birkmeyer NJ, Goodney PP, Stukel TA, et al. Do cancer centers designated by the National Cancer Institute have better surgical outcomes? Cancer. 2005;103:435–41.

Gratwohl A, Brand R, McGrath E, Joint Accreditation Committee of the International Society for Cellular, B. the European Group for, T. Marrow and N. the European Leukemia, et al. Use of the quality management system "JACIE" and outcome after hematopoietic stem cell transplantation. Haematologica. 2014;99:908–15.

Gratwohl A, Brand R, Niederwieser D, et al. Introduction of a quality management system and outcome after hematopoietic stem-cell transplantation. J Clin Oncol. 2011;29:1980–6.

Hartz AJ, Krakauer H, Kuhn EM, et al. Hospital characteristics and mortality rates. N Engl J Med. 1989;321:1720–5.

Loberiza FR, Zhang MJ, Lee SJ, et al. Association of transplant center and physician factors on mortality after hematopoietic stem cell transplantation in the United States. Blood. 2005;105:2979–87.

Marmor S, Begun JW, Abraham J, Virnig BA. The impact of center accreditation on hematopoietic cell transplantation (HCT). Bone Marrow Transplant. 2015;50:87–94.

Snowden JA, McGrath E, Duarte RF, et al. JACIE accreditation for blood and marrow transplantation: past, present and future directions of an international model for healthcare quality improvement. Bone Marrow Transplant. 2017;52:1367–71.

Statistical Methods in HSCT and Cellular Therapies

Simona Iacobelli and Liesbeth C. de Wreede

6.1　Introduction

The analysis of data describing the outcomes of patients who have received an HSCT is not only fundamental to assessing the effectiveness of the treatment but can provide invaluable information on the prognostic role of disease and patient factors. Thus, the appropriate analysis and understanding of such data are of paramount importance. This document provides an overview of the main and well-established statistical methods, as well as a brief introduction of more novel techniques. More insight is provided in the *EBMT Statistical Guidelines* (Iacobelli 2013).

6.2　Endpoints

The outcomes most commonly studied in HSCT analyses are the key events occurring at varying times post HSCT, e.g., engraftment, GVHD, relapse/progression, and death. Besides the clini-

S. Iacobelli (✉)
Department of Biology, University of Rome Tor Vergata, Rome, Italy

EBMT, Leiden, The Netherlands
e-mail: simona.iacobelli@ebmt.org

L. C. de Wreede
Department of Biomedical Data Sciences, Leiden University Medical Center, Leiden, The Netherlands

DKMS Clinical Trials Unit, Dresden, Germany

cal definition of the event of interest, it is important to define the corresponding statistical endpoint and to use a proper method of measuring the occurrence of the event (Guidelines 2.1).

The main distinction is between events that occur with certainty during a sufficiently long observation period (follow-up), like death, and events which are precluded from occurring once another event occurs, e.g., not all patients will experience a relapse of their disease because some die before. We define death without prior relapse (usually called NRM; see Guidelines 2.1.2) as the "competing event" of relapse. The name "NRM" is preferable to TRM, the proper analysis of which requires individual adjudication of causes of death.

Survival endpoints: In addition to death, other examples of events of the first type are the combinations of (negative) events of interest, which in total have 100% probability of occurrence, for example, PFS which considers as failure of the event "either relapse/progression or death." The components of PFS are the two competing events mentioned above, relapse/progression and NRM.

Competing risks endpoints: In addition to relapse/progression and NRM, other examples are death of a specific cause and all intermediate events during a HSCT history (engraftment, GVHD, achievement of CR, CMV infection) including the long-term (secondary malignancy). Notice that the definition of an endpoint requires specifying which are the competing events. Usually, this will be death without prior event of interest, but depending on the disease and the aims of the analysis, other competing events might be included in the analysis, e.g., a second transplantation or other treatment can be considered as competing event for achievement of response.

6.3 Analysis of Time-to-Event Outcomes

Each event of interest may occur at variable times post transplant, so in statistical terms, it has two components—whether it occurs at all and, if it does, when. However, at the end of the follow-up, there can be patients who have not yet had the event of interest but are still at risk for it: their observation times are called "censored." Censoring occurs at different timepoints for different patients. The inclusion of censored data precludes the use of simple statistical methods such as the Chi-Squared or T-test and requires the methods of survival (or competing risks) analysis. The crucial assumption of most methods in survival analysis is that the patients censored at a timepoint are "represented" by those who remain under follow-up beyond that timepoint. In other words, the fact that a patient is censored should not indicate that his/her prognosis is worse or better than the prognosis of a similar

patient who remains under observation. This assumption is called "independent and uninformative" censoring.

6.3.1 Kaplan-Meier Curves

The main method to summarize survival endpoints is the Kaplan-Meier curve (Kaplan and Meier 1958), estimating for each point in time t after HSCT the probability S(t) of surviving beyond that time. This curve is decreasing from 100% and will reach 0% with complete follow-up. A long flat tail of the curve (often called "plateau") is often based on a few censored observations at late times, corresponding to very unreliable estimates of the long-term survival. It is useful to report each S(t) with its 95%CI (confidence interval at 95% level, best obtained using the Greenwood formula) or at least the number of patients still at risk at different timepoints. The median survival time is the minimum time when S(t) is equal to 50% (Fig. 6.1).

6.3.2 Cumulative Incidence Curves

The appropriate method to summarize endpoints with competing risks is the cumulative incidence

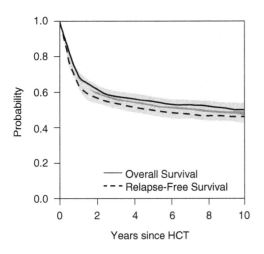
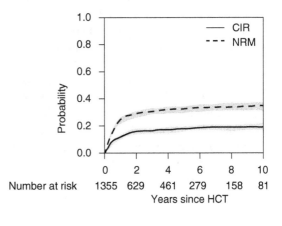

Fig. 6.1 Probability curves of the four main outcomes after HSCT. *CIR* Cumulative Incidence of Relapse. CIR and NRM add up to 1-RFS. Number at risk indicates the number of patients in follow-up who have not experienced an event so far. The grey zones indicate 95% confidence intervals

(CI) curve (Gooley et al. 1999), estimating for each point in time t the probability F(t) of having had the event of interest before that time. This curve is increasing from 0% and will not reach 100% even with complete follow-up if the competing event was observed for some patients. It is always useful to interpret CI curves of competing events together, to understand, e.g., when a category of patients has a small risk of relapse, if this means that they have a good prognosis or that they died too early from complications to experience a relapse (shown by a high NRM curve) (Fig. 6.1).

6.3.3   Comparison of Groups

The main method to compare survival curves for two or more independent groups is the Log-Rank test. This test is based on the comparison of the underlying hazard functions, which express the instantaneous probability of the event at a time t among patients currently at risk. It has good properties in the situation of proportional hazards (PH, described in the next section), but it should be avoided (or considered carefully) when the survival curves cross; with converging curve alternatives like the Wilcoxon Signed-Rank test should be preferred.

In the comparison of cumulative incidence curves, the main method is the Gray test. Also the Log-Rank test can be applied to compare groups in the case of competing risks, when the object of interest is not the cumulative probability of occurrence of the event but its instantaneous probability among the cases at risk at each time, which is called "cause-specific hazard." For the interesting difference of the two approaches to the analysis of competing risks endpoints, see Dignam and Kocherginsky (2008).

We refer to Sects. 1.3 and 1.4 of the Guidelines for remarks on statistical testing and about proper settings for comparisons of groups. Importantly, the simple methods described in this chapter can be applied only to groups defined at or before the time origin (e.g., transplantation); assessing differences between groups defined during the

follow-up requires other approaches, as those described in Sect. 6.4.1 (Guidelines page 14).

6.3.4   Proportional Hazards Regression Analysis

The above tests do not give a summary measure of the difference in outcomes between groups, nor can they be used when the impact of a continuous risk factor (e.g., age) has to be assessed. Furthermore, any comparison could be affected by confounding. These limitations are typically overcome by applying a (multivariable) regression model. The one most commonly used for survival endpoints is the proportional hazards (PH) Cox model (Cox 1972). Results are provided in terms of hazard ratios (HR), which are assumed to be constant during the whole follow-up (Guidelines 4.3.1). The Cox model in its simplest form is thus not appropriate when a factor has an effect that strongly decreases (or increases) over time, but time-varying effects can be accommodated for in more complex models. Effects of characteristics which change during follow-up can be assessed by including them as time-dependent covariates.

For endpoints with competing risks, two methods can be used, which have a different focus: the Cox model can be used to analyse cause-specific hazards, whereas a regression model for cumulative incidence curves was proposed by Fine and Gray (1999).

The use of these regression models requires a sound statistical knowledge, as there are many potential difficulties with the methods both in application and interpretation of results.

6.4   Advanced Methods

Many more advanced methods than the ones described above exist that help to get more insights from the available data. A good application of these needs expert statistical knowledge. The brief introductions given below are primarily meant to help understanding papers where these methods have been applied. For a more in-depth discussion, see, e.g., Therneau and Grambsch (2000).

6.4.1 Multistate Models

The methodology of multistate models (Putter et al. 2007) has been developed to understand the interplay between different clinical events and interventions after HSCT and their impact on subsequent prognosis. Their primary advantage is that sequences of events, such as HSCT, DLI, GVHD, and death, and competing events, such as relapse and NRM, can be modelled simultaneously (see Fig. 6.2 for an example). This is in contrast to analysing composite survival outcomes such as GVHD-free survival where all failures are combined and resolution of GVHD is not considered. Some studies applying this method that offer new insights into the outcomes after HSCT are Klein et al. (2000) about current leukemia-free survival, Iacobelli et al. (2015) about the role of second HSCT and CR for MM patients, and Eefting et al. (2016) about evaluation of a TCD-based strategy incorporating DLI for AML patients.

6.4.2 Random Effect Models

In standard methods, all patients are considered as independent, and each patient only contributes one observation for each endpoint. There are, however, situations when this does not hold, for instance, when patients within the same centre tend to have more similar outcomes than those from another centre or when one patient can experience more than one outcome of the same kind, e.g., infections. In these cases, the outcomes within one "cluster" (a centre or a patient) are more correlated than the outcomes between clusters, which has to be accounted for in the analysis. This is usually done by random effect models, which assume that each cluster shares an unobserved random effect. In survival analysis, these are called frailty models (Therneau and Grambsch 2000, Chap. 9). If the outcome is not an event but a value measured over time, e.g., CD8 counts, the appropriate regression models are called mixed models.

6.4.3 Long-Term Outcomes: Relative Survival/Cure Models

With improved long-term outcomes and increasing numbers of older patients, a substantial number of patients will die from other causes than the disease for which they have been transplanted and the direct and indirect consequences of its treatment. This so-called population mortality can be quantified by methods from relative survival, based on population tables describing mortality of the general population (Pohar Perme et al. 2016).

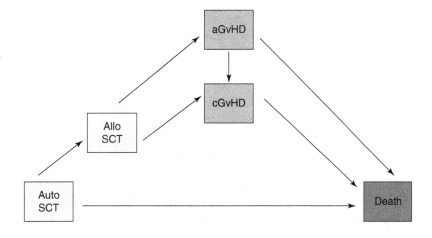

Fig. 6.2 Example of a multistate model. All patients start in state 1 (event-free after HSCT). They can then proceed through the states by different routes. Each arrow indicates a possible transition

Especially for transplanted children, a period with a high risk of mortality can be followed by a very long and stable period where the death risk is (almost) zero. When the focus of an analysis is on the probability of long-term cure, cure models can be used that assess the impact of risk factors on this but only if follow-up is sufficiently long (Sposto 2002).

6.4.4 Propensity Scores

Propensity scores (PS) are useful to compare the outcomes of two treatments in the absence of randomization, to control confounding due to the fact that usually the choice of the treatment depends on patient's characteristics (confounding by indication) (Rosenbaum and Rubin 1983). First, the PS, defined as the probability of receiving one treatment instead of the other, is estimated for each patient. Then PS can be used in various ways (mainly stratification or pair matching), allowing comparison of treatment outcomes among cases with a similar risk profile.

6.4.5 Methods for Missing Values

Missing values in risk predictors are a common problem in clinical studies. The simplest solution is to exclude the patients with missing values from the analysis (complete case analysis). This solution is not optimal, however: firstly, not all information is used (an excluded patient might have other characteristics known), and secondly, this approach can lead to bias if patients with missing values have on average a different outcome from the patients with observed values.

If values can be imputed on the basis of observed values in the dataset, these patients can be retained in the analysis to increase precision of estimates and avoid bias. The method most commonly used is called multiple imputation (White et al. 2011). A major advantage of this method is that it properly takes into account the uncertainty caused by the imputation in the estimates. If data are missing not at random—meaning their values cannot be predicted from the observed variables—multiple imputation can at most decrease the bias but not fully remove it.

Acknowledgements We thank Myriam Labopin, Richard Szydlo and Hein Putter for their contributions to this chapter.

Key Points
- Survival and competing risk endpoints need specific methods.
- Survival analysis methods: Kaplan-Meier, Log-Rank test, Cox model.
- Competing risks methods: Cumulative incidence curve, Gray test, Cox model, and Fine and Gray model.
- Including events/changes of status occurring during follow-up in an analysis requires specific (advanced) methods, like multistate models.

References

Cox DR. Regression models and life tables. J R Stat Soc. 1972;34(Series B):187–220.

Dignam JJ, Kocherginsky MN. Choice and interpretation of statistical tests used when competing risks are present. J Clin Oncol. 2008;26:4027–34.

Eefting M, de Wreede LC, Halkes CJM, et al. Multistate analysis illustrates treatment success after stem cell transplantation for acute myeloid leukemia followed by donor lymphocyte infusion. Haematologica. 2016;101:506–14.

Fine JP, Gray RJ. A proportional hazards models of the subdistribution of a competing risk. J Am Stat Assoc. 1999;94:496–509.

Gooley TA, Leisenring W, Crowley JA, et al. Estimation of failure probabilities in the presence of competing risks: new representations of old estimators. Stat Med. 1999;18:695–706.

Iacobelli S, de Wreede LC, Schönland S, et al. Impact of CR before and after allogeneic and autologous transplantation in multiple myeloma: results from the EBMT NMAM2000 prospective trial. Bone Marrow Transplant. 2015;50:505–10.

Iacobelli S, on behalf of the EBMT Statistical Committee. Suggestions on the use of statistical methodologies in studies of the European Group for Blood and Marrow Transplantation. Bone Marrow Transplant. 2013;48:S1–S37.

Kaplan EL, Meier P. Non-parametric estimation from incomplete observations. J Am Stat Assoc. 1958;53:457–81.

Klein JP, Szydlo RM, Craddock C, et al. Estimation of current leukaemia-free survival following donor lymphocyte infusion therapy for patients with leukaemia who relapse after allografting: application of a multistate model. Stat Med. 2000;19:3005–16.

Pohar Perme M, Estève J, Rachet B. Analysing population-based cancer survival – settling the controversies. BMC Cancer. 2016;16:933.

Putter H, Fiocco M, Geskus RB. Tutorial in biostatistics: competing risks and multi-state models. Stat Med. 2007;26:2389–430.

Rosenbaum PR, Rubin DB. The central role of the propensity score in observational studies for causal effects. Biometrika. 1983;70:41–55.

Sposto R. Cure model analysis in cancer: an application to data from the Children's Cancer group. Stat Med. 2002;21:293–312.

Therneau TM, Grambsch PM. Modeling survival data: extending the Cox model. New York: Springer; 2000.

White IR, Royston P, Wood AM. Multiple imputation using chained equations: issues and guidance for practice. Stat Med. 2011;30:377–99.

Part II
Biological Aspects
Topic leaders: Chiara Bonini and Jürgen Kuball

Biological Properties of HSC: Scientific Basis for HSCT

Alessandro Aiuti, Serena Scala, and Christian Chabannon

7.1 Introduction

Hematopoiesis—from the Greek term for "blood making"—is the adaptive process by which mature and functional blood cells are continuously replaced over the entire lifetime of an individual. Erythrocytes, platelets, and the various subsets of leukocytes all have finite although different life spans. As a consequence, the daily production of red blood cells, platelets, and neutrophils in homeostatic conditions amount to more than 300 billion cells.

In mammals, after the emergence of the first hematopoietic progenitors in extra-embryonic structures such as the yolk sac in mice, cells of

A. Aiuti
San Raffaele Telethon Institute for Gene Therapy (SR-TIGET)/Pediatric Immunohematology and Bone Marrow Transplantation Unit, IRCCS Ospedale San Raffaele, Vita-Salute San Raffaele University, Milan, Italy

S. Scala
San Raffaele Telethon Institute for Gene Therapy (SR-TIGET), IRCCS Ospedale San Raffaele, Milan, Italy

C. Chabannon (✉)
Institut Paoli-Calmettes, Centre de Lutte Contre le Cancer, Marseille, France

Université d'Aix-Marseille, Marseille, France

Inserm BCT-1409, Centre d'Investigations Cliniques en Biothérapies, Marseille, France
e-mail: chabannonc@ipc.unicancer.fr

hematopoietic nature are first detected in the aorto-gonado-mesonephric (AGM) region of the developing embryo (Costa et al. 2012). The site of hematopoiesis then moves to the fetal liver and next to the BM where it remains established until the death of the individual. Extramedullary hematopoiesis in humans denotes a myeloproliferative syndrome.

The considerable knowledge accumulated over more than a century of experimental hematology led to the early understanding that all hematopoietic lineages are derived from a small subpopulation of undifferentiating and self-renewing stem cells. HSC represent the most accurately explored model of somatic stem cells that are present in most if not all tissues and organs, contributing to tissue homeostasis and repair. Existence of a population of HSC also has practical implications in terms of developing innovative therapies aiming at the definitive replacement or enhancement of a function in cells from one or several hematopoietic lineages, including the possibility to establish durable hematopoietic chimerism in recipients of allogeneic HSCT.

7.2 Self-Renewal

A general property of stem cells is self-renewal, assuming that when these cells divide, at least one of the "daughter cells" fully recapitulate the biological properties of the "mother stem cell." Self-renewal of the HSC population prevents exhaustion, while the hematopoietic tissue extensively proliferates and differentiates in steady-state conditions, as well as to repair various damages. Demonstration of self-renewal at the clonal level remains an arduous task, even though high-throughput analytical tools have been adapted. There is a growing body of evidence suggesting aging of the HSC population and decline of stem cell function with age (for a review, see Goodell and Rando 2015; de Haan and Lazare 2018). Appearance of "passenger mutations" in clonal hematopoiesis is one hallmark of aging (Cooper and Young 2017); the significance of such observations remains to be fully elucidated, but obviously raises questions when it comes to solicit elderly individuals to donate HSC for the benefit of a related patient.

7.3 Commitment and Differentiation: New Data Challenge the Historical View of Hematopoietic Hierarchy

The traditional view of HSC differentiation is a hierarchical representation of an inverted tree, where discrete and homogenous populations branch from one another, with successive restrictions in differentiation potentials. This oversimplifying view is increasingly challenged by recent studies reporting on noninvasive genetic experiments and clonal analyses in mice (for a review, see Laurenti and Göttgens 2018; Busch and Rodewald 2016). These studies suggest that hematopoietic differentiation uses different mechanisms under steady-state and stress conditions (Goyal and Zandstra 2015); however, both in steady-state conditions and transplantation models, only a small fraction of HSC contribute to long-term and stable reconstitution without compromising reestablishment of hematopoiesis (Schoedel et al. 2016; Höfer and Rodewald 2016), while most stem cells remain quiescent or proliferate infrequently. Single-cell transcriptional landscapes also suggest that differentiation occurs as a continuous rather than discrete physiological process and that restriction of differentiation is not the result of a "symmetric split" between the myeloid and lymphoid compartments as long thought through the phenotypic identification of "common myeloid progenitors" (CMP) and "common lymphoid progenitors" (CLP).

Commitment to one or several lineages, or conversely restriction in differentiation abilities, results from the expression of a controlled genetic and epigenetic program (Pouzolles et al. 2016; Antoniani et al. 2017; Gottgens, 2015); these mechanisms remain partially understood and thus can only be partially harnessed for in vitro engineering of HSC and their progeny (Rowe et al. 2016). The fate of HSC and their progeny is additionally regulated by extrinsic signals, among which hematopoietic growth factors and cytokines play an important role in survival, proliferation, and amplification (Kaushansky, 2006).

7.4 The Bone Marrow Niches and Maintenance of Stemness (Fig. 7.1)

Recent years have witnessed considerable progress in our understanding of organization and function of the bone marrow microenvironment. HSC establish interactions in the context of microanatomical organizations termed "niches." Progress has been made both in understanding the heterogeneity of niches at and within successive hematopoietic sites and in identifying various categories of cells—either of non-hematopoietic or of hematopoietic origin—that interact with HSC. The various types of bone marrow niches closely associate with the neurovascular network that infiltrates the central bone marrow as well as the endosteal region. The nature of the signaling between these different cell populations is also increasingly deciphered and involves many pathways, some of them unexpected at first (for a review, see Crane et al. 2017; Calvi and Link 2015). Replicating some of these interactions in vitro is key to successful expansion or genetic engineering of isolated HSC. Among the many molecular actors that govern interactions between HSC and the various cells present in niches, the CXCL12 chemokine and its most important

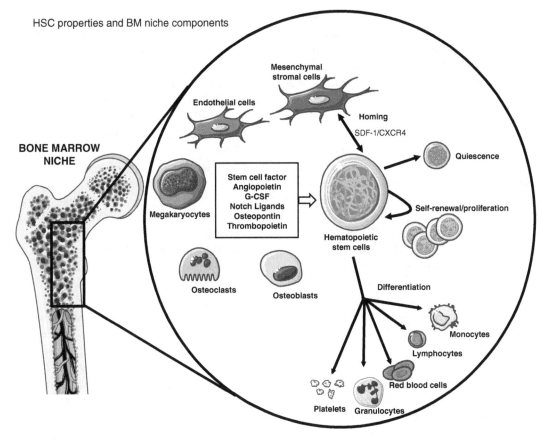

Fig. 7.1 HSC properties and BM niche components

receptor CXCR4 are of particular interest: direct or indirect modulation of this axis is clinically exploited to amplify the compartment of circulating stem cells that exist at low numbers in steady-state conditions.

7.5   Preclinical Models of HSCT

Most of the current knowledge on the biology of HSC and on therapeutic mechanisms of HSCT derives from studies in animal models (Eaves, 2015; Sykes and Scadden 2013). Classical murine transplantation studies showed that single or few engrafting HSC were sufficient and necessary to sustain long-term hematopoiesis in a reconstituted mouse. Human-in-mouse xenografts have become a fundamental tool to study hematopoietic dynamics upon HSCT. The generation of immune-deficient mice bearing a dele-

tion of the interleukin-2 receptor gamma chain on the NOD-SCID background (NSG mice) was instrumental for studying HSC homing, engraftment, lineage differentiation, and serial transplantation capacity. This model has been further modified by introducing human myeloid cytokine genes to increase myeloid differentiation (Doulatov et al. 2012) or loss-of-function mutation in KIT receptor to efficiently support engraftment of human HSC without the need for conditioning therapy (Cosgun et al. 2014). To overcome the lack of human components in the murine BM, humanized-BM niche systems have been recently developed which are based on human stromal cells implanted on specific scaffold or directly injected with extracellular matrix to generate BM micro-ossicles (Di Maggio et al. 2011; Reinisch et al. 2016). These strategies provide novel tools to study the behavior of human HSC in their physiological context and to dissect the role of the niche upon transplantation. However, homing and engraftment parameters in xenografts may be different from the natural setting, and most HSCT models follow recipient mice for few months after transplantations, thus making long-term outcome difficult to assess.

Dogs provide an ideal preclinical modeling system for HSCT studies due to their large body size, life span, and high genetic diversity, which more appropriately recapitulate the human scenario. Preclinical canine modeling has been fundamental for the clinical translation of conditioning regimens and the importance of MHC donor/recipient matching. However, the lack of canine reagents and the logistic difficulties of working with large animal models have precluded widespread availability (Stolfi et al. 2016). Auto-HSCT in nonhuman primates is arguably the experimental model most closely resembling humans; their treatment conditions—including the use of CD34+ cells, mobilization, and conditioning regimens—all parallel those commonly exploited in human transplantation. While the ethical issues and costs have limited their use to selected centers, these animals are able to maintain long-term hematopoiesis up to several years after transplantation allowing the study of HSCT dynamics in a close-to-human fashion (Koelle et al. 2017).

7.6 Gene Transfer/Gene Editing/Gene Therapy Targeting HSC (Fig. 7.2)

Ex vivo HSC gene therapy (GT) is based on the genetic modification of autologous HSC to correct monogenic disorders or to provide novel features to hematopoietic cells for treating infectious diseases or cancers (Naldini, 2011). It is now well established that HSC can be efficiently gene modified to continuously produce a cell progeny expressing the therapeutic gene while maintaining the ability to engraft long-term, for at least 15 years (Cicalese et al. 2016). Potential advantages of this approach over allogeneic HSCT include the lack of GVHD or rejection and the possibility of engineering HSC in order to achieve supra-physiological level of the corrected protein (Naldini, 2011; Aiuti and Naldini 2016).

Currently, integrating vectors derived from retroviruses represent the most efficient platform for engineering HSC and to provide permanent and heritable gene correction. γ-Retroviral vectors (RV) have been used in many clinical applications including GT of inherited blood disorders and cancer therapy. HSC-GT in primary immunodeficiencies was shown to provide clinical benefit, but the use of γ-RV was associated with risks of insertional mutagenesis due to activation of proto-oncogenes with the exception of ADA deficiency (Cicalese et al. 2016). Self-inactivating (SIN)-lentiviral vectors (LV) are currently the tools of choice for most of the HSC-GT applications given their ability to transduce at higher efficiency non-dividing cells, to carry larger and more complex gene cassettes, and to display a safer insertion site (InS) pattern in human HSC (Naldini, 2011). The recent development of designer endonucleases led to the advent of gene targeting approaches. In contrast to viral vectors, which can mediate only one type of gene modification (gene addition), genome-editing technologies can mediate gene addition, gene disruption, gene correction, and other targeted genome modifications (Dunbar et al. 2018). These strategies have the potential to overcome vector InS genotoxicity and to handle diseases due to dominant negative mutations. Despite the great promises, several challenges need to be addressed. Primitive, slow-cycling human BM-derived HSC are very resistant to ex vivo manipulations required for gene targeting, and the current efficiency of gene editing into repopulating HSC may not be suitable for clinical applications requiring high levels of correction (Dunbar et al. 2018; Kohn, 2017).

Thus, there remains a pressing need to develop methods to expand HSC or gene-corrected HSC while maintaining their repopulating capacity. Various cytokines and growth factors derived from BM niche, such as SCF, TPO, and Flt-3 ligand, are able to regulate HSC stemness and differentiation and are commonly used in HSC transduction protocols. However, even efficiently supporting GT, the balance between self-renewal/differentiation still hangs toward differentiation. High-throughput screening of chemical compounds has resulted in the identification of two promising molecules (StemRegenin1, SR1 (Wagner et al. 2016) and a

Gene correction of HSC for cell-based therapies

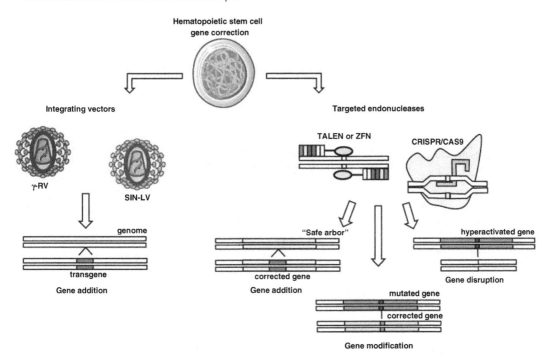

Fig. 7.2 Gene correction of HSC for cell-based therapies

pyrimidole derivative UM171 (Fares et al. 2014)) that are able to achieve great expansion of long-term repopulating HSC. Several small molecules have been identified that may support modest degrees of HSC expansion, but the ideal drug or combination has not yet been reported.

7.7   Studying Dynamics of Hematopoietic Reconstitution upon HSCT (Fig. 7.3)

Upon gene correction, each transduced cell and its progeny become univocally marked by a specific insertion site (InS). The analysis of RV or LV InS has emerged as one of the most effective strategies allowing tracing the activity of genetically engineered hematopoietic cells directly in vivo in animal models as well as in GT-treated patients. Retrieving InS from mature blood cells after HSCT allowed studying the kinetics of blood cell production from individual stem cells within a heterogeneous population (Scala et al. 2016).

In the murine setting, the finding that the vast majority of the InS after transplant were present in either lymphoid or myeloid cells with few InS shared by both lineages led to the concept that murine HSC are heterogeneous and already biased for their fate. The possibility to directly translate these models on human beings is currently under investigation (Lu et al. 2011; Yamamoto et al. 2013).

Clonal tracking studies in nonhuman primates have been pivotal in studying HSCT dynamics in an experimental setting close to humans. The results of these works showed common pattern of hematopoietic reconstitution upon transplantation: clonal fluctuation in the early phases post-HSCT, potentially due to the initial contribution to the hematopoiesis of short-term unilineage progenitors, followed by a recovery of a stable hematopoietic output likely related to the take-over of long-term multipotent HSC contribution. Thus, differently from murine studies, long-term HSC are able to provide multi-lineage engraftment, and there is no evidence of predetermined lineage choice at stem cell level in primates (Koelle et al. 2017; Kim et al. 2014).

Clonal tracking for studying the hematopoietic reconstitution dynamics upon HSCT

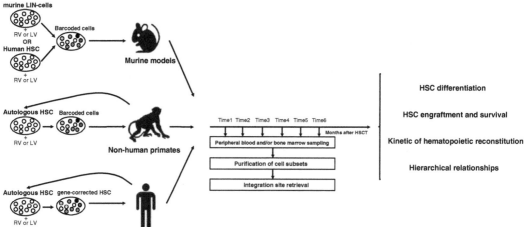

Fig. 7.3 Clonal tracking for studying the hematopoietic reconstitution dynamics upon HSCT

To date, few cutting-edge studies have exploited InS retrieval from GT-treated patients allowing for the first time to study the complexity of hematopoietic system and hematopoietic reconstitution upon HSCT in humans (Biasco et al. 2016; Wang et al. 2010). These studies showed that transplanted gene-repaired HSC are able to engraft and to generate polyclonal multi-lineage output overtime. Longitudinal analyses allowed unveiling that unilineage clones active during the first 6 months after GT tend to be replaced by multilineage long-term clones, indicating HSC-derived activity. Finally, based on the number of InS recaptured overtime, it has been estimated that about 1 in 10^5–10^6 infused gene-corrected cells had the potential to engraft long term. Recently our group unveiled for the first time that primitive HSPC have a distinct role in sustaining human hematopoiesis after transplantation. While MPP are more active in the early phases, long-living HSC are on top of the hematopoietic hierarchy at steady state. Importantly we found that long-term HSC, that were activated in vitro, were capable of homing and resilience upon re-infusion (Scala et al. 2018). These approaches represent a prototypical example of the power of translational studies, providing information relevant on human hematopoietic sys-

tem complementing and expanding the data derived from animal models.

7.8 From Experimental Hematology to Medical Practices and Hematopoietic Cellular Therapies

As already stressed in this brief review, a considerable amount of knowledge has accumulated over years allowing us to understand part of the mechanisms that control HSC behavior and take advantage of this knowledge; many of these observations cross-fertilized other disciplines. A large gap however persists between the technological sophistication of research tools and the rudimentary nature of clinical grade reagents, devices, and laboratory tests. In clinical transplantation or even in the most modern forms of hematopoietic cellular therapies, stem cells remain identified as "CD34+ cells," which can at best be considered as a gross approach to stemness; functional assays are limited to clonogenic cultures in routine practice; flow cytometry-activated cell sorting barely entered the clinical field, and most cell selection procedures rely on immune selection with magnetic beads. Despite these limitations, and as can be seen from the content of the other chapters in this book, HSCT remains as the only example of a worldwide and widely used cell transplant procedure, with many of its underlying conceptual aspects and techniques being used to design innovative and highly personalized somatic cell therapy or gene therapy medicinal products.

Key Points

HSC characteristics

- Self-renewal: ability of HSC to divide maintaining their biological properties
- Multipotency: ability of HSC to generate all mature hematopoietic cell types
- Quiescence: ability of HSC to remain inactive and unresponsive to external stimuli

Models of hematopoietic hierarchy

- Classical model: HSC differentiate into discrete and homogenous populations with successive restrictions in differentiation potentials
- Functional model: HSC differentiate according to hematopoietic state (stressed vs. unperturbed hematopoiesis)
- Progressive model: HSC differentiate through a continuous rather than discrete physiological process as result of a controlled genetic and epigenetic programs

Preclinical models of HSCT

- Murine models: study of HSC homing, engraftment, lineage differentiation, and serial transplantation capacity
- Canine models: validation of conditioning regimens and assessment of MHC donor/recipient matching significance
- Nonhuman primates: evaluation of mobilization procedures, conditioning regimens, and long-term maintenance of hematopoiesis

Ex vivo gene therapy

- Integrating vectors: γ-retroviral vectors (RV) and self-inactivating (SIN)-lentiviral vectors
- Genome editing: zinc-finger nucleases (ZFN), transcription activator-like effector nucleases (TALEN), and clustered, regularly interspaced, short palindromic repeat (CRISPR) nucleases

References

Aiuti A, Naldini L. Safer conditioning for blood stem cell transplants. Nat Biotechnol. 2016;34:721–3.

Antoniani C, Romano O, Miccio A. Concise review: epigenetic regulation of hematopoiesis: biological insights and therapeutic applications. Stem Cells Transl Med. 2017;6:2106–14.

Biasco L, Pellin D, Scala S, et al. In vivo tracking of human hematopoiesis reveals patterns of clonal dynamics during early and steady-state reconstitution phases. Cell Stem Cell. 2016;19:107–19.

Busch K, Rodewald HR. Unperturbed vs. post-transplantation hematopoiesis: both in vivo but different. Curr Opin Hematol. 2016;23:295–303.

Calvi LM, Link DC. The hematopoietic stem cell niche in homeostasis and disease. Blood. 2015;126:2443–52.

Cicalese MP, Ferrua F, Castagnaro L, et al. Update on the safety and efficacy of retroviral gene therapy for immunodeficiency due to adenosine deaminase deficiency. Blood. 2016;128:45–55.

Cooper JN, Young NS. Clonality in context: hematopoietic clones in their marrow environment. Blood. 2017;130:2363–72.

Cosgun KN, Rahmig S, Mende N, et al. Kit regulates HSC engraftment across the human-mouse species barrier. Cell Stem Cell. 2014;15:227–38.

Costa G, Kouskoff V, Lacaud G. Origin of blood cells and HSC production in the embryo. Trends Immunol. 2012;33:215–23.

Crane GM, Jeffery E, Morrison SJ. Adult haematopoietic stem cell niches. Nat Rev Immunol. 2017;17:573–90.

Di Maggio N, Piccinini E, Jaworski M, et al. Toward modeling the bone marrow niche using scaffold-based 3D culture systems. Biomaterials. 2011;32:321–9.

Doulatov S, Notta F, Laurenti E, et al. Hematopoiesis: a human perspective. Cell Stem Cell. 2012;10:120–36.

Dunbar CE, High KA, Joung JK, et al. Gene therapy comes of age. Science. 2018;359:1–10.

Eaves CJ. Hematopoietic stem cells: concepts, definitions, and the new reality. Blood. 2015;125:2605–14.

Fares I, Chagraoui J, Gareau Y, et al. Pyrimidoindole derivatives are agonists of human hematopoietic stem cell self-renewal. Science. 2014;345:1509–12.

Goodell MA, Rando TA. Stem cells and healthy aging. Science. 2015;350:1199–204.

Gottgens B. Regulatory network control of blood stem cells. Blood. 2015;125:2614–21.

Goyal S, Zandstra PW. Stem cells: chasing blood. Nature. 2015;518:488–90.

de Haan G, Lazare S. Aging of hematopoietic stem cells. Blood. 2018;131:479–87.

Höfer T, Rodewald HR. Output without input: the lifelong productivity of hematopoietic stem cells. Curr Opin Cell Biol. 2016;43:69–77.

Kaushansky K. Lineage-specific hematopoietic growth factors. N Engl J Med. 2006;354:2034–45.

Kim S, Kim N, Presson AP, et al. Dynamics of HSPC repopulation in nonhuman primates revealed by a decade-long clonal-tracking study. Cell Stem Cell. 2014;14:473–85.

Koelle SJ, Espinoza DA, Wu C, et al. Quantitative stability of hematopoietic stem and progenitor cell clonal output in transplanted rhesus macaques. Blood. 2017;129:1448–57.

Kohn DB. Historical perspective on the current renaissance for hematopoietic stem cell gene therapy. Hematol Oncol Clin North Am. 2017;31:721–35.

Laurenti E, Göttgens B. Review from haematopoietic stem cells to complex differentiation landscapes. Nature. 2018;553:418–26.

Lu R, Neff NF, Quake SR, et al. Tracking single hematopoietic stem cells in vivo using high-throughput sequencing in conjunction with viral genetic barcoding. Nat Biotechnol. 2011;29:928–33.

Naldini L. Ex vivo gene transfer and correction for cell-based therapies. Nat Rev Genet. 2011;12:301–15.

Pouzolles M, Oburoglu L, Taylor N, et al. Hematopoietic stem cell lineage specification. Curr Opin Hematol. 2016;23:311–7.

Reinisch A, Thomas D, Corces MR, et al. A humanized bone marrow ossicle xenotransplantation model enables improved engraftment of healthy and leukemic human hematopoietic cells. Nat Med. 2016;22:812–21.

Rowe RG, Mandelbaum J, Zon LI, et al. Engineering hematopoietic stem cells: lessons from development. Cell Stem Cell. 2016;18:707–20.

Scala S, Leonardelli L, Biasco L. Current approaches and future perspectives for in vivo clonal tracking of hematopoietic cells. Curr Gene Ther. 2016;16:1–10.

Scala S, Basso-Ricci L, Dionisio F, Pellin D, Giannelli S, Salerio FA, Leonardelli L, Cicalese MP, Ferrua F, Aiuti A, Biasco L. Dynamics of genetically engineered hematopoietic stem and progenitor cells after autologous transplantation in humans. Nat Med. 2018;24(11):1683–90. https://doi.org/10.1038/s41591-018-0195-3.

Schoedel KB, Morcos MNF, Zerjatke T, et al. The bulk of the hematopoietic stem cell population is dispensable for murine steady-state and stress hematopoiesis. Blood. 2016;128:2285–96.

Stolfi JL, Pai C-CS, Murphy WJ. Preclinical modeling of hematopoietic stem cell transplantation—advantages and limitations. FEBS J. 2016;283:1595–606.

Sykes SM, Scadden DT. Modeling human hematopoietic stem cell biology in the mouse. Semin Hematol. 2013;2:1–14.

Wagner JE, Brunstein CG, Boitano AE, et al. Phase I/II trial of stemregenin-1 expanded umbilical cord blood hematopoietic stem cells supports testing as a stand-alone graft. Cell Stem Cell. 2016;18:144–55.

Wang GP, Berry CC, Malani N, et al. Dynamics of gene-modified progenitor cells analyzed by tracking retroviral integration sites in a human SCID-X1 gene therapy trial. Blood. 2010;115:4356–66.

Yamamoto R, Morita Y, Ooehara J, et al. Clonal analysis unveils self-renewing lineage-restricted progenitors generated directly from hematopoietic stem cells. Cell. 2013;154:1112–26.

Biological Properties of Cells Other than HSCs

Attilio Bondanza, Ulrike Koehl, Andrea Hoffmann, and Antoine Toubert

8.1 Introduction

The array of cellular players involved in the biology of HSCT clearly extends beyond HSC themselves and, in the case of transplantation from allogeneic sources, importantly includes cells of the innate and adaptive immune system. Historically, the discovery of the HLA system and the functional characterization of the different immune cell types had a transformational impact on our current understanding of the pathobiological *sequelae* of allo-HSCT (rejection, GVHD, the GVL effect). This body of knowledge coupled to the most recent *exploit* of biotechnology nowadays allows us to design strategies for in vivo stimulation or adoptive transfer of specific immune cell types with the potential to dramatically improve transplantation outcome.

In this chapter, we will review the biological properties of cells other than HSCs that so far have Since apart from vaccination antigen presenting cells and myeloid cells at large have seldom been subject of this type of studies been therapeutically investigated in human allo-HSCT, they will not be discussed here. Conversely, we will briefly touch on mesenchymal stromal cells (MSCs), which, although not classifiable as immune cells *stricto* sensu, have been widely employed in allo-HSCT.

A. Bondanza (✉)
Innovative Immunotherapies Unit, Division of Immunology, Transplantation and Infectious Diseases, University Vita-Salute San Raffaele and Ospedale San Raffaele Scientific Institute, Milan, Italy
e-mail: Bondanza.Attilio@hsr.it

U. Koehl
University Hospital and Fraunhofer IZI, Leipzig, Germany

Hannover Medical School, Hannover, Germany

A. Hoffmann
Department of Orthopaedic Surgery, Laboratory of Biomechanics and Biomaterials, Hannover Medical School, Hannover, Germany

A. Toubert
University Paris Diderot and Hopital Saint Louis, Paris, France

8.2 Conventional or Alpha-Beta T Cells

The majority of mature T cells is characterized by the expression of the $\alpha\beta$ TCR, which endows MHC-restricted recognition of peptides derived from non-self-proteins. Mutually exclusive co-expression of CD8 or CD4 further conveys specificity for MHC class I/MHC class II/peptide complexes, respectively. CD8+ T cells recognize intracellular peptides, mainly derived from viruses or mutated genes, mediating cytotoxicity of infected or transformed cells, thence the name cytotoxic T lymphocytes (CTLs). Conversely, CD4+ T cells recognize extracellular pathogen-derived peptides, providing antigen-specific

specific "help" to bystander immune cells, such as B cells in antibody production and phagocytes in killing of engulfed pathogens. Alloreactivity occurs because of αβ TCR-mediated recognition of mismatched HLAs or of non-HLA polymorphic peptides presented in the context of matched HLAs, e.g., those derived from H-Y (male-specific histocompatibility antigen). The latter are known as minor histocompatibility antigens (mHag) and play a major role in GVHD and the GVL effect after HLA-matched transplantation.

The adoptive transfer of CTLs specific for important opportunistic viruses in allo-HSCT (CMV, EBV, ADV) has been one of the first manipulated cellular immunotherapies to be tested in humans (Bollard and Heslop 2016) and in some EU countries is now available as an off-the-shelf therapy from HLA-matched donors. Conversely, it has been proposed that naïve T cells, i.e., cells that have never encountered their cognate antigen, may be more alloreactive than memory T cells, i.e., antigen-experienced cells that have persisted after clearing the infection. This concept is at the basis of protocols for the depletion of naïve T cells from the graft as a way to prevent GVHD while retaining a strong GVL effect (Bleakley et al. 2015). Promising are also attempts at translating this approach against hematological tumor antigens for treating overt leukemia relapse after allo-HSCT (Chapuis et al. 2013). On a different page, given the overall complexity of immune responses, it is not surprising that during evolution, some immune cell types have evolved with the specific task of immune regulation. T regulatory cells (Tregs) are thymus-derived cells characterized by constitutive expression of the transcription factor FoxP3. Tregs are potent suppressors of alloreactivity and are now being investigated for GVHD management after their ex vivo expansion (Brunstein et al. 2016).

8.3   Unconventional T Cells

Unconventional T cells include T cells expressing the γδ TCR, invariant natural killer T cells (iNKT) cells, and mucosal-associated invariant (MAIT) T cells—which will not be treated here—and are an abundant component of the immune system. Although originating from the thymus, they all share lack of MHC-restricted peptide recognition and mainly reside within epithelial tissues. They have a limited TCR repertoire diversity and get activated quickly, bridging innate to adaptive immunity.

1. A subset of γδ T cells (Vγ2Vδ9) are activated by phosphoantigens, non-peptidic metabolites produced by mammalian cells and intracellular pathogens (*M. tuberculosis*, *M. leprae*, *Listeria* species, *Plasmodium* species) after interacting with intracellular butyrophilin 3A1. Gamma-delta T cells can also recognize stress molecules such as MICA, MICB, and ULBPs through the NK receptor NKG2D. The possibility to expand Vγ2Vδ9 effector T cells in vivo by administering the therapeutic bisphosphonate zoledronate has originated many clinical trials in hematological tumors, also in the context of transplantation (Airoldi et al. 2015).

2. Type I invariant NKT is a distinct population of αβ T cells characterized in humans by the expression of α24-Jα18 preferentially paired to Vβ11. They recognize lipids presented in the context of broadly distributed CD1d (monocytes/macrophages, B cells, epithelial cells). Upon activation, iNKT cells produce immune regulatory cytokines and kill tumor targets. Failure to reconstitute iNKT cells after Allo-HSCT (Rubio et al. 2012) or lower iNKT cells in the graft (Chaidos et al. 2012) has been linked to GVHD and relapse. Alpha-galactosyl ceramide is a marine sponge-derived lipid antigen known to expand iNKT cells in vivo and is currently under investigation in Allo-HSCT (Chen et al. 2017).

8.4   NK Cells

Natural killer (NK) cells belong to the innate immune system and provide immediate reactivity against virally infected, as well as tumor targets. NK cytotoxicity is controlled by a balance of several germ-line encoded inhibitory and activating receptors, such as killer immunoglobulin-like receptors (KIRs) and natural cytotoxicity receptors (Vivier et al. 2011). The importance of NK cells in allo-HSCT has surfaced after the demonstration of their pivotal role in preventing leukemia relapse and decreasing GVHD risk after grafting from HLA-haploidentical donors (Ruggeri et al. 2002). Since then, there has been a growing interest in using both autologous and allogeneic NK cells in patients with leukemia or other high-risk hematological tumors, also in the non-transplant setting (Koehl et al. 2016). These trials have uniformly shown safety and potential efficacy of infused NK cells. Nevertheless, they have also documented the emergence of powerful immune escape mechanisms, raising the question on how to improve NK cell-based therapies (Koehl et al. 2018). Various trials are under way in order to investigate ways to achieve better NK cell cytotoxicity and overcome the immunosuppressive tumor microenvironment, including:

1. Combination of novel checkpoint inhibitors with activated NK cells
2. Bi- or tri-specific antibodies for directly binding NK cells to cancer cells
3. Chimeric antigen receptor (CAR)-modified NK cells for direct targeting of cancer cells

The latter strategy is particularly interesting since CAR-NK cells are expected to retain their natural antitumor reactivity, opening for potentially synergistic effects. The first clinical CAR-NK cell studies targeting CD19 and NKG2D ligands have been initiated (ClinGov. No NCT03056339, NCT01974479, NCT00995137, NCT03415100) and will likely be instrumental to demonstrate proof of concept.

8.5 Mesenchymal Stromal Cells

Mesenchymal stroma cells (MSCs) are multipotent cells capable of differentiating into cells and tissues of the mesodermal lineage (bone, cartilage, and adipose cells) (Pittenger et al. 1999). Apart from their regenerative properties, MSCs have been discovered to secrete a variety of soluble factors and exosomes with paracrine actions. Instead of focusing on MSC regenerative properties, most clinical studies have investigated their immunomodulatory (often immunosuppressive) properties, as well as their trophic influence on tissue repair, especially in GVHD (Fibbe et al. 2013). Interestingly, subsequent to hematopoietic stem cells, MSCs are the second most frequently used cell source for therapeutic applications. Notwithstanding their widespread use, MSCs are currently the stem cell population with the least defined identity and properties (Hoffmann et al. 2017).

Important studies have demonstrated that the physiological counterpart of ex vivo-expanded MSCs can be both CD146+ adventitial reticular cells in the subendothelial layer of microvessels (Tormin et al. 2011) and CD146- pericytes surrounding large vessels (Corselli et al. 2013). MSC biological functions are also highly debated and conflicting results were reported in vitro and, more importantly, in clinical trials (Fibbe et al. 2013). Considerable lack of consensus exists within the field as to how MSCs exert their multipronged effects. This is due to several facts: Firstly, MSCs are isolated from many tissues and by different protocols. Secondly, due to the mode of isolation, these cells present heterogeneous cell populations. Thirdly, protocols for in vitro expansion, including the culture conditions (culture vessels, media, additives, passaging), are different. Fourthly, MSCs have often been reported to survive in vivo only for short time (days). A recent comparison of MSC preparations from eight different centers using BM aspirates as starting material for GMP-guided processes revealed considerable variability between the centers (Liu et al. 2017). Cells from six centers were compared in vivo for bone formation and hematopoiesis support. The quantity of deriving bone was highly variable, and only MSCs from three centers supported hematopoiesis. A critical reappraisal of these cell populations and harmonization of the methods for their isolation and expansion, as well as the development of validated potency assays, is therefore necessary for harnessing their full therapeutic potential.

Key Points

- HSCT rather than a solo play is an orchestral concert, where different cellular players contribute to the overall final result of the symphony.
- Besides obviously HSCs, key contributors are cells of the innate and adaptive immune system. Both have evolved for the key task of self/non-self-discrimination, each however focusing on the recognition of different class of molecules, from proteins to glycolipids.
- The tremendous knowledge in immunobiology acquired in the last few decades has enabled to start exploiting the properties of these cells or ameliorating the outcome of HSCT.

References

Airoldi I, Bertaina A, Prigione I, et al. γδ T-cell reconstitution after HLA-haploidentical hematopoietic transplantation depleted of TCR-αβ+/CD19+ lymphocytes. Blood. 2015;125:2349–58.

Bleakley M, Heimfeld S, Loeb KR, et al. Outcomes of acute leukemia patients transplanted with naive T cell-depleted stem cell grafts. J Clin Invest. 2015;125:2677–89.

Bollard CM, Heslop HE. T cells for viral infections after allogeneic hematopoietic stem cell transplant. Blood. 2016;127:3331–40.

Brunstein CG, Miller JS, McKenna DH, et al. Umbilical cord blood-derived T regulatory cells to prevent GVHD: kinetics, toxicity profile, and clinical effect. Blood. 2016;127:1044–51.

Chaidos A, Patterson S, Szydlo R, et al. Graft invariant natural killer T-cell dose predicts risk of acute graft-versus-host disease in allogeneic hematopoietic stem cell transplantation. Blood. 2012;119:5030–6.

Chapuis AG, Ragnarsson GB, Nguyen HN, et al. Transferred WT1-reactive CD8+ T cells can mediate antileukemic activity and persist in post-transplant patients. Sci Transl Med. 2013;5:174ra27.

Chen Y-B, Efebera YA, Johnston L, et al. Increased Foxp3+Helios+ regulatory T cells and decreased acute graft-versus-host disease after allogeneic bone marrowtransplantation in patients receiving sirolimus and RGI-2001, an activator of invariant natural killer T cells. Biol Blood Marrow Transplant. 2017;23:625–34.

Corselli M, Crisan M, Murray IR, et al. Identification of perivascular mesenchymal stromal/stem cells by flow cytometry. Cytom Part J Int Soc Anal Cytol. 2013;83:714–20.

Fibbe WE, Dazzi F, LeBlanc K. MSCs: science and trials. Nat Med. 2013;19:812–3.

Hoffmann A, Floerkemeier T, Melzer C, Hass R. Comparison of in vitro-cultivation of human mesenchymal stroma/stem cells derived from bone marrow and umbilical cord. J Tissue Eng Regen Med. 2017;11:2565–81.

Koehl U, Kalberer C, Spanholtz J, et al. Advances in clinical NK cell studies: donor selection, manufacturing and quality control. Oncoimmunology. 2016;5:e1115178.

Koehl U, Toubert A, Pittari G. Editorial: tailoring NK cell receptor-ligand interactions: an art in evolution. Front Immunol. 2018;9:351.

Liu S, de Castro LF, Jin P, et al. Manufacturing differences affect human bone marrow stromal cell characteristics and function: comparison of production methods and products from multiple centers. Sci Rep. 2017;7:46731.

Pittenger MF, Mackay AM, Beck SC, et al. Multilineage potential of adult human mesenchymal stem cells. Science. 1999;284:143–7.

Rubio M-T, Moreira-Teixeira L, Bachy E, et al. Early posttransplantation donor-derived invariant natural killer T-cell recovery predicts the occurrence of acute graft-versus-host disease and overall survival. Blood. 2012;120:2144–54.

Ruggeri L, Capanni M, Urbani E, et al. Effectiveness of donor natural killer cell alloreactivity in mismatched hematopoietic transplants. Science. 2002;295:2097–100.

Tormin A, Li O, Brune JC, et al. CD146 expression on primary nonhematopoietic bone marrow stem cells is correlated with in situ localization. Blood. 2011;117:5067–77.

Vivier E, Raulet DH, Moretta A, et al. Innate or adaptive immunity? The example of natural killer cells. Science. 2011;331:44–9.

Histocompatibility

Eric Spierings and Katharina Fleischhauer

9.1 Introduction

Immune-mediated rejection of tissue allografts was first described in 1945 by the British immunologist Peter Medawar, followed by the discovery of the major histocompatibility complex (MHC) carrying the histocompatibility genes by Peter Gorer and George Snell in 1948, and of the human leukocyte antigen (HLA) molecules by Jean Dausset, Jon van Rood, and Rose Payne a decade later (Thorsby 2009). The importance of these discoveries was recognized by the Nobel Prices in Physiology and Medicine to Medawar, Snell, and Dausset in 1960 and 1980, respectively. Since then, the MHC has emerged as the single most polymorphic gene locus in eukaryotes, with 17,695 HLA alleles reported to date in the IMGT/HLA database, Release 3.31.0, 2018/01/19 (Robinson et al. 2015). While the main barrier to successful tissue grafting remain the HLA incompatibilities, also non-HLA polymorphisms have been recognized as important players, in particular minor histocompatibility antigens (mHAg), killer immunoglobulin-like

receptors (KIR), and other polymorphic gene systems (Dickinson and Holler 2008; Gam et al. 2017; Heidenreich and Kröger 2017; Spierings 2014).

9.2 The Biology of Histocompatibility

9.2.1 Major Histocompatibility Antigens

The human MHC is located within ~4 Mbp of DNA on the short arm of chromosome 6 (6p21.3) and contains ~260 genes, many of which with immune-related functions (Trowsdale and Knight 2013). The MHC falls into three main regions, class I, II, and III, containing HLA A, B, and C; HLA DR, DQ, and DP; and complement factor as well as tumor necrosis factor genes, respectively. MHC genes are codominantly expressed and inherited following Mendelian rules, with a resulting 25% probability for two siblings to be genotypically HLA identical, i.e., to have inherited the same MHC from both parents. An additional hallmark of the MHC is linkage disequilibrium (LD), i.e., the nonrandom association of alleles at different HLA loci, and relatively high recombination rates of over 1%, also referred to as "crossing over" (Martin et al. 1995).

E. Spierings
Laboratory for Translational Immunology, University Medical Center, Utrecht, The Netherlands

K. Fleischhauer (✉)
Institute for Experimental Cellular Therapy, University Hospital, Essen, Germany
e-mail: katharina.fleischhauer@uk-essen.de

9.2.2 HLA Class I and II Structure and Function

The classical HLA class I and II molecules are cell surface immunoglobulins (Ig) presenting peptides in their highly polymorphic antigen-binding groove (Madden 1995). HLA class I A, B, and C molecules are heterodimers of a polymorphic α chain of higher molecular weight (MW) than the monomorphic β2 microglobulin (heavy and light chain of 45 kDa and 12 kDa, respectively). The α-chain contains three hypervariable Ig-like domains, two of which form the antigen-binding groove while the third is involved in contacting the CD8 coreceptor on T cells, and the transmembrane region. HLA class I molecules are expressed on all healthy nucleated cells. They present peptides, i.e., protein fragments of mostly intracellular origin generated by proteasomal cleavage and transported to the endoplasmic reticulum via the transporter associated with antigen processing (TAP) (Vyas et al. 2008). Cell surface HLA class I peptide complexes can be recognized by the T cell receptor (TCR) of CD8+ T cells, leading to the activation of cytotoxic and/or cytokine effector functions, or by KIR on natural killer (NK) cells, leading to the inhibition of effector functions. HLA class II DR, DQ, and DP molecules are heterodimers of an α- and a β-chain of similar MW of approximately 30 KDa each, both with a transmembrane part anchored to the cell membrane. Most of the polymorphism is clustered in the β-chain Ig-like domain forming the antigen-binding groove, whose overall structure is similar to that of HLA class I, and the region contacting the CD4 coreceptor on T cells is also located in the β-chain. HLA class II proteins are expressed on professional antigen-presenting cells, as, for example, B cells, macrophages, and dendritic cells. Moreover, HLA class II protein expression on various cell types can be upregulated by proinflammatory cytokines such as IFNγ and TNFα. HLA class II presents peptides generally of extracellular origin generated through degradation of proteins in the phagolysosome (Vyas et al. 2008). Peptide loading onto HLA class II molecules takes place in the dedicated MIIC compartment and is catalyzed by two nonclassical HLA molecules equally encoded in the MHC, HLA DM, and DO. After transport to the cell surface, HLA class II peptide complexes can be recognized by the TCR of CD4+ T cells, leading to the activation of cytokine-mediated helper or regulatory functions. HLA class II receptors on NK cells, analogous to KIR for HLA class I, have not been described to date.

9.2.3 HLA Polymorphism and Tissue Typing

HLA molecules were first detected by serological methods, through the ability of sera from sensitized individuals to agglutinate some but not all leukocytes (hence the term "human leukocyte antigen") (Thorsby 2009). Until the mid-1990s, serological typing was the main method for tissue typing. With the advent of polymerase chain reaction (PCR) techniques, molecular tissue typing took over and unraveled a far greater degree of HLA allelic polymorphism than previously appreciated (Erlich 2012). HLA nucleotide polymorphism is clustered in so-called hypervariable regions (HvR) mainly in exons 2, 3, and 4 of HLA class I and exons 2 and 3 of HLA class II, encoding the functional antigen-binding groove and CD4/CD8 coreceptor-binding regions. Therefore, PCR-based molecular typing focused on these exons, leading to different levels of typing resolution (Table 9.1). With the advent of next-generation sequencing (NGS) for tissue typing purposes (Gabriel et al. 2014), allelic or at least high-resolution typing can be achieved in most cases. Moreover, NGS enables high-throughput sequencing of the entire HLA coding and noncoding regions, unraveling an additional layer of polymorphism with hundreds of new alleles reported to the IMGT/HLA database every month.

9.2.4 T Cell Alloreactivity

The ability of T cells to specifically recognize non-self, allogeneic tissues is called T cell

Table 9.1 HLA typing resolution and appropriate typing methods

HLA typing resolution[a]	Appropriate typing methods[b]
Low (first field)	Serology, SSP, SSOP, others
High (second field)	NGS, SBT
Allelic (all fields)	NGS, SBT
Intermediate	SSP, SSOP, SBT

[a]As defined in (Nunes et al. 2011). *Low:* A serological typing result or DNA-based typing at the first field in the DNA-based nomenclature. *High:* A set of alleles that encode the same protein sequence in the antigen binding site and that exclude alleles not expressed at the cell surface. High resolution thus includes alleles reported with the suffix G (set of alleles with identical nucleotide sequence across the exons encoding the antigen binding site) or the suffix P (set of alleles encoding the same protein sequence at the antigen binding site). *Allelic:* Unique nucleotide sequence for a gene as defined by the use of all of the digits in a current allele name. Intermediate: A level of resolution that falls between high and low resolution, as agreed with the entity requesting the testing. Examples are restriction to common and well-documented (CWD) alleles (Sanchez-Mazas et al. 2017) or reporting by NMDP codes (https://bioinformatics.bethematchclinical.org/hla-resources/allele-codes/allele-code-lists/).
[b]*Serology* complement-dependent cytotoxicity of specific antisera, *SSP* sequence-specific priming, *SSOP* sequence-specific oligonucleotide probing, *Others* additional molecular typing approaches including quantitative PCR and restriction fragment length polymorphism (RFLP), *SBT* sequencing-based typing (Sanger sequencing), *NGS* next-generation sequencing

alloreactivity. It can be either direct or indirect. Direct T cell alloreactivity is targeted to intact mismatched HLA peptide complexes expressed on the cell surface of allogeneic cells and can be mediated by both naïve and memory T cells (Archbold et al. 2008). Indirect T cell alloreactivity refers to the recognition of peptides derived by proteasomal cleavage from mismatched HLA and presented in the antigen-binding groove of self HLA molecules (Gokmen et al. 2008). These peptides are also referred to as Predicted Indirectly ReCognizable HLA Epitopes (PIRCHE, see Sect. 9.3.3) (Geneugelijk and Spierings 2018). A special form of indirect T cell alloreactivity is the recognition of foreign peptides not deriving from mismatched HLA but from any other expressed polymorphic gene and presented by self HLA molecules. These peptides are referred to as minor histocompatibility antigens (mHAg) (Spierings 2014). mHAg are the

only targets of T cell alloreactivity in HLA-matched hematopoietic cell transplantation (HSCT) and are mainly recognized by naïve T cells. T cell alloreactivity is the main mediator of both the major benefit and the major toxicity of allogeneic HSCT, represented by immune control of residual malignant disease (graft versus leukemia; GvL) and immune attack of healthy tissues (graft versus host disease; GvHD), respectively.

Key Points

- HLA molecules are encoded by highly polymorphic genes in the human MHC and play a crucial role for peptide antigen recognition by T cells.
- HLA tissue typing can be performed at different levels of resolution, the highest being attainable only by NGS-based methods, which are unraveling an unprecedented degree of polymorphism in the MHC.
- Alloreactive T cells can recognize non-self HLA molecules on healthy and malignant cells after Allo-HSCT, mediating both toxic GvHD and beneficial GvL.

9.3 HLA Matching in Allogeneic HSCT

9.3.1 Donor Types

In HLA identical sibling HSCT, patient and donor have inherited the same parental MHCs, an event occurring with a likelihood of 25% according to Mendelian rules. Genotypic HLA identity should be confirmed by family studies for all six HLA loci (to exclude recombination). Haploidentical donors share only one MHC haplotype while the other haplotype is different. These donors are available for more than 90% of patients and can be found in parents or offsprings (100% likelihood), siblings (50% likelihood), as well as the extended family. Also HLA haploidentity should be confirmed by family studies wherever possible. Unrelated donors (UD) can be found among over 30 million volunteers enrolled in the worldwide registries or from over 700,000 banked cord blood units. The probability to find a volunteer UD matched for 8/8 HLA A, B, C, and DRB1 alleles varies according to the ethnic group of the patient between 30% and over 90% (Gragert et al. 2014). For UD HSCT, HLA identity should be confirmed at the highest resolution level possible (allelic, high, or intermediate resolution, Table 9.1), to be agreed between the transplant center and the tissue typing laboratory.

9.3.2   Clinical Impact of HLA Mismatches

The clinical relevance of histocompatibility for the outcome of HSCT is significantly influenced by different patient-, donor-, and transplant-related factors (Table 9.2). The most striking example for the impact of these confounding factors is the advent of haploidentical HSCT, in which successful transplantation across an entire mismatched haplotype was rendered possible by extensive T cell depletion of the graft and, more recently, by innovative schemes of pharmacological GvHD prophylaxis (Slade et al. 2017). On the other hand, haploidentical HSCT has been associated with a particular form of immune escape relapse characterized by the selective genomic loss of the mismatched HLA haplotype, with important implications for treatment strategies (Vago et al. 2012). In UD HSCT, high-resolution matching for 8/8 HLA A, B, C, and DRB1 alleles has been shown to be associated with the best clinical outcomes, with an approximately 10% decrease in survival probabilities for every (antigenic or allelic) HLA mismatch at these four loci (Lee et al. 2007). On the other hand, the impact of HLA disparity was shown to be significantly reduced by advanced disease status at transplant, again demonstrating the inextricable link between HLA mismatches and confounding factors. The notion that there will be no "one-size-fits-all" solution to the question on

Table 9.2 Confounding factors of HLA/non-HLA immunogenetics and HSCT outcome

Confounding factor[a]	
Patient related	Age, sex, ABO, CMV serostatus, diagnosis, disease status
Donor related	Age, sex, ABO, CMV serostatus
Transplant related	Conditioning, GvHD prophylaxis, stem cell source, and composition

[a]The impact of HLA matching is additionally confounded by non-HLA immunogenetic factors and vice versa

the impact of histocompatibility in HSCT has to be taken into account when critically interpreting studies in this complex field.

9.3.3   Models of High-Risk/ Nonpermissive HLA Mismatches

HLA mismatches that are clinically less well tolerated than others are referred to as high risk or nonpermissive. This is based on the observation that limited T cell alloreactivity is generally sufficient for the beneficial effect of GvL without inducing clinically uncontrollable GvHD, while intolerable toxicity can be induced by excessive T cell alloreactivity leading to severe treatment refractory GvHD. Therefore, high-risk or nonpermissive HLA mismatches are those associated with excessive T cell alloreactivity compared to their low-risk or permissive counterparts. Different models have been developed over the past years for their identification (Table 9.3). They rely on the presence of shared or nonshared T cell epitope (TCE) groups between mismatched HLA DPB1 alleles (Fleischhauer and Shaw 2017), genetically controlled expression levels of mismatched HLA C or DPB1 alleles in the patient (Petersdorf et al. 2014, 2015), specific high-risk HLA C and DPB1 allele mismatch combinations identified by retrospective statistical association between mismatch status and clinical outcome (Fernandez-Vina et al. 2014; Kawase et al. 2009), and the total number of PIRCHEI (presented by HLA class I) and PIRCHEII (presented by HLA class II) as a measure of the potential level of indirect alloreactivity after transplantation (Geneugelijk and

Table 9.3 Models of high-risk/nonpermissive HLA mismatches

Model	HLA locus, donor type, and clinical association
T cell epitope (TCE) groups[a]	HLA-DPB1; 8/8 UD; mortality and acute GvHD
Expression levels[b]	HLA C and DPB1; 7–8/8 UD; acute GvHD
Mismatch combinations[c]	HLA C and DPB1; 7–8/8 UD; mortality, acute GvHD and relapse
PIRCHE[d]	HLA C and DPB1; 8/8 UD; acute GvHD

[a]*TCE groups:* HLA DPB1 mismatches involving alleles from the same (permissive) or different (nonpermissive) TCE groups (Fleischhauer and Shaw 2017)
[b]*Expression levels:* HLA C or DPB1 mismatches involving a high-expression allele in the patient, as predicted by noncoding single nucleotide expression polymorphisms (Petersdorf et al. 2014, 2015)
[c]*Mismatch combinations*, high-risk allele mismatches defined by statistical associations (Fernandez-Vina et al. 2014; Kawase et al. 2009)
[d]*PIRCHE*, predicted indirectly recognizable HLA epitope numbers as predicted by online tools (Geneugelijk and Spierings 2018)

Spierings 2018). It should be noted that HLA DPB1 mismatches are present in over 80% of 8/8 matched UD HSCT, and models for high-risk or nonpermissive mismatches at this locus are therefore of particular practical relevance. The PIRCHE model is attractive since it is potentially applicable to any HLA-mismatched donor transplantation including <8/8 matched UD and haploidentical HSCT; on the other hand, clinical evidence for its validity in HSCT has so far been obtained only on relatively limited transplant cohorts. As stated above (Sect. 9.3.2), it is crucial that any of these or future models be tested in independent cohorts of sufficient statistical size and that they be continuously revalidated as clinical transplant practice and hence potential confounding factors evolve.

9.3.4 Guidelines for UD Selection by Histocompatibility

Consensus guidelines for donor selection have been established in many countries both in Europe and overseas, through the collaboration between donor registries and national immunogenetic societies. The general recommendation is the selection of an 8/8 HLA A, B, C, and DR (in Europe often 10/10, i.e., including the HLA DQ locus) matched UD if an HLA identical sibling is not available, followed by a 7/8 (or 9/10) UD or a haploidentical donor. Avoidance of high-risk or nonpermissive HLA mismatches according to any of the models outlined in Table 9.3 is usually regarded as optional, with particular emphasis on the avoidance of nonpermissive HLA DPB1 TCE mismatches since the TCE model is the only one to have been validated in different independent clinical studies to date (Fleischhauer and Shaw 2017). Also the inclusion of some of the non-HLA immunogenetic factors outlined in Sect. 9.4 can be considered, in particular with regard to donor KIR typing in haploidentical HSCT (Heidenreich and Kröger 2017).

Key Points

- HSCT donor types (in parenthesis the % probability of their identification for a given patient) include genotypically HLA identical siblings (25%), HLA haploidentical family donors (>90%), UD (30–90%), and cord blood donors (>80%).
- HLA typing strategies including family studies for related donors and typing resolution level for UD should be agreed between the transplant center and the tissue typing laboratory.
- The clinical relevance of HLA matching for the outcome of HSCT is critically dependent on numerous patient-, donor-, and transplant-related factors.
- In UD HSCT, survival probability decreases by 10% with every mismatch at HLA A, B, C, and DRB1, in patients transplanted at early disease stage.
- Models for high-risk nonpermissive HLA mismatches eliciting excessive T cell alloreactivity with intolerable toxicity include structural TCE, expression levels, specific allele

combinations, and PIRCHE. All these and future models need to be tested in independent cohorts of sufficient statistical size and be continuously revalidated as clinical transplant practice evolves.

- Consensus guidelines established at the national level between donor registries and immunogenetic societies aid in the selection of HSCT donors.

9.4 Non-HLA Immunogenetic Factors

9.4.1 Overview

HLA alleles are the most but not the only polymorphic genes in humans. Overall, interindividual gene variability by single nucleotide polymorphism (SNP) or copy-number variation (CNV) affects 0.5% of the 3×10^9 bp in the human genome. Although most of these polymorphisms are probably nonfunctional, some of them can give rise to polymorphic proteins that can be mHAg as described in Sect. 9.2.2, affect the expression of different genes including those encoding immunologically active cytokines, or act themselves as immune ligands or receptors relevant to transplantation biology. Among the latter, the KIR gene locus on the long arm of human chromosome 19 displays considerable polymorphism, with 907 alleles reported to the IPD/KIR database, Release 2.7.0, July 2017 (Robinson et al. 2005). Similar to high-risk or nonpermissive HLA mismatches, the role of non-HLA polymorphism in allo-HSCT is still incompletely defined. It is impossible to give a comprehensive overview of all non-HLA factors under study, and the list of factors listed in Table 9.4 and discussed in Sect. 9.4.2 is only a selection based on existing evidence for their clinical impact in certain transplant settings.

Table 9.4 Non-HLA immunogenetic factors and HSCT outcome

Non-HLA factor	Clinical outcome association
mHAg[a]	GvHD and relapse
KIR[b]	Relapse and mortality
MIC[c]	GvHD, relapse, and transplant-related mortality
Others[d]	GvHD and transplant-related mortality

[a]*Minor histocompatibility antigens* (Spierings 2014)
[b]*Killer Ig-like receptors* (Heidenreich and Kröger 2017; Shaffer and Hsu 2016)
[c]*MHC class I-related chain* (Isernhagen et al. 2016)
[d]*Cytokine, chemokine, and immune response gene polymorphisms* including tumor necrosis factor, interleukin (IL)10, the IL1 gene family, IL2, IL6, interferon γ, tumor growth factor β and their receptors, NOD-like receptors (NOD2/CARD15), toll-like receptors, micro-RNAs (Dickinson and Holler 2008; Gam et al. 2017; Chen and Zeiser 2018)

9.4.2 Clinical Impact of Non-HLA Immunogenetic Factors

mHAg are the only targets of T cell alloreactivity in HLA identical HSCT (see Sect. 9.2.2) and as such play an important role for both GvHD and GvL (Spierings 2014). This dual function is related to their different modes of tissue and cell expression, i.e., hematopoietic system restricted or broad. Broadly expressed mHAg can cause both GvHD and GvL, and donor-recipient matching for these mHAg is therefore desirable yet virtually impossible due to their large number, with many of them probably currently undefined. In contrast, mHAg restricted to hematopoietic cells are more prone to induce selective GvL. The latter are being explored as targets for HSCT-based immunotherapy of hematological malignancies, in which mHAg-specific responses are specifically enhanced to promote GvL.

KIR are predominantly expressed by NK cells and recognize certain HLA class I specificities on target cells. KIR have either long inhibitory or short activating cytoplasmic domains and are stochastically coexpressed on NK cells. The eventual outcome of KIR interaction (or lack thereof) with its HLA class I ligand (inhibition or activation) is a complex process that depends on the relative number of inhibitory or activatory KIR and on the state of education of the NK cell. Educated NK cells from individuals expressing the cognate HLA ligand are strongly reactive against cells missing that ligand. This "missing self" reactivity is at the basis for the potent GvL effect attributed to NK cells in the setting of HLA-mismatched transplantation, in particular haploidentical HSCT (Heidenreich and Kröger 2017). Depending on the donor KIR gene asset, a role for NK cell-mediated GvL has also been postulated in the HLA-matched setting (Shaffer and Hsu 2016). Based on all this evidence, KIR typing is increasingly being adopted as an additional criterion for donor selection.

MHC class I chain-related (MIC) A and B are nonclassical MHC class I genes. MICA encodes a ligand for NKG2D, an activating NK receptor. The SNP Val/Met at position 129 of the MICA protein results in isoforms with high (Met) and low affinities (Val) for NKG2D. Consequently, various studies suggest a role for this SNP in SCT outcome, including GvHD, relapse and survival (Isernhagen et al. 2016).

Immune response gene polymorphisms have also been reported to contribute to the risks associated with HSCT (Dickinson and Holler 2008; Gam et al. 2017; Chen and Zeiser 2018). They often comprise SNPs in cytokine or chemokine-coding genes or their regulatory elements such as micro-RNAs (miRNAs). These variations in both the donor and the recipient can have a significant impact on transplant outcome and the development of GvHD; however, their relative role in different transplant settings is not yet fully elucidated.

Key Points

- Non-HLA immunogenetic factors that have been associated with clinical outcome of HSCT include polymorphic mHAg, KIR, MIC, and immune response genes.
- Hematopoietic tissue-specific mHAg are being exploited for specific cellular immunotherapy of hematologic malignancies.

- Polymorphic KIR are responsible for "missing self" recognition by alloreactive NK cells mediating selective GvL after HSCT, and KIR genotyping is therefore increasingly included into donor selection algorithms.

References

Archbold JK, Ely LK, Kjer-Nielsen L, et al. T cell allorecognition and MHC restriction–a case of Jekyll and Hyde? Mol Immunol. 2008;45:583–98.

Chen S, Zeiser R. The role of microRNAs in myeloid cells during graft-versus-host disease. Front Immunol. 2018;9:4.

Dickinson AM, Holler E. Polymorphisms of cytokine and innate immunity genes and GVHD. Best Pract Res Clin Haematol. 2008;21:149–64.

Erlich H. HLA DNA typing: past, present, and future. Tissue Antigens. 2012;80:1–11.

Fernandez-Vina MA, Wang T, Lee SJ, et al. Identification of a permissible HLA mismatch in hematopoietic stem cell transplantation. Blood. 2014;123:1270–8.

Fleischhauer K, Shaw BE. HLA-DP in unrelated hematopoietic cell transplantation revisited: challenges and opportunities. Blood. 2017;130:1089–96.

Gabriel C, Fürst D, Fae I, et al. HLA typing by next-generation sequencing–getting closer to reality. Tissue Antigens. 2014;83:65–75.

Gam R, Shah P, Crossland RE, Norden J, et al. Genetic association of hematopoietic stem cell transplantation outcome beyond histocompatibility genes. Front Immunol. 2017;8:380.

Geneugelijk K, Spierings E. Matching donor and recipient based on predicted indirectly recognizable human leucocyte antigen epitopes. Int J Immunogenet. 2018;45:41–53.

Gokmen MR, Lombardi G, Lechler RI. The importance of the indirect pathway of allorecognition in clinical transplantation. Curr Opin Immunol. 2008;20:568–74.

Gragert L, Eapen M, Williams E, et al. HLA match likelihoods for hematopoietic stem-cell grafts in the U.S. registry. N Engl J Med. 2014;371:339–48.

Heidenreich S, Kröger N. Reduction of relapse after unrelated donor stem cell transplantation by KIR-based graft selection. Front Immunol. 2017;8:41.

Isernhagen A, Malzahn D, Bickeboller H, Dressel R. Impact of the MICA-129Met/Val dimorphism on NKG2D-mediated biological functions and disease risks. Front Immunol. 2016;7:588.

Kawase T, Matsuo K, Kashiwase K, et al. HLA mismatch combinations associated with decreased risk of relapse: implications for the molecular mechanism. Blood. 2009;113:2851–8.

Lee SJ, Klein J, Haagenson M, et al. High-resolution donor-recipient HLA matching contributes to the success of unrelated donor marrow transplantation. Blood. 2007;110:4576–83.

Madden DR. The three-dimensional structure of peptide-MHC complexes. Annu Rev Immunol. 1995;13:587–622.

Martin M, Mann D, Carrington M. Recombination rates across the HLA complex: use of microsatellites as a rapid screen for recombinant chromosomes. Hum Mol Gen. 1995;4:423–8.

Nunes E, Heslop H, Fernandez-Vina MA, et al. Definitions of histocompatibility typing terms. Blood. 2011;118:e180–3.

Petersdorf EW, Gooley TA, Malkki M, et al. HLA-C expression levels define permissible mismatches in hematopoietic cell transplantation. Blood. 2014;124:3996–4003.

Petersdorf EW, Malkki M, O'HUigin C, et al. High HLA-DP expression and graft-versus-host disease. N Engl J Med. 2015;373:599–609.

Robinson J, Halliwell JA, Hayhurst JD, et al. The IPD and IMGT/HLA database: allele variant databases. Nucleic Acids Res. 2015;43:D423–31.

Robinson J, Waller MJ, Stoehr P, Marsh SG. IPD–the immuno polymorphism database. Nucleic Acids Res. 2005;33:D523–6.

Sanchez-Mazas A, Nunes JM, Middleton D, et al. Common and well-documented HLA alleles over all of Europe and within European sub-regions: a catalogue from the European Federation for Immunogenetics. HLA. 2017;89:104–13.

Shaffer BC, Hsu KC. How important is NK alloreactivity and KIR in allogeneic transplantation? Best Pract Res Clin Haematol. 2016;29:351–8.

Slade M, Fakhri B, Savani BN, Romee R. Halfway there: the past, present and future of haploidentical transplantation. Bone Marrow Transplant. 2017;52:1–6.

Spierings E. Minor histocompatibility antigens: past, present, and future. Tissue Antigens. 2014;84:374–60.

Thorsby E. A short history of HLA. Tissue Antigens. 2009;74:101–16.

Trowsdale J, Knight JC. Major histocompatibility complex genomics and human disease. Anuu Rev Genomics Hum Genet. 2013;14:301–23.

Vago L, Toffalori C, Ciceri F, Fleischhauer K. Genomic loss of mismatched human leukocyte antigen and leukemia immune escape from haploidentical graft-versus-leukemia. Semin Oncol. 2012;39:707–15.

Vyas JM, Van der Veen AG, Ploegh HL. The known unknowns of antigen processing and presentation. Nat Rev Immunol. 2008;8:607–18.

Clinical and Biological Concepts for Mastering Immune Reconstitution After HSCT: Toward Practical Guidelines and Greater Harmonization

Jürgen Kuball and Jaap Jan Boelens

10.1 Introduction/Background

The main mechanisms of action resulting in a long-term cure, but also in many life-threatening side effects after HSCT, are mediated by the rapidly reconstituting immune repertoire, which depends on the conditioning regimen, cell dose and graft composition, as well as the type of immune suppression. However, knowledge of these mechanisms is limited, due to many variations in clinical programs, including the specific type of transplantation procedure, as well as a lack of standardized immune monitoring after HSCT.

To date, only the process of donor selection has been significantly impacted by new biological insights, but little attention has been given to the design of the cell product in terms of numbers and composition, to avoid variations between different patients. In addition, high variations between patients in the clearance of agents used during the conditioning are rarely investigated. Given the dearth of prospective clinical studies addressing these important concepts, and the fact that such studies will most likely never be performed, due to the lack of interest from pharmaceutical companies, we aim to initiate a consensus discussion. Our goal is to harmonize the intervention HSCT by exploring how individual differences between patients and overall transplantation strategies impact the final effector mechanisms of HSCT, namely, a timely and well-balanced immune reconstitution.

10.2 Impact of Conditioning Regimens on Immune Reconstitution and Outcomes: Pharmacokinetics-Pharmacodynamics (PK-PD), Individualized Dosing

Various groups have recently demonstrated that agents administered as part of the conditioning regimen, as well as after HSCT, will influence both short-term and long-term immune reconstitution (Soiffer and Chen 2017; Admiraal et al. 2015). These agents may, therefore, have an unknown effect on also other cell-based therapeutics. In the context of HSCT, "predictable" immune reconstitution is important when studying maintenance therapies with novel drugs, DLI,

J. Kuball (✉)
Department of Hematology, UMC,
Utrecht, The Netherlands

Laboratory of Translational Immunology, UMC,
Utrecht, The Netherlands
e-mail: J.H.E.Kuball@umcutrecht.nl

J. J. Boelens
Laboratory of Translational Immunology, UMC,
Utrecht, The Netherlands

Memorial Sloan Kettering Cancer Center,
New York, NY, USA

and advanced cell therapy interventions. Therefore, it is essential to understand the impact of the agents used on the immune reconstitution. Comprehensive pharmacokinetic (PK) and pharmacodynamic (PD) information can help to illuminate the effects that exposure of agents in the conditioning have on immune reconstitution and subsequent outcomes (e.g., GvHD, relapse and non-relapse mortality).

The recent discovery that the pharmacokinetics of serotherapy (e.g., ATG and ATLG) is highly dependent on receptor load (represented by absolute lymphocyte count; ALC) before the first dosing is one example. In adults, receptor load was the only predictor for ATG clearance, while in pediatric patients (<40 kg), weight also influenced clearance. While prospective validation trials of novel ATG nomograms currently include patients linked to defined transplantation regimens, initial recommendations for dosing serotherapy on lymphocyte count rather than body weight seem to be reasonable, e.g., within the context of T cell-replete reduced conditioning regimens (Admiraal et al. 2015) (Table 10.1). From a post hoc analysis of a recent randomized controlled trial allowing three different types of regimens, we learned that different regimens had the reverse effects of ATLG on the outcomes, resulting in overlapping curves for the primary endpoint, chronic-GvHD-free, leukemia-free survival (Soiffer et al. 2017).

Serotherapy is not the only agent in a conditioning regimen with variable PK that can have a dramatic impact on the chances for survival. In a recent retrospective cohort analysis that included more than 650 pediatric and young adult patients, cumulative exposure to BU was found to influence outcomes (Bartelink et al. 2016). The optimal BU exposure, for the main outcome of EFS, was found to be independent of indication, combination (BU/FLU, BU/CY, or BU/CY/MEL), age, and donor source. BU/FLU within the optimal BU exposure (80–100 mg*h/L) was associated with the highest survival chances and lowest toxicity compared to other combinations. More recently, fludarabine exposure was also found to influence survival (in an ATG-FLU/BU: Boelens et al. 2018). These studies further illustrate that pharmacokinetic variations in individuals can have significant effects on survival. Historically, and still in daily practice, a variety of conditioning regimens are used, which complicates comparisons of HSCT outcomes across different centers and even within trials.

10.3 Graft Composition as an Additional Predictor for Immune Reconstitution and Clinical Outcomes

Although transplant physicians carefully monitor the levels of many drugs, such as CSA or antibiotics, an additional opportunity to further harmonize the transplantation procedure arises from the surprising clinical observation that substantial cell dose variations are currently accepted across patients. The hesitation to monitor cell numbers in the graft or after HSCT, and to act on them, is of course partially driven by the confusing magnitude of immunological subsets, the narrow nature of many immunological programs with a lack of consensus on immune monitoring, and also rather limited immunological education across the majority of transplant physicians. However, currently available retrospective and prospective studies can provide guidance. A retrospective EBMT study indicated that T cell numbers vary frequently between 50 and

Table 10.1 Suggested novel ATG dosing nomograms based on PK-PD modeling for (non-)myelo-ablative settings in pediatrics and adults[a]

Setting	Dosing on	Target AUC after HSCT (AU*d/mL) and donor source	Starting day
Pediatrics; MAC Admiraal et al. (2015)	Weight ALC Cell source	<20 for cord blood <50 for bone marrow	9
Adults: Non-MAC Admiraal et al. (2017)	ALC	60–90 for peripherally mobilized stem cells	9

ALC absolute lymphocyte count, *AUC* area under the curve
[a]Level C evidence (retrospective studies)

885 × 10⁶/kg and the highest quartile in CD34+ cells, as well as T cells associate with an inferior clinical outcome (5). As we cannot expect in the future randomized trials addressing the impact of different graft compositions in T cell-replete transplantations on clinical outcomes, avoiding higher numbers of CD34 and T cells within the highest quartile might be reasonable (Czerw et al. 2016). Higher numbers of NKT cells (Malard et al. 2016) and γδT cells (Perko et al. 2015) in the graft have been reported to associate with favorable immune reconstitution, and a positive clinical outcome, most likely due to their impact on controlling GVHD (Du et al. 2017) and acting on CMV, as well as on leukemia (Scheper et al. 2013; de Witte et al. 2018). However, these variables are more difficult to control in daily clinical practice. Direct ex vivo graft engineering provides an elegant solution to further control immune subsets in the graft and the consecutive immune reconstitution. It also allows for the standardization of cell numbers, as well as subsets per patient, e.g., selecting CD34-positive stem cells alone has been reported to associate with less chronic GVHD, while the graft versus leukemia effect is maintained (Pasquini et al. 2012). As the next generation of graft engineering, depletion of αβT cells has been reported to associate with lower frequencies of infection and very low GVHD rates (Locatelli et al. 2017).

10.4 Immune Monitoring

10.4.1 Immune Cell Phenotyping

The most important questions that arise when monitoring immune therapeutic interventions are:

1. How many cells within each leukocyte subset are present in patients at different stages of disease, before immune intervention?
2. What is the immune composition of the graft?
3. Which immune subsets are reconstituting at what points in time?

4. What is the functional response of these cells to additional immunotherapeutic or drug interventions after transplantation (Table 10.1)?

These questions are particularly important in an era when post-HSCT pharmaceutical maintenance interventions and DLI or the administration of other ATMPs (advanced therapy medicinal products) have become daily practice for many different disease categories (Soiffer and Chen 2017).

Flow cytometry is often available for comprehensive immune phenotyping, usually in accredited laboratories within transplant centers. Markers identifying the most common leukocyte subsets are broadly used and can therefore be considered as a "standard" panel: CD45 (lymphocytes), CD3 (T cells), CD19 (B cells), αβTCR, γδTCR, and CD16/CD56 (NK) cells. In some centers/studies, this panel has been extended to identify the differentiation and activation state of subsets of T (T-helper, regulatory T cells), B, and NK(T) cells, as well as cells from the myeloid lineage (monocytes, dendritic cell subsets). This knowledge is important because the success of cell-based immunotherapies, as well as agents modulating the immune system after transplantation, will significantly depend on the presence or absence of different immune subsets. Mastering the diversity might allow for the definition of subpopulations who would benefit from checkpoint-inhibitor treatment after HSCT, as well as characterize patients who would be at high risk for GVHD, while currently this intervention is considered to be very toxic (Davids et al. 2016). Also, other subsets may be suitable as biomarkers to predict clinical efficacy. Given the potential impact of sorafenib on post-HSCT outcomes through the induction of IL15 (Mathew et al. 2018), additional immune subsets associating with improved leukemia control need to be identified. In another study, high baseline frequencies of peripheral blood dendritic cells (DC) correlated with a clinical response to high-dose IL-2 (Finkelstein et al. 2010). These data emphasize the importance of DC in endogenous and therapy-induced antitumor immunity and arguably warrant the incorporation of DC markers in immune-monitoring panels.

Taken together, a variety of specialized subsets may have potential as predictive markers for clinical efficacy, but they require more sophisticated staining protocols, making more cumbersome staining techniques less broadly applicable for harmonized panels across centers or in multicenter clinical trials. Furthermore, it is important to note that trials using whole blood assays may produce different percentages of cell subsets when compared with studies using PBMCs. The same is true when comparing freshly isolated PBMCs with biobanked material, which has been subjected to freeze/thaw procedures that affect expression levels of various markers. Even when the same samples are collected, variations can be introduced by the selection of antibody clones, combination of clones and fluorochromes, and the gating strategies. In sum, minimizing the variability in sample handling and the pre-analysis phase is critical for standardization.

10.4.2 Immune Monitoring: Secretome Analyses

Measuring the production of cytokines, chemokines, and growth factors and their profiles (i.e., the secretome) represents an integral part of immunomonitoring during immunotherapeutic treatments. These biomarkers may distinguish diverse disease/response patterns, identify surrogate markers of efficacy, and provide additional insight into the therapeutic mode of action. Peripheral blood is often the only source for protein analysis, which may lack the sensitivity to reflect local responses in affected tissues. As examples, proteins, such as interleukin-6, granulocyte-macrophage colony-stimulating factor (GM-CSF), hepatocyte growth factor (HGF), ST2 (suppressor of tumorigenicity), and soluble IL-2a, have been suggested as potential biomarkers for GvHD, whereas increased levels of TNF-a and IL-6 are associated with robust immune responses to viral reactivation (de Koning et al. 2016).

The most commonly used methods to identify these markers include antibody-based ELISA or multiplex platforms, such as protein microarrays, liquid chromatography-mass spectrometry (LC-MS), electro-chemiluminescence, and bead-based multiplex immunoassays (MIA). Again, different technologies and reagents (e.g., antibodies and recombinants for standard curves) may lead to different concentrations and dramatic variability in results, depending on how the pre-analytic samples are handled (e.g., differences in processing and storage, including duration of storage). Cytokine levels differ considerably between serum and plasma samples obtained from the same donor, due to release of platelet-associated molecules into serum. Moreover, the type of anticoagulant used in plasma isolation and time- and/or temperature-sensitive changes need to be considered (Keustermans et al. 2013). These phenomena underscore the need for extensive documentation with respect to all biomarker analysis before any conclusions can be made when comparing patient cohorts treated at multiple sites.

10.5 Summary

The failure or success of HSCT is significantly impacted by the patient's immune status. However, only a minority of HSCT programs systematically consider individualized drug monitoring during conditioning, graft design, and immune monitoring as key for patient surveillance, in order to maximally control and capture essential details of the intervention HSCT. Therefore, guidelines are needed to further harmonize the procedure HSCT as well as standardized immune monitoring to allow for distillation of key features for success and failure. First, careful recommendations for individualized drug dosing as well as graft compositions can be made based on available data sets. However, it will be key to register within the new cellular therapy registry of EBMT additional details of drug dosages, graft compositions, as well as immune reconstitution, to capture clinical variations in programs, as well as defined immune reconstitutions. This will enable a retrospective

Table 10.2 Panels under consideration in the panel discussion of the CTIWP (Greco et al. 2018)[a]

	General		Advanced
Graft composition	αβT γδT Treg B NK/NKT	αβTCR, CD45RO/RA, CD3, CD4, CD8, CD27 γδTCR, CD45RO/RA, CD3, CD27 CD45, CD4, CD25, CD127, FoxP3 CD45, CD19, CD38, CD27, IgM/G/D, CD21 CD45, CD3, CD56, TCRα24/β11)	Intracellular cytokines after PMA/ionomycin stimulation Specific TCR by multimer approach
Cell phenotyping pre- and post transplantation	αβT γδT Treg B NK/NKT DC/mono	αβTCR, CD45RO/RA, CD3, CD4, CD8, CD27 γδTCR, CD45RO/RA, CD3, CD27 CD45, CD4, CD25, CD127, FoxP3 CD45, CD19, CD38, CD27, IgM/G/D, CD21 CD45, CD3, CD56, TCRα24/β11) CD11c, HLA-DR, CD14, CD16, CD1c, CD141, CD303	Intracellular cytokines after PMA/ionomycin stimulation Specific TCR by multimer approach αβTCR and γδTCR repertoire
Secretome	–		Multiplex panel (e.g., IL-7, ST2, TNF-a, IL-6, HGF, IL-2R, IL-8, GM-CSF, etc.)
Cell function	–		NK cell lyses T cell proliferation upon antigens and mitogens B cell maturation
PK	BU, FLU, ATG, Campath (if part of conditioning)		Trial drug
MRD	qPCR (targets expressed, flow cytometry)		Next-generation sequencing
Viral load	CMV, EBV, HV6, adenovirus		–

[a]General parameters that could be included in harmonized immune-monitoring protocols across most studies/centers and advanced parameters that may be of great value in specific studies and that can only be performed in specialized immunology labs or analyzed in a central laboratory

increase in insight into daily clinical practice, and its impact on immune reconstitution, as well as clinical outcome. Also, clinical trials should adopt such consensus measurements. Nevertheless, the markers and phenotypes studied in one setting may not be considered relevant in another, supporting the definition of a set of general recommended protocols and a set of add-on trial-specific parameters (Table 10.2). A consensus panel is currently prepared by the cellular therapy and immunobiology working party (CTIWP) of EBMT (Greco et al. 2018). A harmonization procedure to achieve a more balanced immune reconstitution might have a more profound impact on patient survival than any other novel maintenance therapy (Admiraal et al. 2017; Boelens et al. 2018) and allow for a better success rate for novel drugs tested as maintenance therapy.

Key Points

- The failure or success of HCT is significantly impacted by the patient's immune status.
- Harmonizing individualized drug monitoring during conditioning, graft design, and immune monitoring is key for patient surveillance and needs to be registered within the new cellular therapy registry of EBMT.
- A harmonization procedure to achieve a more balanced immune reconstitution might have a more profound impact on patient survival than any other novel maintenance therapy and allow for a better success rate for novel drugs tested as maintenance therapy.

References

Admiraal R, van Kesteren C, Jol-van der Zijde CM, et al. Association between anti-thymocyte globulin exposure and CD4+ immune reconstitution in paediatric haemopoietic cell transplantation: a multicentre, retrospective pharmacodynamic cohort analysis. Lancet Haematol. 2015;2:e194–203.

Admiraal R, Nierkens S, de Witte MA, et al. Association between anti-thymocyte globulin exposure and survival outcomes in adult unrelated haemopoietic cell transplantation: a multicentre, retrospective, pharmacodynamic cohort analysis. Lancet Haematol. 2017;4:e183–91.

Bartelink IH, Lalmohamed A, van Reij EM, et al. Association of busulfan exposure with survival and toxicity after haemopoietic cell transplantation in children and young adults: a multicentre, retrospective cohort analysis. Lancet Haematol. 2016;3:e526–36.

Boelens JJ, Admiraal R, Kuball J, Nierkens S. Fine-tuning antithymocyte globulin dosing and harmonizing clinical trial design. J Clin Oncol. 2018;36:1175–6.

Czerw T, Labopin M, Schmid C, et al. High CD3+ and CD34+ peripheral blood stem cell grafts content is associated with increased risk of graft-versus-host disease without beneficial effect on disease control after reduced-intensity conditioning allogeneic transplantation from matched unrelated donors for acute myeloid leukemia - an analysis from the Acute Leukemia Working Party of the European Society for Blood and Marrow Transplantation. Oncotarget. 2016;7(19):27255–66.

Davids MS, Kim HT, Bachireddy P, et al. Ipilimumab for patients with relapse after allogeneic transplantation. N Engl J Med. 2016;375:143–53.

de Koning C, Plantinga M, Besseling P, et al. Immune reconstitution after allogeneic hematopoietic cell transplantation in children. Biol Blood Marrow Transplant. 2016;22:195–206.

de Witte MA, Sarhan D, Davis Z, et al. Early reconstitution of NK and gammadelta T cells and its implication for the design of post-transplant immunotherapy. Biol Blood Marrow Transplant. 2018;24(6):1152–62.

Du J, Paz K, Thangavelu G, et al. Invariant natural killer T cells ameliorate murine chronic GVHD by expanding donor regulatory T cells. Blood. 2017;129:3121–5.

Finkelstein SE, Carey T, Fricke I, et al. Changes in dendritic cell phenotype after a new high-dose weekly schedule of interleukin-2 therapy for kidney cancer and melanoma. J Immunother. 2010;33:817–27.

Greco R, Ciceri F, Noviello M, et al. Immune monitoring in allogeneic hematopoietic stem cell transplant recipients: a survey from the EBMT-CTIWP. Bone Marrow Transplant. 2018;53:1201–5.

Keustermans GC, Hoeks SB, Meerding JM, et al. Cytokine assays: an assessment of the preparation and treatment of blood and tissue samples. Methods. 2013;61:10–7.

Locatelli F, Merli P, Pagliara D, et al. Outcome of children with acute leukemia given HLA-haploidentical HSCT after alphabeta T-cell and B-cell depletion. Blood. 2017;130:677–85.

Malard F, Labopin M, Chevallier P, et al. Larger number of invariant natural killer T cells in PBSC allografts correlates with improved GVHD-free and progression-free survival. Blood. 2016;127:1828–35.

Mathew NR, Baumgartner F, Braun L, et al. Sorafenib promotes graft-versus-leukemia activity in mice and humans through IL-15 production in FLT3-ITD-mutant leukemia cells. Nat Med. 2018;24:282–91.

Pasquini MC, Devine S, Mendizabal A, et al. Comparative outcomes of donor graft CD34+ selection and immune suppressive therapy as graft-versus-host disease prophylaxis for patients with acute myeloid leukemia in complete remission undergoing HLA-matched sibling allogeneic hematopoietic cell transplantation. J Clin Oncol. 2012;30:3194–201.

Perko R, Kang G, Sunkara A, et al. Gamma delta T cell reconstitution is associated with fewer infections and improved event-free survival after hematopoietic stem cell transplantation for pediatric leukemia. Biol Blood Marrow Transplant. 2015;21:130–6.

Scheper W, van Dorp S, Kersting S, et al. Gammadelta T cells elicited by CMV reactivation after Allo-SCT cross-recognize CMV and leukemia. Leukemia. 2013;27:1328–38.

Soiffer RJ, Chen YB. Pharmacologic agents to prevent and treat relapse after allogeneic hematopoietic cell transplantation. Blood Adv. 2017;1:2473–82.

Soiffer RJ, Kim HT, McGuirk J, et al. Prospective, randomized, double-blind, phase III clinical trial of anti-T-lymphocyte globulin to assess impact on chronic graft-versus-host disease-free survival in patients undergoing HLA-matched unrelated myeloablative hematopoietic cell transplantation. J Clin Oncol. 2017;35:4003–11.

Part III
Methodology and Clinical Aspects
Topic leaders: Arnon Nagler and Nicolaus Kröger

Evaluation and Counseling of Candidates

Enric Carreras and Alessandro Rambaldi

11.1 Evaluation of Candidates and Risk Factors for HSCT

Enric Carreras

11.1.1 Introduction

The evaluation of candidates and the analysis of individual risk factors for HSCT permit to establish four fundamental aspects:

1. The HSCT indication
2. To inform the patient properly
3. To choose the best donor, conditioning, and post-HSCT IS
4. To evaluate the results of the transplant in large series

E. Carreras
Spanish Bone Marrow Donor Registry,
Josep Carreras Foundation and Leukemia Research
Institute, Barcelona, Catalunya, Spain

Hospital Clinic Barcelona, Barcelona University,
Barcelona, Spain

A. Rambaldi(✉)
Department of Hematology-Oncology,
Azienda Socio Sanitaria Territoriale Papa Giovanni
XXIII, Bergamo, Università Statale di Milano,
Milano, Italy
e-mail: alessandro.rambaldi@unimi.it

11.1.2 Candidates' Evaluation Work Flow

11.1.2.1 First Visit

The most relevant aspects to take into account in this first visit are:

- Medical history (past and present) and physical examination (see Sect. 11.1.2.4).
- Review of diagnostic tests (in referred patients).
- Revaluate HLA typing of patient and potential donors (if allo-HSCT).
- Preliminary information on:
  - Therapeutic options and results
  - HSCT procedure
  - Possible complications and side effects (see specific chapters in Part V)
- Schedule reevaluation of the current status of the disease (see Sect. 11.1.3).
- Schedule visits with radiation therapist (if TBI), dentist, gynecologist, blood bank (list of blood/platelet donors), HSCT unit supervisor nurse, etc.
- Signature of the informed consent for HSCT and for procurement of HSC (if auto-HSCT).

11.1.2.2 Visit Preharvesting (Auto-HSCT)

- Assess the results of complementary explorations.
- Complete information on the procedure.

- If PBSC, assess the status of venous accesses. Program CVC (if necessary) and mobilization schedule.
- If BM: preanesthetic visit.
- Program manipulation of HSCT (if applicable) and/or cryopreservation.

11.1.2.3 Last Visit Before Admission

- Final and complete patient information (see Sect. 11.1.2.5).
- Evaluate reevaluation studies performed (see Sect. 11.1.3).
- Schedule admission and conditioning treatment.
- If necessary, program CVC placement.
- If allo-HSCT: confirm that the donor's evaluation is correct and there are no contraindications for donation (see Chap. 12).
- If auto-HSCT: confirm that the cryopreserved cellularity is correct.
- Submit donor and recipient information to the blood bank (group, CMV serology, previous transfusions, etc.).
- If TBI: confirm that the dosimetry has been carried out and the RT has been programmed.
- Confirm storage of patient and donor samples for serotheque and cellular library.

11.1.2.4 Medical History

Collect information on:

Medical background; childhood illnesses and vaccines; allergies and adverse drug reactions; surgical interventions (previous anesthesia); medications not related to the basic process; previous transfusion history, family tree, and family history valuable; in women, menarche/menopause, pregnancy and childbirth, contraceptive methods, date last rule, and gynecological checkups

Travel to malaria, trypanosomiasis, and HTLV-I/II endemic areas

Previous relevant infections

Data about the current illness:

- Start date and initial symptomatology
- Diagnostic methodology used (staging)
- Chemotherapy and radiotherapy treatments (doses and dates)
- Complications from such treatments
- Result of these treatments
- Recurrences and their treatment

- Transfusions received
- Current state of the disease

Social aspects

- Smoking, alcoholism, and other drug use
- Sexual habits
- Availability of accommodation close to the center and means of transport
- Support family members
- Ethnic, cultural, and intellectual aspects

11.1.2.5 Information to Provide (See Detailed Information in Counseling Section)

Ask the patient (privately) which escorts he or she wishes to have present in this session. For adolescents follow the rules of each country respecting the right of information. Transmit as much information as possible in writing. She/he must be informed about:

- Most frequent early and late complications (see specific chapters in Parts V and VI) including graft failure, GI complications, alopecia, SOS/VOD, acute GVHD, early infections, chronic GVHD, late infections, relapse of the disease, infertility, endocrine complications, neoplasms, and other secondary.
- Treat specifically serious complications (ICU admissions) and possibility of death. Inform about the advance directive registry. Agreeing with the patient on an interlocutor in case at some point they may not be able to make decisions.
- Estimated duration of admission, approximate day of admission.
- Most frequent complications on discharge, outpatient follow-up, likelihood of readmission, and need for caregivers at discharge.

11.1.3 Complementary Explorations

All the following studies must be performed within 30 days prior to the HSCT except the assessment of baseline disease status (7–15 days) and the pregnancy test (7 days):

- CBC and basic coagulation; complete biochemistry (including ferritin); blood type and

Rh/irregular antibodies; dosage of Igs; serology CMV, EBV, VHS, VVZ, toxoplasma, syphilis, HBsAg, HBcAb, and anti-HBsAb (HTLV-I/II, and Chagas disease according to the patient's origin); NAT for HCV, HBV, and HIV; pregnancy test

- Chest x-ray; respiratory function tests (including FEV1 and DLCO); electrocardiogram; echocardiogram or isotopic ventriculography (depending on previous treatment)
- Reevaluation of the disease (MRD) (see specific chapters in part IX)
- Dental evaluation; gynecological evaluation; psychological/psychiatric evaluation
- Nutritional assessment
- HLA typing (recheck) (see Chap. 9)

11.1.4 Risk Assessment

11.1.4.1 Individual Risk Factors

There are a group of variables that have a prognostic value in all predictive models

Variables	High risk
Age	Older. Do not use as a single criterion. Relative importance
General condition	Karnofsky index <80%
Disease	Not in remission. See specific chapters
Type of donor	Others than HLA-identical siblings
HLA compatibility	Any HLA-A, HLA-B, HLA-C, and DRB1 difference
CMV serology	Different serology than the donor
Donor	Age >35–40 years For male recipient, female donor (especially if multiparous)
Interval diagnosis-HSCT	Prolonged (relevant in CML and SAA)
Comorbidities	See HCT-CI model
Iron overload	Present
Experience of the center	Non-JACIE/FACT accredited centers

11.1.4.2 Predictive Models

Disease Risk Index (DRI) (Armand et al. 2012, 2014)

Prognostic index based in the disease and its status at HSCT. It doesn't take into account factors as age or comorbidities. This score index classi-

Table 11.1 Disease risk index (Armand 2012, 2014)

Risk	Disease
Low	AML with favorable cyt., CLL, CML, indolent B-cell NHL
Intermediate	AML intermediate cyt., MDS intermediate cyt., myeloproliferative neoplasms, MM, HL, DLBCL/transformed indolent B-NHL, MCL, T-cell lymphoma nodal
High	AML adverse cyt, MDS adverse cyt, T-cell lymphoma extranodal

Risk	Stage
Low	CR1, CR≥2, PR1, untreated, CML CP, PR≥2 (if RIC)
High	PR≥2 (if MAC), induction failure, active relapse, CML AP or BP

Disease risk	Stage risk	Overall risk	OS at 4 years
Low	Low	Low	64% (56–70%)
Low	High	Intermediate	46% (42–50%)
Intermediate	Low		
Intermediate	High	High	26% (21–31%)
High	Low		
High	High	Very high	6 (0–21%)

Adapted from Armand (2012). *Cyt.* cytogenetics

fies the disease in four prognostic groups and anticipates overall survival, progression-free survival, cumulative incidence of relapse, and cumulative incidence of non-relapse mortality (see Table 11.1).

EBMT Risk Score (Gratwohl et al. 1998, 2009)

This predictive score, validated with 56,505 patients, permits to predict approximately the 5-year probability of OS and the TRM for the main diseases (see Tables 11.2, 11.3, and 11.4).

EBMT risk score is also useful to predict OS and TRM in patients receiving a second HSCT (Rezvani et al. 2012) and in those receiving a TCD HSCT (Lodewyck et al. 2011).

Some authors have introduced modifications in this risk score (including the concept of disease stage) to improve its predictivity (Terwey et al. 2010; Hemmati et al. 2011). Similarly, it has been associated with the HCT-CI (Barba et al. 2014).

This score has been validated by many groups and for many diseases (AML, ALL, PMF, CLL, and CML, among others).

Table 11.2 EBMT risk score (Gratwohl 2009)

Variables	Value of variables	Points
Age	<20 years	0
	20–40 years	1
	>40 years	2
Disease status[a]	Early	0
	Intermediate	1
	Advanced	2
Interval diagnosis-HSCT[b]	<12 months	0
	≥12 months	1
Donor	HLA-identical sibling	0
	Unrelated donor	1
Gender donor – recipient	Female to male	1
	Other combinations	0

Adapted from Gratwohl (2009)

[a]Do not apply in patients with SAA. Early = AL in CR1; MDS in CR1 or untreated; CML in 1st chronic phase; NHL/MM untreated or in CR1. Intermediate = AL in CR2; CML in other status than accelerated phase or blastic phase; MDS in CR2 or in PR; NHL/MM in CR2, PR, or stable dis. Late = AL in other stages; CML in blastic crisis; MDS in all other stages; NHL/MM in all other stages

[b]Do not apply to patients in CR1

Table 11.3 Probability (%) of TRM at 5 years applying the EBMT risk score

Points	0	1	2	3	4	5	6–7
AML	14	20	25	30	36	40	41
ALL	15	23	24	30	40	47	53
CML	15	22	30	38	45	52	55
AA	18	26	40	49	52		
MDS	25	28	30	35	38	46	50
MM			29	35	40	42	52
NHL	15	24	28	30	34	36	38

Extracted from Gratwohl (2009)

Table 11.4 Probability (%) of OS at 5 years applying the EBMT risk score

Points	0	1	2	3	4	5	6–7
AML	68	59	52	38	30	23	18
ALL	66	52	43	38	22	16	14
CML	76	72	60	51	39	26	14
AA	81	72	60	49	45		
MDS	56	52	46	40	35	28	25
MM			48	40	36	22	17
NHL	75	59	50	48	43	40	38

Extracted from Gratwohl (2009)

HCT-Comorbidity Index (HCT-CI) (Sorror et al. 2005)

Developed in Seattle in 2005. It is an adaptation to the HSCT of the classical Charlson Comorbidity Index (CCI). Validated in several cohorts and widely used. The score analyzes 17 comorbidities as well as their degree (see Table 11.5).

Given the impact of age on outcomes, the authors modified the model (Sorror et al. 2014), including a 1-point score for patients aged 40. This modification significantly improved the predictive capacity of the model. Consequently, the patients could be classified in three different risk groups (0 points, low risk; 1–2 points, intermediate risk; 3 or more, high risk) that clearly correlated with 2-year NRM.

Other authors re-stratified the HCT-CI index (flexible HCT-CI) as low risk, 0–3 points; intermediate risk, 4–5 points; and high risk, >5 points, being this classification a better predictor for NRM. In RIC setting, the 100-day and 2-year NRM incidence in these risk categories was 4%, 16%, and 29% and 19%, 33%, and 40%, respectively. They do find this predictive NRM value using neither the original HCT-CI nor the PAM or CCI models. Regarding the 2-year OS, this flexible HCT-CI score was also associated with the highest predictive hazard ratio (Barba et al. 2010).

HCT-CI has also been validated in CD34+ selected HSCT (Barba et al. 2017) and associated with the EBMT risk score that permits a better stratification (Barba et al. 2014).

Pretransplantation Assessment of Mortality (PAM) Score (Parimon et al. 2006; Au et al. 2015)

Developed in Seattle in 2006 but underused and poorly validated. It combines eight variables from patients and HSCT. Only useful for assessing mortality at 2 years.

Variables included age, type of donor, risk of disease, intensity of conditioning, DLCO, FEV1, creatinine, and ALT.

EBMT Machine Learning Algorithm (Shouval et al. 2015)

Based in an alternating decision tree able to detect variables associated with the primary

Table 11.5 HSCT-comorbidity index including age variable (Sorror 2005, 2014)

Comorbidity/definition	Points
Age ≥ 40 years	1
Arrhythmia Atrial fibrillation, flutter, sick sinus node syndrome, or ventricular arrhythmias	1
Cardiac Coronary heart disease, congestive heart failure, IAM, FEVE ≤50%	1
Inflammatory bowel disease Crohn's disease or ulcerative colitis that has required treatment	1
Diabetes Requiring insulin or oral antidiabetic medication in the 4 weeks prior to HSCT	1
Cerebrovascular CVA or TIA or cerebral thrombosis	1
Psychiatric Depression or anxiety or others requiring ongoing treatment (not on demand)	1
Mild liver Chronic hepatitis, elevated bilirubin <1.5 × NV or AST/ALT <2.5 × NV Previous HBV or HCV infection	1
Obesity BMI >35 kg/m^2	1
Previous infection Infection in admission requiring continuation of treatment beyond day 0	1
Moderate lung DLCO and/or FEV1 66–80% or minimal stress dyspnea	2
Rheumatology Systemic lupus, rheumatoid arthritis, polymyositis, polymyalgia rheumatica, connective tissue disease	2
Peptic ulcer Endoscopic or radiological diagnosis (does not score if only reflux or gastritis)	2
Renal Creatinine >176 mcmol/L, dialysis, or previous kidney transplant	2
Previous tumor[a] Neoplasia at some point (excludes non-melanoma skin tumor)	3
Heart valve Diagnosed (except mitral prolapse)	3
Severe pulmonary DLCO and/or FEV1 ≤%, dyspnea at rest or oxygen at home	3
Severe liver disease Bilirubin ≥0.5 for VN or AST or ALT ≥0.5 for VN or cirrhosis	3

[a]A most recent version also includes in this category hematological/tumors of a different lineage to that which motivates the transplant (e.g., lymphoma in an AML patient but not previous MDS in AML patient)

outcome, assigning weights and ignoring redundancies. This score was developed to analyze the NRM at day +100 in patients with acute leukemia but also predict NRM, LFS, and OS at 2 years.

The variables included in the model are age, Karnofsky (≥80; <80), diagnostic (AML; ALL), disease stage (CR1; CR2; all other stages), interval diagnostic-HSCT (<142 days; ≥142 days), donor-recipient CMV status (both (sero +); both (sero -); any other combination), donor type (MSD; MUD), conditioning (MAC; RIC), and annual allo-HSCT performed in the center (<20; ≥21). The total +100 NRM and 2-year NRM, LFS, and OS could be obtained through a web page: http://bioinfo.lnx.biu.ac.il/~bondi/web1.html.

Recently this algorithm has also been validated by an independent set of data from GITMO (Shouval et al. 2017).

11.1.4.3 Predictive Capacity of These Models

Unfortunately, all these models have a relatively low predictive capacity, and none of them stand out more than the rest.

Author	Predictive/s model/s	Predictive capacity
Sorror et al. (2005)	HCT-CI	0.65
Xhaard (2008)	rHCT-CT, PAM	0.49, 0.57
Gratwohl (2009)	EBMT	0.63
Barba et al. (2010)	fHCT-CI, PAM	0.67, 0.63
Barba et al. (2014)	HCT-CI, EBMT	0.60, 0.54
Versluis (2015)	(HCT-CI-EBMT)	0.58, 0.58 (0.64)

Courtesy of P. Barba, MD. rHCT-CI = reduced model, without PFTs; fHSCT = flexible model (modified scale)

11.1.5 Practical Applications of Risk Assessment

Election of the conditioning	In patients with a high risk of NRM following one of the mentioned risk scores, a RIC should be considered
Relative contraindications	Uncontrolled infection, severe or chronic liver disease (excluding cirrhosis), severe disturbances in heart function (FEV <40%), respiratory (DLCO <40%) or renal (creatinine clearance <30 mL/min)
Absolute contraindications	Pregnancy Cirrhosis. Even compensated cirrhosis receiving RIC have a high likelihood of hepatic decompensation (Hogan et al. 2004)

Key Points

- The evaluation of a candidate must be carried out according to a preestablished work plan designed by each institution. The use of standardized procedures reduces the risk of errors or omissions
- Several pretransplant variables (such as age) have a clear impact on the results of the procedure but, when assessed in isolation, are highly insufficient to predict the results
- Predictive models (DRI, EBMT risk score, HCT-CI, PAM) allow a much more realistic approach to the real possibilities of a given candidate and adapt the procedure to their needs

11.2 Counseling of Candidates

Alessandro Rambaldi

11.2.1 Introduction

Allo-HSCT is a potentially curative treatment modality for otherwise incurable diseases. Unfortunately, after transplantation patients may experience not only the persistence or recurrence of their own disease but also some dramatic clinical complications and toxicities, including death. The clinical indications to transplant have been addressed in the section "indications" of this book, but in general, when the allo-HSCT is advised, the strength of the indication (the likelihood to be cured by transplant), the patient fitness, and his/her personal commitment to transplant must be carefully evaluated for each candidate.

Obviously, a first distinction must be done between patients with a neoplastic versus a non-neoplastic disease, and the transplant option should be progressively discussed with the patient during the course of the disease, particularly in the case of hematologic malignancies. Many professionals should concur to illustrate the patients the curative potential of an allo-HSCT and to help understanding the severe complications that can eventually develop. It is clear that different indications remarkably affect the way a patient is advised. However, there is a time when the transplant option must be formally presented and advised. Therefore, evaluation of each transplant candidate must be based on well-predefined formal standard operating procedures to collect exhaustive clinical, instrumental, and laboratory data that may lead to a robust definition of the risks and benefits related to allo-HSCT. All in all, the counseling is to tailor such evaluation to the individual patients (Shouval et al. 2015), according to both objective data and subjective data such as patient propensity and fear of side effects. At the end of this process, the patient should be aware of the rationale, the benefit and the toxicity associated with each step, and component of the transplant procedure. In this chapter, I will hereby summarize the main topics I cover with my patients when they come to my office to discuss the option of the allo-HSCT.

11.2.2 Understanding the Benefit and Risk of Allogeneic Transplant

Patients must be informed that allo-HSCT is a therapeutic option that is always proposed with the intent to achieve a permanent cure of the underlying disease, but despite this premise, disease progression or relapse may eventually happen. The indication to allo-HSCT depends not only on the disease characteristics but also on patient-related factors such as age and comorbidities (Sorror et al. 2007) so that the transplant proposal is the result of an accurate and wise evaluation of both these factors (Sorror et al. 2013; Wang et al. 2014).

The patient should understand the specific risk/benefit balance associated with a conventional versus a transplant-based proposal, and this may be remarkably different if he has been diagnosed with a non-neoplastic disease such as thalassemia or sickle cell anemia, a bone marrow failure syndrome like aplastic anemia, or a blood cancer, such as an acute leukemia. Even when allo-HSCT may in theory represent the most efficacious treatment modality to get a permanent cure of a specific disease, an accurate description of the available alternatives must be presented. This is particularly important when the non-transplant options, albeit not curative, may have the chance to keep the patient alive for a long time (Samuelson Bannow et al. 2018) or, even more importantly, when the conventional treatment may lead to a definitive cure such as in the case of some patients with acute leukemia with intermediate-risk genetic factors or those achieving a deep molecular remission after conventional chemotherapy (Cornelissen and Blaise 2016).

11.2.3 Understanding the Transplant Procedure: The Donor, the Conditioning Regimen, and the Clinical Complications

Once the indication to transplant has been confirmed, patients and their relatives must be informed on how the transplant is performed. Patients should understand that identifying a stem cell donor is an absolute prerequisite to perform a transplant. Accordingly, patients should be informed about the human leukocyte antigen (HLA) genetic system, its specificity for each individual, how it is inherited by parents according to the Mendelian laws, and what is the probability to find a compatible donor in the family group. Understanding the HLA system is crucial to explain why the use of a HLA family-matched sibling donors is considered standard and when such a sibling is not available; an international search has to be performed to identify a HLA-compatible unrelated donor. It is important to underline that more than 30 million of potentially available donors are registered by the World Marrow Donor Association (WMDA), and the probability to find a compatible donor is between 50 and 80% according to the ethnical origin of each patient.

Once such matched unrelated donor is identified, this type of transplant is considered a standard of care, and its clinical outcome is fully comparable to what was observed when using an HLA-identical sibling. In patients for whom a MSD or a MUD is not available, the patient should be informed that two additional options are available, namely, the use of HSC obtained by a family mismatched donor (commonly defined as haploidentical because sharing only one of the patient's HLA haplotypes) or a banked cord blood units. Patients should understand how the HLA diversity between patient and donor has been overcome by specific programs of in vitro or in vivo manipulation of the graft.

Patients should be reassured that the incidence and severity of GvHD, the most important side effect of allo-HSCT, seems not to be higher than observed with MUD. In addition, patients should know that many single-arm studies reported that transplants performed with these alternative stem cell sources proved to be effective and safe even when offered to patients of advanced age and/or with existing accompanying illnesses or when the disease was refractory to conventional treatment. All in all, at the present time, the clinical outcome of these alternative types of transplants compares reasonably well with those achieved with MUD. Therefore, the decision to use this type of stem cell source only when an HLA-matched donor is not available is mostly related to the lack of randomized clinical trials that are planned to be performed in the near future.

The goal of an allo-HSCT is to eradicate the patient's hematopoiesis either neoplastic or normal. This is achieved by the delivery of the conditioning regimen and by the lifelong in vivo effect played by the donor's immune system. Most often, high doses of chemotherapy and/or radiation are included in the preparations although remarkable differences exist depending on the disease needing transplant and patient tolerance. The patient should understand that the intensity of the conditioning regimen may be particularly important in the case of hematologic malignancies when the aim to remove most of the neoplastic cells present in the patient's body is the first goal. However, to avoid at least part of the treatment toxicity, the intensity of the preparative regimen can be down-modulated leading to the definition of this preparative regimen as non-myeloablative or reduced intensity. The depletion of the patient bone marrow stem cells induces a prolonged pancytopenia and the need of donor-derived healthy stem cells to grow and establish a new blood cell production system.

The allogeneic HSC, collected from the donor's BM or PB or a frozen CBU, are infused through the central venous catheter into the bloodstream: HSCT is not a surgical procedure and it is very similar to receiving a blood transfusion. The stem cells find their way into the bone marrow and begin reproducing and growing new, healthy blood cells. It is very important to explain how the donor immune system will develop progressively after transplantation and will either exert a crucial beneficial role against residual neoplastic cells or restore the immune competence against infections, but it could mediate the most harmful GvHD effect against the patient.

After the transplant, supportive care is given to prevent and treat infections, side effects of treatments, and complications. Prolonged anemia, thrombocytopenia, and leukopenia can be dangerous and even life-threatening. A low platelet count can be potentially associated with bleeding in the lungs, GI tract, and brain. Leukopenia, including either a defect of neutrophils and lymphocytes, leads to the development of frequent infections, the most common clinical complications after transplantation. Infections can include not only bacterial, most likely when the patient has a severe bone marrow suppression, but also viral and fungal pathogens. Infections can require an extended hospital stay, prevent or delay engraftment, and/or cause permanent organ damage. On average the time to hematologic engraftment (recovery of the neutrophil and platelet function) is about 2–3 weeks, but a protective recovery of the immune system can take months and sometimes years. High doses of chemotherapy and radiation can cause remarkable toxicities that include but not limited to severe mucositis (inflammation of the mouth and GI tract) that favors bacterial translocation with related infections and GvHD and multi-organ failure mainly the lung, heart, liver, and kidney.

A particular attention should be paid to risk of graft failure that can occur early or late after transplantation. A graft failure is more frequent in some diseases such as myelofibrosis or as the results of infections or when the stem cell content of the graft is insufficient to guarantee a durable engraftment. A graft rejection can also happen after reduced intensity conditioning regimen (when the immune system of the host is not completely eradicated and can actively reject the donor stem cells).

Finally, and most importantly, patients must be aware of what GvHD is, when and how it may develop, and why it represents the most serious complication of a HSCT, being not only life-threatening but also the principal reason of a long-lasting poor quality of life. Transplant candidates should be aware that GvHD is the negative counterpart of the deep interaction of the donor immune system within patient body that at the same time may lead to definitive cure of an otherwise incurable disease. In other words, when transplant is advised, patients must realize that they are accepting the possible onset of a chronic, often invalidating, autoimmune disease. GVHD can appear at any time after transplant. GvHD is conventionally distinguished in an acute form that usually develops within the first 100 days after transplant and the chronic form that occurs later in the transplant course. Patients who develop acute GVHD are more likely to also develop the chronic form of GVHD. Patients must understand the importance of their compliance to all the treatments given post transplant to prevent GvHD and how this is instrumental for a successful transplant. GvHD occurs when the donor's immune system reacts against the recipient's tissue. At variance to what happens after a solid organ transplant where the patient's immune system is driven to reject only the transplanted organ, in GVHD, the donor immune system can react against many different organs of the recipient. This is why the new cells do not recognize the tissues and organs of the recipient's body as self. Over time, thanks to the effect of immune suppressive drugs, a progressive tolerance can develop. The most common sites for GVHD are the GI tract, liver, skin, and lungs.

Key Points

Counseling of patients should be carefully performed to inform candidates that:

- Disease and patient's specific characteristics are equally important to advise transplant
- Allo-HSCT is performed to cure otherwise incurable diseases
- Despite transplant, disease persistence or relapse may occur
- Transplant can severely compromise the quality of life of patients
- Transplant is a form of immunotherapy requiring long-term follow-up care
- Logistics are important to ensure adequate care and assistance

11.2.4 Logistics

After discharge for the transplant ward, patients are followed up in the outpatient clinic two to three times per week until day +100. Patients should be helped to realize how complex is the transplant procedure and that the time spent in the hospital represents only the first part of the treatment program. All allo-HSCT patients should ideally stay within 1 h of the hospital until it is about 3 months from the day of the transplant. Patients and their families should also realize that the overall recovery time varies from person to person and in general this process takes about 1 year to be satisfactory. Allogeneic transplantation is therefore a long-lasting immunotherapy, and the interaction between the donor immune system and the patient requires a careful and prolonged medical assistance, quite often long life.

References

Armand P, Gibson CJ, Cutler C, et al. A disease risk index for patients undergoing allogeneic stem cell transplantation. Blood. 2012;120:905–13.

Armand P, Kim HT, Logan BR, et al. Validation and refinement of the disease risk index for allogeneic stem cell transplantation. Blood. 2014;123:3664–71.

Au BK, Gooley TA, Armand P, et al. Reevaluation of the pretransplant assessment of mortality score after allogeneic hematopoietic transplantation. Biol Blood Marrow Transplant. 2015;21:848–54.

Barba P, Piñana JL, Martino R, et al. Comparison of two pretransplant predictive models and a flexible HCT-CI using different cut off points to determine low-, intermediate-, and high-risk groups: the flexible HCT-CI Is the best predictor of NRM and OS in a population of patients undergoing allo-RIC. Biol Blood Marrow Transplant. 2010;16:413–20.

Barba P, Martino R, Pérez-Simón JA, et al. Combination of the hematopoietic cell transplantation comorbidity index and the European Group for blood and marrow transplantation score allows a better stratification of high-risk patients undergoing reduced-toxicity allogeneic hematopoietic cell transplantation. Biol Blood Marrow Transplant. 2014;20:66–72.

Barba P, Ratan R, Cho C, et al. Hematopoietic cell transplantation comorbidity index predicts outcomes in patients with acute myeloid leukemia and myelodysplastic syndromes receiving CD34(+) selected grafts for allogeneic hematopoietic cell transplantation. Biol Blood Marrow Transplant. 2017;23:67–74.

Cornelissen JJ, Blaise D. Hematopoietic stem cell transplantation for patients with AML in first complete remission. Blood. 2016;127:62–70.

Gratwohl A, Hermans J, Goldman JM, et al. Risk assessment for patients with chronic myeloid leukaemia before allogeneic blood or marrow transplantation. Chronic Leukemia Working Party of the European Group for Blood and Marrow Transplantation. Lancet. 1998;352:1087–92.

Gratwohl A, Stern M, Brand R, et al. Risk score for outcome after allogeneic hematopoietic stem cell transplantation: a retrospective analysis. Cancer. 2009;115:4715–26.

Hemmati PG, Terwey TH, le Coutre P, et al. A modified EBMT risk score predicts the outcome of patients with acute myeloid leukemia receiving allogeneic stem cell transplants. Eur J Haematol. 2011;86:305–16.

Hogan WJ, Maris M, Storer B, et al. Hepatic injury after nonmyeloablative conditioning followed by allogeneic hematopoietic cell transplantation: a study of 193 patients. Blood. 2004;103:78–84.

Lodewyck T, Oudshoorn M, van der Holt B, et al. Predictive impact of allele-matching and EBMT risk score for outcome after T-cell depleted unrelated donor transplantation in poor-risk acute leukemia and myelodysplasia. Leukemia. 2011;25:1548–54.

Parimon T, Au DH, Martin PJ, Chien JW. A risk score for mortality after allogeneic hematopoietic cell transplantation. Ann Intern Med. 2006;144:407–14.

Rezvani K, Kanfer EJ, Marin D, Gabriel I, et al. EBMT risk score predicts outcome of allogeneic hematopoietic stem cell transplantation in patients who have failed a previous transplantation procedure. Biol Blood Marrow Transplant. 2012;18:235–40.

Samuelson Bannow BT, Salit RB, Storer BE, et al. Hematopoietic cell transplantation for myelofibrosis: the dynamic international prognostic scoring system plus risk predicts post-transplant outcomes. Biol Blood Marrow Transplant. 2018;24:386–92.

Shouval R, Labopin M, Bondi O, et al. Prediction of allogeneic hematopoietic stem-cell transplantation mortality 100 days after transplantation using a machine learning algorithm: a European Group for Blood and Marrow Transplantation Acute Leukemia Working Party retrospective data mining study. J Clin Oncol. 2015;33:3144–51.

Shouval R, Bonifazi F, Fein J, et al. Validation of the acute leukemia-EBMT score for prediction of mortality following allogeneic stem cell transplantation in a multi-center GITMO cohort. Am J Hematol. 2017;92:429–34.

Sorror ML. How I assess comorbidities before hematopoietic cell transplantation. Blood. 2013;121:854–63.

Sorror ML, Maris MB, Storb R, et al. Hematopoietic cell transplantation (HCT)-specific comorbidity index: a new tool for risk assessment before allogeneic HCT. Blood. 2005;106:2912–9.

Sorror ML, Giralt S, Sandmaier BM, et al. Hematopoietic cell transplantation specific comorbidity index as an outcome predictor for patients with acute myeloid leukemia in first remission: combined FHCRC and MDACC experiences. Blood. 2007;110:4606–13.

Sorror ML, Storb RF, Sandmaier BM, et al. Comorbidity-age index: a clinical measure of biologic age before allogeneic hematopoietic cell transplantation. J Clin Oncol. 2014;32:3249–56.

Terwey TH, Hemmati PG, Martus P, et al. A modified EBMT risk score and the hematopoietic cell transplantation-specific comorbidity index for pretransplant risk assessment in adult acute lymphoblastic leukemia. Haematologica. 2010;95:810–8.

Versluis J, Labopin M, Niederwieser D, et al. Prediction of non-relapse mortality in recipients of reduced intensity conditioning allogeneic stem cell transplantation with AML in first complete remission. Leukemia. 2015;29:51–7.

Wang HT, Chang YJ, Xu LP, Liu DH, Wang Y, Liu KY, Huang XJ. EBMT risk score can predict the outcome of leukaemia after unmanipulated haploidentical blood and marrow transplantation. Bone Marrow Transplant. 2014;49:927–33.

Xhaard A, Porcher R, Chien JW, et al. Impact of comorbidity indexes on non-relapse mortality. Leukemia. 2008;22:2062–9.

Donor Selection for Adults and Pediatrics

Francis Ayuk and Adriana Balduzzi

12.1 Introduction

It is known that multiple factors impact on transplantation outcome; the heaviest ones are disease-related (disease refractoriness, phase, clonal abnormalities, etc. in malignancies and disease type and associated rejection risk in non-malignant diseases) and patient-related (age, comorbidities, infectious diseases/colonization, etc.). Moreover, donor-related issues and stem cell source may influence the extent of disease control and transplant-related mortality.

The availability of a suitable stem cell graft is an absolute prerequisite for the performance of allo-HSCT. Beyond donor-recipient histocompatibility, other factors such as stem cell source, donor age and gender, donor-recipient CMV status, and ABO compatibility may play a role on transplant outcome.

In this chapter we discuss results of studies investigating these factors and conclude with an algorithm for donor selection. Issues which are peculiar to pediatric recipients are also analyzed and discussed.

F. Ayuk
Department of Stem Cell Transplantation,
University Medical Center Hamburg-Eppendorf
(UKE), Hamburg, Germany

A. Balduzzi (✉)
Outpatient Hematology and Transplant Department,
Clinica Pediatrica, Università degli Studi di Milano
Bicocca, Ospedale San Gerardo, Monza, Italy
e-mail: abalduzzi@fondazionembbm.it

12.2 Donor HLA Compatibility
(See Chap. 9)

The outcome of HSCT depends in part on the matching between the donor and the recipient for the human leukocyte antigens (HLA), encoded by a group of genes on chromosome 6; genes and products are labelled as major histocompatibility complex (MHC). The HLA system is the most polymorphic genetic region known in the human genome. A set of HLA gene alleles, called haplotype, is inherited from each parent; therefore, the probability that a child inherited and shares both parental haplotypes with a full sibling is 25%. Such HLA-identical sibling is still considered an optimal donor.

The most relevant genes for transplantation belong to class I (HLA-A, HLA-B, and HLA-Cw) and class II (HLA-DR, HLA-DQ, and HLA-DP). HLA compatibility with the donor is usually defined by high-resolution typing (four digits) for ten alleles, HLA-A, HLA-B, HLA-C, HLA-DR, and HLA-DQ (Petersdorf 2013), even though there is an increasing evidence supporting the relevance of DPB1 matching (reviewed by Fleischhauer and Shaw 2017).

The concept of "compatibility" for CB donor-recipient pairs is still under debate. Any CB unit which was 6/6 or 5/6 matched was labelled HLA compatible (MD), in the past as defined by low-resolution typing at A and B loci and high-resolution typing at the DRB1 locus; more recently, high resolution for at least A, B,

C, and DRB1 loci is requested, and progressively the same criteria used for volunteer donors are considered to define CB HLA matching (Eapen et al. 2017).

12.3 Donor Selection for Adult Patients

12.3.1 Donor Type (Summarized in Fig. 12.1)

12.3.1.1 Matched Related Siblings and Unrelated Donors

Donor-recipient histocompatibility is one of the key variables in allo-HSCT. An HLA-identical sibling donor is generally considered the best donor for allo-HSCT; however less than a third of patients will have one available. Unrelated donor registries worldwide now include more than about 30 million volunteer donors, most of them in North America and Europe (www.bmdw.org). The probability of finding a fully MUD (8/8 or 10/10) varies on average between 16% and 75% (Gragert et al. 2014; Buck et al. 2016) depending on ethnicity, with lowest and highest probabilities in patients of African and European descent,

respectively. Increasing ethnic diversity will with time further limit the chances of finding a fully matched unrelated donor.

Till date no randomized trial has compared outcome of transplants from different donors. However, one prospective (Yakoub-Agha et al. 2006) and several retrospective analyses indicate that outcomes after MSD and fully MUD (8/8 or 10/10) HSCT are comparable (Schetelig et al. 2008; Szydlo et al. 1997; Arora et al. 2009; Ringden 2009; Gupta et al. 2010; Woolfrey et al. 2010; Saber et al. 2012). Increase in donor-recipient HLA disparity in HLA-A, HLA-B, HLA-C, or HLA-DRB1 is associated with poorer outcome after unrelated donor transplantation (Lee et al. 2007; Shaw et al. 2010; Woolfrey et al. 2011; Horan et al. 2012; Fürst et al. 2013; Pidala et al. 2014; Verneris et al. 2015). The overall decrease in survival can be explained by the increase in NRM with no positive effect on relapse. Disparities in HLA-DQB1 as well as C-allele disparities in C*03:03 vs 03:04 have been reported to be permissive with no negative effects on outcome (Lee et al. 2007; Fürst et al. 2013; Morishima et al. 2015; Pidala et al. 2014; Crivello et al. 2016). Disparities in HLA-DPB1 are observed in the majority of HLA-A, HLA-B, HLA-C, and HLA-DQB1

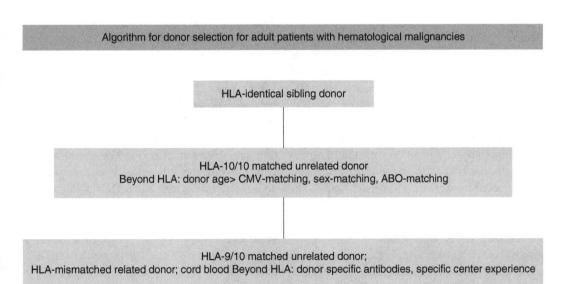

Fig. 12.1 Algorithm for donor selection

(10/10) MUD transplants. Nonpermissive mismatches in DPB1 defined according to T-cell epitope matching (Zino et al. 2004; Crocchiolo et al. 2009; Fleischhauer et al. 2012; Pidala et al. 2014; Oran et al. 2018) or allele cell-surface expression levels (Petersdorf et al. 2015) are associated with poorer outcome compared to full matches or permissive mismatches. Associations of permissive DPB1 mismatches with lower relapse incidence are currently being explored (Fleischhauer and Beelen 2016; Fleischhauer and Shaw 2017).

12.3.1.2 Haploidentical Related Donors

Improvements in transplant technology including pre-transplant ATG (Huang et al. 2006), PT-CY (Luznik et al. 2008), and alpha-beta TCD (Bertaina et al. 2014) have led to improved outcome and rapidly increasing use of haploidentical related donor transplantation (Passweg et al. 2014). Several retrospective comparison studies have reported similar outcome for haploidentical and MUD transplants (summarized by Fuchs 2017). The results of prospective comparative trials are eagerly awaited.

12.3.2 Role of Non-HLA Donor Characteristics

Besides donor-recipient histocompatibility, donor age is now considered one of, if not the most relevant, the non-HLA donor characteristics in unrelated donor HSCT (Kollman et al. 2001, 2016; Wang et al. 2018) with a 2-year survival being 3% better when a donor 10 years younger is selected (Shaw et al. 2018). These findings have impacted daily practice such that the percentage of selected donors under 30 years of age has increased from 36% in the period 1988–2006 to 51% in 1999–2011 up to 69% in 2012–2014 (Kollman et al. 2016).

Matching for patient/recipient CMV serostatus also seems to be a determinant of transplant outcome with best outcome seen in seronegative patients receiving seronegative grafts (Ljungman 2014; Kalra et al. 2016; Shaw et al. 2017).

The impact of sex mismatch on outcome is more controversial, possibly reflecting different definitions of sex mismatch, which has been considered only for male recipients (Gratwohl et al. 2009, 2017; Nakasone et al. 2015) or for both male and female in others (Kollman et al. 2016). Interestingly, all three studies confining sex mismatch to male recipients reported a significant impact for this variable, albeit possibly dependent on conditioning regimen.

The impact of ABO (blood group) compatibility on outcome has been reported to be modest and seems to have further diminished in recent years probably due to changes in transplant practice including less frequent use of bone marrow grafts (Seebach et al. 2005; Kollman et al. 2016; Shaw et al. 2018).

The impact of non-HLA donor characteristics may be less conspicuous in matched and mismatched related donor transplantations using PT-CY. It must however be taken into consideration that the close association of donor age and donor-patient relation on the one hand with patient age on the other hand makes these analyses more complex (McCurdy et al. 2018; Robinson et al. 2018). Larger patient cohorts and prospective studies are required for more definite conclusions.

12.3.3 Donor Choice According to Stem Cell Source

The three graft sources for allo-HSCT are BM, PBSC, and CB. In matched related donor and unrelated donor HSCT, survival outcome has been similar for BM and PBSC. However hematological recovery is more rapid and graft rejection less frequent after PB compared to BM HSCT, while the incidence of chronic GvHD and, to a lesser extent, acute GvHD tends to be higher after PB HSCT (Bensinger et al. 2001; Couban et al. 2002; Schmitz et al. 2002; Couban et al. 2016; Anasetti et al. 2012). In allo-HSCT for nonmalignant diseases, in particular for SAA, BM is still the preferred stem cell source in high-income countries, despite improvements in outcome after PB HSCT (Schrezenmeier et al. 2007;

Chu et al. 2011; Bacigalupo et al. 2012; Kumar et al. 2016).

Traditionally BM has been used as stem cell source for haploidentical HSCT with PT-CY (Luznik et al. 2008), while GCSF-stimulated BM has been used for haploidentical HSCT with ATG (Huang et al. 2006) and PBSC for haploidentical HSCT with alpha-beta T-cell depletion (Bertaina et al. 2014). There are no prospective studies comparing different stem cell sources within these strategies. When PT-CY is used, PBSC seems to be associated with a higher risk of acute and chronic GvHD and lower risk of relapse in patients with leukemia (Bashey et al. 2017).

The use of umbilical CB grafts continues to decrease with the rise in numbers of haploidentical transplants performed (Passweg et al. 2014). Due to the limited number of stem cells per unit, CB grafts have been more frequently used in pediatric HSCT and will be discussed in that section and in the specific CB Chapter.

12.3.4 Anti-HLA Antibodies

The abovementioned improvements in transplant technology have led to an increased use of grafts from HLA-mismatched donors. Detection of donor-specific anti-HLA antibodies in the patients' serum has been associated with increased risk of graft failure and also poorer survival of those patients with graft failure (Ciurea et al. 2015) after haploidentical HSCT. The risk of graft failure and overall mortality may however also depend on the type and intensity of TCD used. The EBMT recently published a consensus guideline on detection and treatment of donor-specific antibodies in haploidentical HSCT (Ciurea et al. 2018).

12.4 Donor Selection for Pediatric Patients

Donor selection criteria may vary between adult and pediatric recipients. According to the "motto" of the Pediatric Disease Working Party, "children are not small adults," besides the size, what makes HSCT in children different is mainly related with indications and the biology of a growing individual.

12.4.1 Pediatric Recipient Size

In terms of size, the recipient weight may vary between few Kg in most patients transplanted for immunodeficiencies and a full adult size in some adolescents. The recommended cell dose in the graft is shown in Table 12.1 (Gluckmann 2012). The lower the recipient weight, the smaller is the amount of the requested absolute count in the graft, which makes the harvest easier, often matching the transplant center requests. An appropriate cell dose in the graft yields a lower risk of rejection, which is actually lowest in pediatrics. On the other hand, the lower amount of cells requested to ensure engraftment in children makes CB a more valuable source than in adults.

12.4.2 Indications

In terms of indications, according to the EBMT, nowadays 46% of the patients younger than 18 years who undergo HSCT are affected with non-malignant diseases (Passweg et al. 2014), which are mainly inherited disorders, namely, immunodeficiencies, hemoglobinopaties, inborn errors of

Table 12.1 Number of cells according to stem cell source

	Volume collected	Med CD34 content	Med CD3 content	Target cell dose
Bone marrow	10–20 mL/kg	$2–3 \times 10^6$/kg[a]	25×10^6/kg	$>2 \times 10^8$ TNC/kg
Peripheral blood	150–400 mL	8×10^6/kg	250×10^6/kg	$5–10 \times 10^6$ CD34+/kg
Umbilical cord blood	80–160 mL	0.2×10^6/kg	2.5×10^6/kg	$>3 \times 10^7$ TNC/kg

[a]Per kg recipient body weight

metabolism, and congenital bone marrow failures. As nonmalignant diseases do not benefit of any alloreactivity, the closest HLA matching (possibly "10 out of 10" HLA alleles) is recommended. On the contrary, a small degree of HLA incompatibility is tolerated in malignancies, as the detrimental effect of HLA disparity, triggering higher risk of GvHD and consequent higher risks of toxicity and mortality, might be counterbalanced by the so-called "graft-versus-leukemia" or "graft-versus-tumor" effect, which is the alloreactivity of immunocompetent donor cells potentially eradicating residual malignant cells in the patient and playing a role in the prevention of malignant disease recurrence.

12.4.3 Donor Type

Due to the decreasing size of modern families in the so-called Western countries, HLA-identical siblings are available in less than 25% of the children in need of a transplant, as shown by the few studies performing a "randomization by genetic chance," based on the availability of an HLA-identical sibling or not (Balduzzi et al. 2005). As a consequence, 75% of the patients may need to run a search for an unrelated donor.

Eligibility criteria for HSCT in malignant diseases varied overtime, resulting from the balance between the outcome of frontline and relapse chemotherapy protocols and the outcome of transplantation, which partially depends on the degree of compatibility within each donor-recipient pair. Similarly, the eligibility for transplantation in nonmalignant diseases increased as the safety profile of the procedure improved. Some patients are considered eligible for transplantation only in case an HLA-identical sibling is available; as the risk profile of the patient worsens, a broader degree of HLA mismatching is considered acceptable.

Within the International BFM Study Group, regardless of their relationship with their recipient, donors are defined as HLA-matched (MD) if the donor-recipient pairs are fully matched

(10/10) or have a single allelic or antigenic disparity (9/10) or are defined mismatched donor (MMD) if the donor-recipient pairs have two (8/10) or more allelic or antigenic disparities, up to a different haplotype (Peters et al. 2015). Any donor who is not an HLA-identical sibling or a MD, as defined above, is considered a MMD. Both MD and MMD could be either related or unrelated to their recipient. A related donor who is not an HLA-identical sibling is actually regarded as a MD, and GvHD prophylaxis is planned accordingly (Peters et al. 2015).

Recently, results from a BFM study showed that transplantation from a "10 or 9 out of 10" matched donor, either related or unrelated, was not inferior to transplantation from an HLA-identical sibling in terms of EFS, OS, and CIR in pediatric patients with ALL (Peters et al. 2015). As a consequence eligibility criteria for HSCT might be reviewed and extended to those for MSD HSCT, at least in ALL, and, possibly, considered for other malignant diseases. Therefore, an unrelated donor search activation and transplantation might be recommended in the future virtually for every child for whom an allo-HSCT is indicated. Disparities within donor-recipient pairs are progressively accepted as the risk profile of the patient increases.

Unfortunately some inherited disorders, in particular sickle cell disease (Gluckman et al. 2017) or other recessively inherited disease, which incidence is highly increased by a parental blood relation, have higher incidences in non-Caucasian ethnicities, which are less represented within stem cell donor banks. The consequence is that well-matched donors often lack when a perfect matching is crucial; progresses in haploidentical HSCT broadened its indications and may overcome this issue.

Depending on each transplant center experience, MMD might be preferred, carrying the advantage of prompt donor availability and flexible schedule and bringing higher degree of alloreactivity, potentially associated with lower relapse risk. HSCT from MMD is widely recommended when timing adjustment is crucial, as in advanced disease phase in malignancies and in case of post transplant relapse.

12.4.4 Haploidentical Donors in Pediatrics

Successful haploidentical HSCT mainly evolved in pediatrics over the last two decades from ex vivo T-cell depletion by CD34+-positive selection, to CD34+-negative selection, up to selective CD3 αβ depletion, to allow other cells in the graft, potentially protecting from viral infections (Handgretinger et al. 2001; Klingebiel et al. 2010). In pediatrics, an improved immune recovery after TCR αβ-depleted haploidentical HSCT (Lang et al. 2015), a similar outcome between TCR αβ-depleted and matched sibling and matched unrelated donors HSCT in children with acute leukemia (Locatelli et al. 2017) and in non-malignant diseases (Bertaina et al. 2014), was recently reported and confirmed by a multicenter phase I/II study (Lang et al. 2017). Moreover, some reports of PT-CY in pediatric show promising results (Jaiswal et al. 2016; Sawada et al. 2014; Wiebking et al. 2017).

One of the parents mostly serves as a donor in haploidentical donors for pediatric recipients. The choice between the mother and the father is still debated. Better survival was shown in patients transplanted from the mother than from the father (51% vs 11%; $P < 0.001$), due to both reduced incidence of relapse and TRM, with a protective effect on the risk of failure (HR 0.42; $P = 0.003$), possibly explained by transplacental leukocyte trafficking during pregnancy, inducing long-term, stable, reciprocal microchimerism in mother and child (Stern et al. 2008).

As donor-derived alloreactive NK cells have been shown to play a key role in the eradication of leukemic cells, favorable NK matching should guide donor selection (Stringaris and Barrett 2017; Mavers and Bertaina 2018). Moreover, anti-HLA antibodies should be checked and accounted for to guide donor selection.

12.4.5 Stem Cell Source

BM is usually recommended as stem cell source. A donor with a body weight allowing for a graft containing at least 3×10^8 nucleated cells/kg recipient body weight and 3×10^6 CD34+ cells/kg body weight should be selected, in order to yield more than 95% neutrophil engraftment chances at a median of 21 days in the setting of hematological malignant diseases (Simonin et al. 2017).

It is rare in pediatrics to require PB just in order to obtain an adequate amount of cells to ensure engraftment, as the absolute cell dose needed rarely overcomes the maximum amount which could be harvested from a donor. As higher numbers of CD3 cells are obtained in PB grafts, it is recommended not to exceed an amount of 10×10^8 CD3+ cells/kg recipient body weight.

The increased risk of chronic GvHD, and possibly acute, after PBSC transplantation, as compared to BM, is commonly reported. In a recent European retrospective study, including 2584 pediatric patients transplanted from 2003 to 2012 for ALL, both TRM and chronic GvHD appeared significantly higher after PBSC, as compared with other SC sources, despite the overall survival was similar for both stem cell sources (Simonin et al. 2017). In the prospective ALL-SCT-BFM 2003 study, the same OS was reported, and no difference could be demonstrated in TRM, acute GvHD, and relapse, whichever the stem cell source in the two cohorts of patients transplanted from HLA-identical siblings and other matched donors. Nevertheless, within patients transplanted from HLA-identical siblings, the cumulative incidence of chronic GvHD was higher in PB compared with BM recipients (Peters et al. 2015).

Reinforced GvHD prophylaxis may be recommended when PBSC are used, mainly when no serotherapy is included as for GvHD prophylaxis, as in most protocols in the HLA-identical sibling setting in malignancies (Simonin et al. 2017).

Nowadays, in the ongoing prospective ALL-I-BFM HSCT trial (FORUM), the algorithm for choosing stem cell source recommends BM as the first choice. To date, there is no demonstration for a better GVL effect after PB HSCT in the pediatric population.

Due to the increased risk of cGvHD after PB transplant, which is almost consistent among investigators, it is definitely recommended to avoid PB in nonmalignant disorders.

From the first CB transplantation performed for a Fanconi anemia patient in 1987, CB appeared as a useful and an efficient stem cell source, due to two major features: high proliferative capacity, allowing engraftment despite 1-log fewer cells, and immune plasticity, allowing a wider HLA disparity within each donor recipient pair (Gluckman et al. 1989).

The possibility to adopt less stringent HLA-matching criteria enlarged the availability of grafts to at least 90% of the pediatric patients in need of an allogeneic transplant (Eapen et al. 2017). According to Eurocord consortium recommendations, unrelated CB with two or less HLA disparities typed in low resolution (i.e., two digit) for class I (A and B loci) and high resolution (i.e., four-digit) for class II (DRB1 locus) and with more than 2.5×10^7 nucleated cell dose/kg or 2×10^5 CD34+ cells/kg are suitable for engraftment (Gratwohl et al. 2009). Recent studies from both Eurocord, NetCord, EBMT, and CIBMTR recommend high-resolution HLA typing for A, B, C, and DRB1 and a maximum of 1 or 2 mismatched loci with a cellularity of 3×10^7 TNC/kg or higher (Eapen et al. 2014).

Two prospective studies could demonstrate no benefit of double CB in pediatric patients transplanted for malignant diseases (Wagner et al. 2014; Michel et al. 2016).

12.4.6 Other Donor-Recipient-Related Factors

Besides HLA compatibility and stem cell source, also donor age, gender, female parity, weight,

ABO blood group, and viral serological status should be considered in the decision-making process for donor selection, whenever more than one donor were available, which may not be often the case (Wang et al. 2018).

Most studies report that a young donor is better than an older one. Few studies also report that a male donor is better for a male recipient and better than a multiparous woman for any recipient, even though this finding is not consistent through the literature. The donor gender effect may be mild and need larger series of patients to be demonstrated (Friedrich et al. 2018). Unfavorable weight disparity, with donors weighing less than their recipient, should be avoided, when possible (Styczynski et al. 2012). CMV-IgG, as well as EBV-positive patients, should be grafted from CMV- and EBV-positive donors, respectively (Jeljeli et al. 2014; Bontant et al. 2014). ABO matching is usually preferred, especially instead of a major or even minor incompatibility (Booth et al. 2013). Donor location might also be considered, as oversea deliveries increase the time elapsing between collection and infusion, thus reduce cell viability and potentially jeopardize engraftment. More recently, KIR genotyping would allow to identify alloreactive donors who may contribute to prevent relapse also in the non-haploidentical setting (Mavers and Bertaina 2018).

Even though it is mainly clear which variant should be preferred within each variable, there is no consensus regarding the hierarchical order by which the factors above should be combined. In a recent survey within the Pediatric Diseases Working Party of the EBMT, the features above were listed in the following order of importance, on the average, but evaluations widely differed among responders:

1. HLA compatibility, with 10/10 better than 9/10 or worse matching
2. CMV serological status of positive donors in case of positive recipients
3. BM as stem cell source
4. Donor age, being preferable a younger donor compared with an older one

5. Donor gender, with a male donor preferred, particularly for a male recipient
6. ABO major compatibility
7. Donor center location
8. ABO minor compatibility (unpublished data)

Moreover, the presence of anti-HLA antibodies directed to any mismatched HLA alleles should be ruled out, mainly in heavily transfused nonmalignant diseases, such as hemoglobinopaties or bone marrow failures (Ciurea et al. 2018).

Key Points

- An HLA-identical sibling is considered a donor of first choice.
- For patients with hematological malignancies, transplantation from fully HLA-MUD (8/8 or 10/10) is not inferior to transplantation from HLA-identical siblings in terms of EFS.
- The choice of alternative donors (haploidentical related donors, cord blood, mismatched unrelated donors) depends on center experience, urgency of transplant procedure, and detection of donor-specific anti-HLA antibodies.
- For pediatric patients and patients with nonmalignant disorders, BM is the preferred stem cell source.
- For adult patients with hematological malignancies, survival outcome after HSCT with PBSC and BM is comparable.
- In URD transplantation, donor age is probably the most relevant non-HLA donor factor.

References

Anasetti C, Logan BR, Lee SJ, et al. Peripheral-blood stem cells versus bone marrow from unrelated donors. N Engl J Med. 2012;367:1487–96.

Arora M, Weisdorf DJ, Spellman SR, et al. HLA-identical sibling compared with 8/8 matched and mismatched unrelated donor bone marrow transplant for chronic phase chronic myeloid leukemia. J Clin Oncol. 2009;27:1644–52.

Bacigalupo A, Socie G, Schrezenmeier H, et al. Bone marrow versus peripheral blood as the stem cell source for sibling transplants in acquired aplastic anemia: survival advantage for bone marrow in all age groups. Haematologica. 2012;97:1142–8.

Balduzzi A, Valsecchi MG, Uderzo C, et al. Chemotherapy versus allogeneic transplantation for very-high-risk childhood acute lymphoblastic leukaemia in first complete remission: comparison by genetic randomisation in an international prospective study. Lancet. 2005;366:635–42.

Bashey A, Zhang MJ, McCurdy SR, et al. Mobilized peripheral blood stem cells versus unstimulated bone marrow as a graft source for T-cell-replete haploidentical donor transplantation using post-transplant cyclophosphamide. J Clin Oncol. 2017;35:3002–9.

Bensinger WI, Martin PJ, Storer B, et al. Transplantation of bone marrow as compared with peripheral-blood cells from HLA-identical relatives in patients with hematologic cancers. N Engl J Med. 2001;344:175–81.

Bertaina A, Merli P, Rutella S, et al. HLA-haploidentical stem cell transplantation after removal of αβ+ T and B cells in children with nonmalignant disorders. Blood. 2014;124:822–6.

Bontant T, Sedláček P, Balduzzi A, et al. Survey of CMV management in pediatric allogeneic HSCT programs, on behalf of the inborn errors, infectious diseases and pediatric diseases working parties of EBMT. Bone Marrow Transplant. 2014;49:276–9.

Booth GS, Gehrie EA, Bolan CD, Savani BN. Clinical guide to ABO-incompatible allogeneic stem cell transplantation. Biol Blood Marrow Transplant. 2013;19:1152–8.

Buck K, Wadsworth K, Setterholm M, et al. High-Resolution Match Rate of 7/8 and 9/10 or Better for the Be The Match Unrelated Donor Registry. Biol Blood Marrow Transplant. 2016;22:759–63.

Chu R, Brazauskas R, Kan F, et al. Comparison of outcomes after transplantation of G-CSF-stimulated bone marrow grafts versus bone marrow or peripheral blood grafts from HLA-matched sibling donors for patients with severe aplastic anemia. Biol Blood Marrow Transplant. 2011;17:1018–24.

Ciurea SO, Thall PF, Milton DR, et al. Complement-binding donor-specific anti-HLA antibodies and risk of primary graft failure in hematopoietic stem cell transplantation. Biol Blood Marrow Transplant. 2015;21:1392–8.

Ciurea SO, Cao K, Fernadez-Vina M, et al. The European Society for Blood and Marrow Transplantation (EBMT) consensus guidelines for the detection and treatment of donor-specific anti-HLA antibodies (DSA) in haploidentical hematopoietic cell transplantation. Bone Marrow Transplant. 2018;53:521–34.

Couban S, Simpson DR, Barnett MJ, et al. A randomized multicenter comparison of bone marrow and peripheral blood in recipients of matched sibling allogeneic transplants for myeloid malignancies. Blood. 2002;100:1525–31.

Couban S, Aljurf M, Lachance S, et al. Filgrastim-stimulated bone marrow compared with filgrastim-mobilized peripheral blood in myeloablative sibling allografting for patients with hematologic malignancies: a randomized Canadian Blood and Marrow Transplant Group Study. Biol Blood Marrow Transplant. 2016;22:1410–5.

Crivello P, Heinold A, Rebmann V, et al. Functional distance between recipient and donor HLA-DPB1 determines nonpermissive mismatches in unrelated HCT. Blood. 2016;128:120–9.

Crocchiolo R, Zino E, Vago L, et al. Gruppo Italiano Trapianto di Midollo Osseo, Cellule Staminale Ematopoietiche (CSE) e Terapia Cellulare; Italian Bone Marrow Donor Registry. Nonpermissive HLA-DPB1 disparity is a significant independent risk factor for mortality after unrelated hematopoietic stem cell transplantation. Blood. 2009;114:1437–44.

Eapen M, Klein JP, Ruggeri A, et al. Impact of allele level HLA matching on outcomes after myeloablative single unit umbilical cord blood transplantation for hematologic malignancy. Blood. 2014;123:133–4.

Eapen M, Wang T, Veys PA, et al. Allele-level HLA matching for umbilical cord blood transplantation for non-malignant diseases in children: a retrospective analysis. Lancet Haematol. 2017;4:e325–33.

Fleischhauer K, Beelen DW. HLA mismatching as a strategy to reduce relapse after alternative donor transplantation. Semin Hematol. 2016;53:57–64.

Fleischhauer K, Shaw BE. HLA-DP in unrelated hematopoietic cell transplantation revisited: challenges and opportunities. Blood. 2017;130:1089–96.

Fleischhauer K, Shaw BE, Gooley T, et al. Effect of T-cell-epitope matching at HLA-DPB1 in recipients of unrelated-donor haemopoietic-cell transplantation: a retrospective study International Histocompatibility Working Group in hematopoietic cell transplantation. Lancet Oncol. 2012;13:366–74.

Friedrich P, Guerra-García P, Stetson A, et al. Young female donors do not increase the risk of graft-versus-host disease or impact overall outcomes in pediatric HLA-matched sibling hematopoietic stem cell transplantation. Biol Blood Marrow Transplant. 2018;24:96–102.

Fuchs EJ. Related haploidentical donors are a better choice than matched unrelated donors: point. Blood Adv. 2017;1:397–400.

Fürst D, Müller C, Vucinic V, et al. High-resolution HLA matching in hematopoietic stem cell transplantation: a retrospective collaborative analysis. Blood. 2013;122:3220–9.

Gluckman E, Broxmeyer HA, Auerbach AD, et al. Hematopoietic reconstitution in a patient with Fanconi's anemia by means of umbilical-cord blood from an HLA-identical sibling. N Engl J Med. 1989;321:1174–8.

Gluckman E, Cappelli B, Bernaudin F, et al. Sickle cell disease: an international survey of results of HLA-identical sibling hematopoietic stem cell transplantation. Blood. 2017;129:1548–56.

Gluckmann E (2012) Choice of the donor according to HLA typing and stem cell source. EBMT handbook.

Gragert L, Eapen M, Williams E, et al. HLA Match likelihoods, for hematopoietic stem-cell grafts in the U.S. registry. N Engl J Med. 2014;371:339–48.

Gratwohl A, Stern M, Brand R, et al. European Group for Blood and Marrow Transplantation and the European Leukemia Net. Risk score for outcome after allogeneic hematopoietic stem cell transplantation: a retrospective analysis. Cancer. 2009;115:4715–26.

Gratwohl A, Sureda A, Cornelissen J, et al. Alloreactivity: the Janus-face of hematopoietic stem cell transplantation. Leukemia. 2017;31:1752–9.

Gupta V, Tallman MS, He W, et al. Comparable survival after HLA-well-matched unrelated or matched sibling donor transplantation for acute myeloid leukemia in first remission with unfavorable cytogenetics at diagnosis. Blood. 2010;116:1839–48.

Handgretinger R, Klingebiel T, Lang P, et al. Megadose transplantation of purified peripheral blood CD34(+) progenitor cells from HLA-mismatched parental donors in children. Bone Marrow Transplant. 2001;27:777–83.

Horan J, Wang T, Haagenson M, et al. Evaluation of HLA matching in unrelated hematopoietic stem cell transplantation for nonmalignant disorders. Blood. 2012;120:2918–24.

Huang XJ, Liu DH, Liu KY, et al. Haploidentical hematopoietic stem cell transplantation without in vitro T-cell depletion for the treatment of hematological malignancies. Bone Marrow Transplant. 2006;38:291–7.

Jaiswal SR, Chakrabarti A, Chatterjee S, et al. Haploidentical peripheral blood stem cell transplantation with post-transplantation cyclophosphamide in children with advanced acute leukemia with fludarabine-, busulfan-, and melphalan-based conditioning. Biol Blood Marrow Transplant. 2016;22:499–504.

Jeljeli M, Guérin-El Khourouj V, Porcher R, et al. Relationship between cytomegalovirus (CMV) reactivation, CMV-driven immunity, overall immune recovery and graft-versus-leukaemia effect in children. Br J Haematol. 2014;166:229–39.

Kalra A, Williamson T, Daly A, et al. Impact of donor and recipient cytomegalovirus serostatus on outcomes of antithymocyte globulin-conditioned hematopoietic cell transplantation. Biol Blood Marrow Transplant. 2016;22:1654–63.

Klingebiel T, Cornish J, Labopin M, et al. Results and factors influencing outcome after fully haploidentical hematopoietic stem cell transplantation in children with very high-risk acute lymphoblastic leukemia: impact of center size: an analysis on behalf of the Acute Leukemia and Pediatric Disease Working Parties of the European Blood and Marrow Transplant group. Blood. 2010;115:3437–46.

Kollman C, Howe CW, Anasetti C, et al. Donor characteristics as risk factors in recipients after transplantation of bone marrow from unrelated donors: the effect of donor age. Blood. 2001;98:2043–51.

Kollman C, Spellman SR, Zhang MJ, et al. The effect of donor characteristics on survival after unrelated donor transplantation for hematologic malignancy. Blood. 2016;127:260–7.

Kumar R, Kimura F, Ahn KW, et al. Comparing outcomes with bone marrow or peripheral blood stem cells as graft source for matched sibling transplants in severe aplastic anemia across different economic regions. Biol Blood Marrow Transplant. 2016;22:932–40.

Lang P, Feuchtinger T, Teltschik HM, et al. Improved immune recovery after transplantation of TCRαβ/CD19-depleted allografts from haploidentical donors in pediatric patients. Bone Marrow Transplant. 2015;50(Suppl 2):S6–10.

Lang PL, Schlegel PG, Meisel R, et al. Safety and efficacy of Tcr alpha/beta and CD19 depleted haploidentical stem cell transplantation following reduced intensity conditioning in children: results of a prospective multicenter phase I/II clinical trial. Blood. 2017;130:214.

Lee SJ, Klein J, Haagenson M, et al. High-resolution donor-recipient HLA matching contributes to the success of unrelated donor marrow transplantation. Blood. 2007;110:4576–83.

Ljungman P. The role of cytomegalovirus serostatus on outcome of hematopoietic stem cell transplantation. Curr Opin Hematol. 2014;21:466–9.

Locatelli F, Merli P, Pagliara D, et al. Outcome of children with acute leukemia given HLA-haploidentical HSCT after αβ T-cell and B-cell depletion. Blood. 2017;130:677–85.

Luznik L, O'Donnell PV, Symons HJ, et al. HLA-haploidentical bone marrow transplantation for hematologic malignancies using nonmyeloablative conditioning and high-dose, posttransplantation cyclophosphamide. Biol Blood Marrow Transplant. 2008;14:641–50.

Mavers M, Bertaina A. High-risk leukemia: past, present, and future role of NK cells. J Immunol Res. 2018 Apr;15:2018.

McCurdy SR, Zhang MJ, St Martin A, et al. Effect of donor characteristics on haploidentical transplantation with posttransplantation cyclophosphamide. Blood Adv. 2018;2:299–307.

Michel G, Galambrun C, Sirvent A, et al. Single- vs double-unit cord blood transplantation for children and young adults with acute leukemia or myelodysplastic syndrome. Blood. 2016;127:3450–7.

Morishima Y, Kashiwase K, Matsuo K, et al. Biological significance of HLA locus matching in unrelated donor bone marrow transplantation. Japan Marrow Donor Program. Blood. 2015;125:1189–97.

Nakasone H, Remberger M, Tian L, et al. Risks and benefits of sex-mismatched hematopoietic cell transplantation differ according to conditioning strategy. Haematologica. 2015;100:1477–85.

Oran B, Saliba RM, Carmazzi Y, et al. Effect of nonpermissive HLA-DPB1 mismatches after unrelated allogeneic transplantation with in vivo T-cell depletion. Blood. 2018;131:1248–57.

Passweg JR, Baldomero H, Peters C, et al. European Society for Blood and Marrow Transplantation EBMT. Hematopoietic SCT in Europe: data and trends in 2012 with special consideration of pediatric transplantation. Bone Marrow Transplant. 2014;49:744–50.

Peters C, Schrappe M, von Stackelberg A, et al. Stem-cell transplantation in children with acute lymphoblastic leukemia: a prospective international multicenter trial comparing sibling donors with matched unrelated donors-The ALL-SCT-BFM-2003 trial. J Clin Oncol. 2015;33:1265–74.

Petersdorf EW. The major histocompatibility complex: a model for understanding graft-versus-host disease. Blood. 2013;122:1863–72.

Petersdorf EW, Malkki M, O'hUigin C, et al. High HLA-DP expression and graft-versus host disease. N Engl J Med. 2015;373:599–609.

Pidala J, Lee SJ, Ahn KW, et al. Nonpermissive HLA-DPB1 mismatch increases mortality after myeloablative unrelated allogeneic hematopoietic cell transplantation. Blood. 2014;124:2596–606.

Robinson TM, Fuchs EJ, Zhang MJ, et al. Related donor transplants: has posttransplantation cyclophosphamide nullified the detrimental effect of HLA mismatch? Blood Adv. 2018;2:1180–6.

Saber W, Opie S, Rizzo JD, et al. Outcomes after matched unrelated donor versus identical sibling hematopoietic cell transplantation in adults with acute myelogenous leukemia. Blood. 2012;119:3908–16.

Sawada A, Shimizu M, Isaka K, et al. Feasibility of HLA-haploidentical hematopoietic stem cell transplantation with post-transplantation cyclophosphamide for advanced pediatric malignancies. Pediatr Hematol Oncol. 2014;31:754–64.

Schetelig J, Bornhauser M, Schmid C, et al. Matched unrelated or matched sibling donors result in comparable survival after allogeneic stem-cell transplantation in elderly patients with acute myeloid leukemia: a report from the cooperative German Transplant Study Group. J Clin Oncol. 2008;26:5183–91.

Schmitz N, Beksac M, Hasenclever D, et al. Transplantation of mobilized peripheral blood cells to HLA-identical siblings with standard-risk leukemia. Blood. 2002;100:761–7.

Schrezenmeier H, Passweg JR, Marsh JC, et al. Worse outcome and more chronic GVHD with peripheral blood progenitor cells than bone marrow in HLA-matched sibling donor transplants for young patients with severe acquired aplastic anemia. Blood. 2007;110:1397–400.

Seebach JD, Stussi G, Passweg JR, et al. ABO blood group barrier in allogeneic bone marrow transplantation revisited. Biol Blood Marrow Transplant. 2005;11:1006–13.

Shaw BE, Arguello R, Garcia-Sepulveda CA, Madrigal JA. The impact of HLA genotyping on survival following unrelated donor haematopoietic stem cell transplantation. Br J Haematol. 2010;150:251–8.

Shaw BE, Mayor NP, Szydlo RM, et al. Recipient/donor HLA and CMV matching in recipients of T-cell-depleted unrelated donor haematopoietic cell transplants. Bone Marrow Transplant. 2017;52:717–25.

Shaw BE, Logan BR, Spellman SR, et al. Development of an unrelated donor selection score predictive of survival after HCT: donor age matters most. Biol Blood Marrow Transplant. 2018;24:1049–56.

Simonin M, Dalissier A, Labopin M, et al. More chronic GvHD and non-relapse mortality after peripheral blood stem cell compared with bone marrow in hematopoietic transplantation for paediatric acute lymphoblastic leukemia: a retrospective study on behalf of the EBMT Paediatric Diseases Working Party. Bone Marrow Transplant. 2017;52:1071–3.

Stern M, Ruggeri L, Mancusi A, et al. Survival after T cell-depleted haploidentical stem cell transplantation is improved using the mother as donor. Blood. 2008;112:2990–5.

Stringaris K, Barrett AJ. The importance of natural killer cell killer immunoglobulin-like receptor mismatch in transplant outcomes. Curr Opin Hematol. 2017;24:489–95.

Styczynski J, Balduzzi A, Gil L, et al. Risk of complications during hematopoietic stem cell collection in pediatric sibling donors: a prospective European Group for Blood and Marrow Transplantation Pediatric Diseases Working Party study. Blood. 2012;119:2935–42.

Szydlo R, Goldman JM, Klein JP, et al. Results of allogeneic bone marrow transplants for leukemia using donors other than HLA-identical siblings. J Clin Oncol. 1997;15:1767–77.

Verneris MR, Lee SJ, Ahn KW, et al. HLA mismatch is associated with worse outcomes after unrelated donor reduced-intensity conditioning hematopoietic cell transplantation: an analysis from the Center for International Blood and Marrow Transplant Research. Biol Blood Marrow Transplant. 2015;21:1783–9.

Wagner JE, Eapen M, Carter S, et al. One-unit versus two-unit cord-blood transplantation for hematologic cancers. N Engl J Med. 2014;371:1685–94.

Wang Y, Wu DP, Liu QF, et al. Donor and recipient age, gender and ABO incompatibility regardless of donor source: validated criteria for donor selection for haematopoietic transplants. Leukemia. 2018;32:492–8.

Wiebking V, Hütker S, Schmid I, et al. Reduced toxicity, myeloablative HLA-haploidentical hematopoietic stem cell transplantation with post-transplantation cyclophosphamide for sickle cell disease. Ann Hematol. 2017;96:1373–7.

Woolfrey A, Lee SJ, Gooley TA, et al. HLA-allele matched unrelated donors compared to HLA-matched sibling donors: role of cell source and disease risk category. Biol Blood Marrow Transplant. 2010;16:1382–7.

Woolfrey A, Klein JP, Haagenson M, et al. HLA-C antigen mismatch is associated with worse outcome in unrelated donor peripheral blood stem cell transplantation. Biol Blood Marrow Transplant. 2011;17:885–92.

Yakoub-Agha I, Mesnil F, Kuentz M, et al. Allogeneic marrow stem-cell transplantation from human leukocyte antigen-identical siblings versus human leukocyte antigen-allelic-matched unrelated donors (10/10) in patients with standard-risk hematologic malignancy: a prospective study from the French Society of Bone Marrow Transplantation and Cell Therapy. J Clin Oncol. 2006;24:5695–702.

Zino E, Frumento G, Marktel S, et al. A T-cell epitope encoded by a subset of HLA-DPB1 alleles determines nonpermissive mismatches for hematologic stem cell transplantation. Blood. 2004;103:1417–24.

Conditioning

Arnon Nagler and Avichai Shimoni

13.1 Overview

HSCT is a therapeutic procedure that can cure and/
or prolong life in a broad range of hematologic disorders including malignant and nonmalignant
pathologies. Conditioning is the preparative regimen that is administered to the patients undergoing
HSCT before the infusion of the stem cell grafts.
Historically, the pre-HSCT conditioning had to:

1. Eradicate the hematologic malignancy in case
   of malignant indication for HSCT.
2. Provide sufficient IS to ensure engraftment
   and to prevent both rejection and GVHD.
3. Provide stem cell niches in the host BM for
   the new stem cells.

The third purpose is controversial as it was demonstrated in animal models that with mega doses of
HSC and repeated administrations engraftment can
be achieved without conditioning.

A. Nagler (✉)
Department of Medicine, Tel Aviv University,
Tel-Hashomer, Israel

Hematology Division, BMT and Cord Blood Bank,
Chaim Sheba Medical Center, Tel-Hashomer, Israel
e-mail: arnon.nagler@sheba.health.gov.il

A. Shimoni
Bone Marrow Transplantation, Chaim Sheba Medical
Center, Tel-Aviv University, Tel Hashomer, Israel

From the theoretic point of view, the conditioning consisted of two components:

1. Myelo-depletion which targets the host stem
   cells
2. Lymphodepletion which targets the host lymphoid system, respectively

Some of the compounds used in the conditioning are more myeloablative (MA) in nature, for
example, MEL or BU, while some are more lym-
phodepleting like FLU or CY. The pretransplant
conditioning may include TBI or in rare and specific instances other types of irradiations like TLI
that is applied, for example, in haplo-HSCT, or
TAI that was used in the past in Fanconi anemia.
Alternatively, the pre-HSCT conditioning can be
radiation-free including only chemotherapy. In
recent years, serotherapy, specific targeted novel
compounds, and MoAb and radiolabeled Ab
started to be incorporated into specific disease-
oriented conditioning regimens.

Not just the constituents but also the schedule
(days) of administration and doses may differ in
the various conditioning regimen protocols. The
pretransplantation conditioning regimens depend
on the type of the HSC donor. For example, in
auto-HSCT, the pre-HSCT conditioning consisted
of chemotherapy alone, and in some transplant
centers, it may include also irradiation, while, in
allo-HSCT from unrelated or mismatched donors

as well as in HSCT from alternative donors, the pre-HSCT conditioning usually includes serotherapy with ATG or ALEM (Campath; anti-CDW52 MoAb). Similarly, the intensity of the conditioning is traditionally higher in unrelated and mismatched transplants as well as in transplants from alternative donors in comparison to transplants from HLA MSD. The pre-HSCT conditioning regimen takes into account also the specific disease for which the HSCT is being performed, more so in auto-HSCT than in the allogeneic setting aiming to include an effective anti-disease-specific chemotherapy, for example, MEL for MM or BCNU and CY in lymphoma.

Other factors to be taken into account while choosing the optimal conditioning for a specific patient besides the disease he is afflicted with and the type of donor are age, comorbidities, and organ-specific toxicity risk. The conditioning protocols also differ between pediatrics and adults as in pediatric more emphasis should be given to growth and puberty issues. It also differs between nonmalignant and malignant disorders; the former are not just more frequent in pediatrics, but of major importance is the fact that in nonmalignant indications, there is no need for the GVL, and a main goal is to ensure absolutely no GVHD.

Historically, the conditioning protocols were MA in nature, and the two most popular ones were the CY/TBI (TBI 12Gy followed by IV CY 60 mg/kg × 2 days) and the BU/CY protocol (BU 4 mg/kg × 4 days and CY 60 mg/kg × 2 days). However, MAC is associated with significant organ- and transplant-related toxicity (TRT), limiting allo-HSCT to younger patients in good medical conditioning, typically up to age of 55 and 50 years old in allo-HSCT from sibling and URD, respectively. During the past two decades, non-MA (NMA), RIC, and reduced toxicity conditioning (RTC) regimens have been developed aiming in reducing the organ and TRM while keeping the anti-malignant effect and allowing allo-HSCT in elderly and medically infirm patients. These are relatively nontoxic and tolerable regimens designed not to maximally eradicate the malignancy but rather to provide sufficient IS to achieve engraftment and to allow induction of GVL as the primary treatment.

Furthermore, special conditioning protocols have been developed for allo-HSCT from alternative donors including from MMUD, CB donors, and haploidentical family-related donors. These relatively new pre-HSCT conditioning typically includes new drug formulations like IV BU, compounds from the oncology field that are newcomers in HSCT like TREO or TT, new compounds like clofarabine (CLO), or new schedules sequentially administrating novel chemotherapy combination (FLAMSA) to be followed by RIC containing reduced doses of TBI.

13.2 Total Body Irradiation

TBI is a major constituent of MAC regimens. Historically, TBI combined with CY has been the standard regimen used to condition patients with acute leukemia prior to HSCT. TBI is typically given at a dose of 12 Gy (Thomas et al. 1982). Higher doses of TBI up to 14.25 Gy resulted in improved antileukemic effect, but this was counterbalanced by increased toxicity and TRM (Clift et al. 1990). TBI provides both MA and IS ensuring engraftment in combination with optimal antileukemic effect. It provides homogeneous dose distribution in the whole body including sanctuaries for systemic chemotherapy such as the CNS and testicles. Fractionation of 12 Gy TBI in six doses of 2 Gy delivered twice a day over 3 days became the standard over time (Thomas et al. 1982).

The Acute Leukemia Working Party (ALWP) of the EBMT recently showed that 12 Gy fractionated TBI dose delivered either in two fractions or in one fraction per day over 3 or 4 days prior to HSCT resulted in similar outcome, in both ALL and AML patients (Belkacemi et al. 2018). Dose fractionation and dose rate have been shown to be of importance determining both efficacy and toxicity which includes mucositis, interstitial pneumonia, SOS/VOD, hemorrhagic cystitis, and long-term toxicity including growth retardation, endocrine problems, cataracts, and secondary malignancies.

As for mode of TBI administration across Europe, the ALWP of the EBMT performed a questionnaire-based study focusing on technical practices across 56 EBMT centers and 23 countries demonstrating an extremely high heterogeneity of fractionation schedules. The total doses delivered ranged between 8 and 14.4 Gy with dose per fraction varying between 1.65 and 8 Gy. The dose rate at the source ranged between 2.25 and 37.5 Gy/min. This resulted in 40 different reported schedules, to which variations in beam energy, dosimetry, in vivo techniques, and organ shielding disparities had to be added (Giebel et al. 2014). Regarding TBI-mediated antileukemic effect, most studies have shown the equivalence of chemotherapy-based MAC mostly BU/CY and CY/TBI conditioning for AML (Nagler et al. 2013). In contrast, despite the absence of consensus, TBI has remained the first choice in many centers for ALL (Cahu et al. 2016).

13.3 Myeloablative Non-TBI-Containing Conditioning

The MAC are a high-dose chemotherapy mostly alkylating agent-based regimens used in both auto- and allo-HSCT. They cause by definition profound and prolong cytopenia that lasts up to 21 days and necessitates stem cell graft in order to recover (Bacigalupo et al. 2009). Historically, BU/CY is the prototype of chemotherapy-based MAC. It was developed by the Johns Hopkins group as early as 1983 as an alternative to TBI in an effort to reduce the incidence of long-term radiation-induced toxicities and improve the planning of HSCT in institutions lacking easy availability of linear accelerators (Tutschka et al. 1987). A considerable number of studies have shown the equivalence of BU/CY and CY/TBI for allo-HSCT in AML (Nagler et al. 2013) and recently also in ALL (Mohty et al. 2010) although most centers still use TBI-based MAC as the preferred pre-HSCT conditioning for ALL in fit patients with low comorbidities.

The original studies used oral BU that has an erratic and unpredictable absorption with wide inter- and also intra-patient variability with the risk of increased toxicity mainly SOS/VOD in patients with a high area under the curve of BU

plasma concentration versus time, while low BU concentrations may be associated with a higher risk of graft rejection and relapse (Hassan 1999). The common solution was monitoring of BU levels and dose adjustments that allowed for better control of the dose administered and reduction of the abovementioned risks (Deeg et al. 2002). The development of the IV BU with more predictable pharmacokinetics, achieving tight control of plasma levels, and less need for plasma level testing and dose adjustments significantly reduced BU-mediated SOS/VOD and TRM (Nagler et al. 2014).

Some other MAC regimens include MEL in combination with BU (Vey et al. 1996), while others incorporated VP (Czyz et al. 2018). Subsequently, in an attempt to further reduce regimen-related toxicity, CY was replaced with FLU, a nucleoside analog with considerable IS properties that also has a synergizing effect with alkylators by inhibiting DNA repair. The combination of BU and FLU used in patients with AML was found to have more favorable toxicity profile with similar efficacy. Recently a well-designed two-arm study compared BU/CY to BU/FLU, demonstrating a significant reduction of TRM in the FLU/BU arm with no difference in RI (Rambaldi et al. 2015). Recently, other alkylators like TT (Eder et al. 2017) and CLO (Chevallier et al. 2012) have been incorporated into MAC protocols for both AML and ALL in an attempt to reduce risk of relapse with equivalent results to TBI-containing conditioning protocols.

13.4 Nonmyeloablative, Reduced Intensity and Reduced Toxicity Conditioning

NMA and RIC have been widely introduced over the past 20 years in an attempt to reduce organ toxicity and TRM allowing HSCT in elderly and medically infirm patients not eligible for standard MAC (Slavin et al. 1998). In addition, RTC based on FLU and MA alkylating agent doses were designed to allow safer administration of dose-intensive therapy. Multiple such protocols have been reported over the years with somewhat overlapping dose intensity and to a certain extent unclear categorization among NMA versus RIC and RTC.

A group of experts had an attempt to define and dissect the conditioning regimen intensity based on the expected duration and reversibility of cytopenia after HSCT (Bacigalupo et al. 2009). MAC was defined as a conditioning regimen that results in irreversible cytopenia in most patients, and stem cell support after HSCT is required. Truly NMA regimens cause minimal cytopenia and can theoretically be given without stem cell support. RIC regimens cause profound cytopenia and should be given with stem cells, but cytopenia may not be irreversible. The original NMA conditioning protocols were the TBI 2 Gy in combination with MMF and CSA (the so-called Seattle protocol that subsequently incorporated FLU 90 mg because of high non-engraftment in the original protocol) (McSweeney et al. 2001) and the FLAG conditioning protocol (FLU, Ara-C, idarubicin, and G-CSF) pioneered in MD Anderson (Giralt et al. 1997).

Additional very popular protocol is the FLU/BU conditioning regimen we pioneered in Jerusalem initially with oral but subsequently with the IV formulation of BU that is given 2–4 days determining the intensity of the conditioning being NMA, RIC/RTC, and MAC, respectively (Kharfan-Dabaja et al. 2014). Overall multiple studies indicated that the conditioning dose intensity is highly correlated with outcome after HSCT. Increased dose intensity is associated with reduced RI but also with higher NRM (Aoudjhane et al. 2005). For example, few studies compared the FLU/BU RIC to another frequently used RIC regimen, namely, the FLU/MEL protocol demonstrating lower RI but higher toxicity with the FLU/MEL protocol which is more intense (Shimoni et al. 2007). Subsequently TREO (L-threitol-1,4-bis-methanesulfonate, dihydroxybusulfan) with activity against both on committed and noncommitted stem cells as well as potent IS properties (Danylesko et al. 2012) was combined with FLU as an effective conditioning regimen pre-HSCT for both myeloid and lymphatic malignancies with a favorable toxicity

profile with little extramedullary toxicity (Nagler et al. 2017).

Overall outcome comparing these low-intensity conditioning protocols versus MAC was determined by the net effect of the opposing effects, i.e., reduction in TRM, while higher RI, leading to similar LFS and OS with patient age, comorbidities, and disease status at transplantation being significant prognostic factors. Retrospective comparative trials showed that while outcome may be similar with the various regimens in patients given HSCT in remission, NMA/RIC are inferior when HSCT is given in advanced disease, due to high RI. These observations were confirmed in some of the long-term studies but not in others (Shimoni et al. 2016). Interestingly, no disadvantage was observed for the low-intensity protocols in comparison to MAC even in high-risk disease like AML with monosomal karyotype or secondary leukemia (Poiré et al. 2015). RTC regimens are typically with more intensive antileukemic activity but limited toxicity and thus better tolerated by patients not eligible for myeloablative conditioning (Shimoni et al. 2018).

New novel conditioning protocols that may be categorized in this family of conditioning although no consensus was established are the regimens that incorporate CLO and TT and especially the TBF regimen (TT, BU, FLU) (Saraceni et al. 2017). Another worth mentioning conditioning that was developed for high-risk leukemia with encouraging results is the FLAMSA conditioning which comprised sequential chemotherapy including FLU, Ara-C, and amsacrine followed by RIC pre-allo-HSCT (Malard et al. 2017). Only few randomized studies compared head-to-head MAC to RIC or RTC regimens mostly confirming the above findings. A French well-designed two-arm study compared BU/FLU to TBI (low dose)/FLU demonstrating less RI with the BU/FLU regimen but higher TRM resulting in similar LFS and OS (Blaise et al. 2013). Similarly, a German randomized study compared RIC regimen of four doses of 2 Gy of TBI and 150 mg/m^2 FLU versus MAC of six doses of 2 Gy of TBI and 120 mg/kg CY demonstrating reduced toxicity in the RIC arm but similar RI, TRM, LFS, and OS between both study arms (Bornhäuser et al. 2012). These results were recently confirmed with longer follow-up.

Finally, a recent CTN phase III randomized trial compared MAC (BU/CY, FLU/BU, or CY/TBI) with RIC (FLU/BU or FLU/MEL) in patients with AML and MDS (Scott et al. 2017). RIC resulted in lower TRM but higher RI compared with MAC, with a statistically significant advantage in RFS and a trend to an advantage in OS with MAC. Another randomized study comparing RIC and MAC in patients with MDS demonstrated similar 2-year RFS and OS with no difference between the two conditioning regimens (Kröger et al. 2017). As for the issue of higher risk of RI post RIC, novel immunological and pharmacologic approaches are being currently explored (as will be discussed in Chap. 69). Treatment options include second HSCT or DLI with similar results (Kharfan-Dabaja et al. 2018).

13.5   Conditioning Regimens for Allo-HSCT from Alternative Donors: MMUD, CB, and Haploidentical

Historically, these types of allo-HSCT were the most challenging ones with relatively high incidence of non-engraftment and high TRM. Notably, recent development in the field of transplantation including novel conditioning regimens resulted in major improvement in the results of allo-HSCT from alternative donors with the haplo-HSCT being of the most interest (Lee et al. 2017). A key component of the conditioning regimen for MMUD and haplo-HSCT is ATG, recently reviewed for the ALWP of the EBMT (Baron et al. 2017). In previous well-designed randomized clinical trials in allo-HSCT from URD and in a single study also from MSD, ATG was demonstrated to reduce GVHD and TRM without jeopardizing the GVL effect, and

thus there is no increase in RI (Baron et al. 2017). In contrast and somewhat still puzzling in CBT, ATG is a negative factor associated with decreased OS and EFS rates and a high incidence of NRM (Pascal et al. 2015).

In an analysis performed by Eurocord, the MAC regimen for CBT included TBI 12 Gy—or BU—with or without FLU, TBI 12 Gy + CY, and more recently TBF (TT, BU, FLU) (Ruggeri et al. 2014). Comparing these regimens in single (s) (with >2.5 × 10^7 cells/kg) and double (d) CBT resulted in similar outcomes, NRM and RI incidence, which were not statistically different among the groups. LFS was 30% for sUCBT using TBI- or BU-based MAC compared with 48% for sUCBT TBF and 48% for dUCBT ($P = 0.02$ and $P = 0.03$, respectively), and it was not statistically different between sUCBT with TBF and dUCBT. They concluded that the choice of TBF conditioning regimen for sUCBT may improve results, and whether this regimen may be effective in dUCBT should be further analyzed (Ruggeri et al. 2014). In the haploidentical setting, the field moved from T-depleted to T-repleted haplo-HSCT and in recent years from ATG-based anti-GVHD prophylaxis to PT-CY pioneered by the Baltimore group (reviewed in Lee et al. 2017). Initial conditioning protocols in the Baltimore approach were RIC with BM grafts, but subsequently MAC regimens and PB grafts were introduced. In recent years, the TBF condoning is increasingly used for haplo-HSCT in Europe. Similarly, the PT-CY strategy for GVHD prophylaxis is being adopted to allo-HSCT from MUD, MMUD, and sibling donors (Ruggeri et al. 2018). In general comparing RIC to MAC for MMUD, CBT, and haplo-HSCT demonstrated in large similar transplantation global outcome for RIC versus MAC with some differences in the various alternative donors (Baron et al. 2016). For example, in the allo-HSCT from MMUD in patients >50 years, RIC resulted in reduced TRM and better LFS and OS in comparison to MAC, while in those <50 years, no difference was observed (Savani et al. 2016). In CBT, RIC resulted in a higher RI and a lower NRM, translating to comparable LFS, GVHD and relapse-free survival (GRFS), and OS (Baron et al. 2016). In the haplo-setting, no significant difference was observed (Rubio et al. 2016).

13.6   Preparative Conditioning for Autologous HSCT

Auto-HSCT are performed mainly for malignant lymphoma and MM. The most popular conditioning protocol for auto-HSCT in lymphoma is BEAM (BCNU, VP, Ara-C, and MEL) (Mills et al. 1995) or BEAC (with CY instead of MEL), while some centers substitute the BCNU with TT (the so-called TEAM or TECAM protocol), especially in patients with pulmonary problems in order to prevent the BCNU-mediated lung toxicity. Others tried to replace the BCNU by bendamustine (the so-called BeEAM protocol). Adding anti-CD20 radiolabeled MoAb like yttrium-90-ibritumomab tiuxetan (Zevalin) to the condition improved results in some studies, but a large randomized multicenter study with 131I-tositumomab (Bexxar) was negative (Vose et al. 2013).

As for auto-HSCT in MM, high-dose MEL has been shown to be superior to TBI/MEL. Recently some centers incorporated IV BU into the auto-HSCT in MM, while others included BOR. The numbers of auto-HSCT in acute leukemia went down in the last two decades in parallel to the increase in the numbers of allo-HSCT with RIC and from alternative donors (Gorin et al. 2015). The most popular preparative regimen for AML is BU/CY. Recently on behalf of the ALWP of the EBMT, we demonstrated that BU/MEL is a better preparative regimen as compared to BU/CY with lower RI, better LFS and OS, and no difference in TRM. Similar results were obtained in the subgroup of patients with high-risk AML. Patients with negative MRD before auto-HSCT did better (Gorin et al. 2017).

Key Points

- Conditioning regimens are integral and important part of HSCT enabling engraftment and provide an antitumor effect.
- The conditioning regimen pretransplantation should take into consideration patient and disease characteristics including age, comorbidities, disease status, and most probably measurable residual disease.
- Conditioning regimens may include irradiation, chemotherapy, serotherapy, monoclonal antibodies, and targeted therapy which varied in different malignancies and types of donors.
- The dose intensity of the pre-HSCT conditioning varied between MAC, RTC, RIC, and NMA in decreasing intensity order.
- The NMA and RIC significantly reduced transplant-related organ toxicity and mortality enabling transplant in elderly and medically infirm patients.
- The conditioning regimens for allo-HSCT from cord blood and haploidentical donors are somewhat specific.

References

Aoudjhane M, Labopin M, Gorin NC, et al. Comparative outcome of reduced intensity and myeloablative conditioning regimen in HLA identical sibling allogeneic haematopoietic stem cell transplantation for patients older than 50 years of age with acute myeloblastic leukaemia: a retrospective survey from the Acute Leukemia Working Party (ALWP) of the European Group for Blood and Marrow Transplantation (EBMT). Leukemia. 2005;19:2304–12.

Bacigalupo A, Ballen K, Rizzo D, et al. Defining the intensity of conditioning regimens: working definitions. Biol Blood Marrow Transplant. 2009;15:1628–33.

Baron F, Ruggeri A, Beohou E, et al. RIC versus MAC UCBT in adults with AML: a report from Eurocord, the ALWP and the CTIWP of the EBMT. Oncotarget. 2016;7:43027–38.

Baron F, Mohty M, Blaise D, et al. Anti-thymocyte globulin as graft-versus-host disease prevention in the setting of allogeneic peripheral blood stem cell transplantation: a review from the Acute Leukemia Working Party of the European Society for Blood and Marrow Transplantation. Haematologica. 2017;102:224–34.

Belkacemi Y, Labopin M, Giebel S, et al. Single dose daily fractionated is not Inferior to twice a day fractionated total body irradiation prior to allogeneic stem cell transplantation for acute leukemia: a useful practice simplification resulting from the Sarasin Study. Int J Radiat Oncol Biol Phys. 2018;102:515–26.

Blaise D, Tabrizi R, Boher JM, et al. Randomized study of 2 reduced-intensity conditioning strategies for human leukocyte antigen-matched, related allogeneic peripheral blood stem cell transplantation: prospective clinical and socioeconomic evaluation. Cancer. 2013;119:602–11.

Bornhäuser M, Kienast J, Trenschel R, et al. Reduced-intensity conditioning versus standard conditioning before allogeneic haemopoietic cell transplantation in patients with acute myeloid leukaemia in first complete remission: a prospective, open-label randomised phase 3 trial. Lancet Oncol. 2012;13:1035–44.

Cahu X, Labopin M, Giebel S, et al. Impact of conditioning with TBI in adult patients with T-cell ALL who receive a myeloablative allogeneic stem cell transplantation: a report from the acute leukemia working party of EBMT. Bone Marrow Transplant. 2016;51:351–7.

Chevallier P, Labopin M, Buchholz S, et al. Clofarabine-containing conditioning regimen for allo-SCT in AML/ALL patients: a survey from the Acute Leukemia Working Party of EBMT. Eur J Haematol. 2012;89:214–9.

Clift RA, Buckner CD, Appelbaum FR, et al. Allogeneic marrow transplantation in patients with acute myeloid leukemia in first remission: a randomized trial of two irradiation regimens. Blood. 1990;76:1867–71.

Czyz A, Labopin M, Giebel S, et al. Cyclophosphamide versus etoposide in combination with total body irradiation as conditioning regimen for adult patients with Ph-negative acute lymphoblastic leukemia undergoing allogeneic stem cell transplant: on behalf of the ALWP of the European Society for Blood and Marrow Transplantation. Am J Hematol. 2018;93:778–85.

Danylesko I, Shimoni A, Nagler A. Treosulfan-based conditioning before hematopoietic SCT: more than a BU look-alike. Bone Marrow Transplant. 2012;47:5–14.

Deeg HJ, Storer B, Slattery JT, et al. Conditioning with targeted busulfan and cyclophosphamide for hemo-poietic stem cell transplantation from related and unrelated donors in patients with myelodysplastic syndrome. Blood. 2002;100:1201–7.

Eder S, Canaani J, Beohou E, et al. Thiotepa-based conditioning versus total body irradiation as myeloablative conditioning prior to allogeneic stem cell transplantation for acute lymphoblastic leukemia: a matched-pair analysis from the Acute Leukemia Working Party of the European Society for Blood and Marrow Transplantation. Am J Hematol. 2017;92:997–1003.

Giebel S, Miszczyk L, Slosarek K, et al. Extreme heterogeneity of myeloablative total body irradiation techniques in clinical practice: a survey of the Acute Leukemia Working Party of the European Group for Blood and Marrow Transplantation. Cancer. 2014;120:2760–5.

Giralt S, Estey E, Albitar M, et al. Engraftment of allogeneic hematopoietic progenitor cells with purine analog-containing chemotherapy: harnessing graft-versus-leukemia without myeloablative therapy. Blood. 1997;89:4531–6.

Gorin NC, Giebel S, Labopin M, et al. Autologous stem cell transplantation for adult acute leukemia in 2015: time to rethink? Present status and future prospects. Bone Marrow Transplant. 2015;50:1495–502.

Gorin NC, Labopin M, Czerw T, et al. Autologous stem cell transplantation for adult acute myelocytic leukemia in first remission-Better outcomes after busulfan and melphalan compared with busulfan and cyclophosphamide: a retrospective study from the Acute Leukemia Working Party of the European Society for Blood and Marrow Transplantation (EBMT). Cancer. 2017;123:824–31.

Hassan M. The role of busulfan in bone marrow transplantation. Med Oncol. 1999;16:166–76.

Kharfan-Dabaja MA, Labopin M, Bazarbachi A, et al. Comparing i.v. BU dose intensity between two regimens (FB2 vs FB4) for allogeneic HCT for AML in CR1: a report from the Acute Leukemia Working Party of EBMT. Bone Marrow Transplant. 2014;49:1170–5.

Kharfan-Dabaja MA, Labopin M, Polge E, et al. Association of second allogeneic hematopoietic cell transplant vs donor lymphocyte infusion with overall survival in patients with acute myeloid leukemia relapse. JAMA Oncol. 2018. https://doi.org/10.1001/jamaoncol.2018.2091.

Kröger N, Iacobelli S, Franke GN, et al. Dose-reduced versus standard conditioning followed by allogeneic stem-cell transplantation for patients with myelodysplastic syndrome: a prospective randomized phase III study of the EBMT (RICMAC trial). J Clin Oncol. 2017;35:2157–64.

Lee CJ, Savani BN, Mohty M, et al. Haploidentical hematopoietic cell transplantation for adult acute myeloid leukemia: a position statement from the Acute Leukemia Working Party of the European Society for Blood and Marrow Transplantation. Haematologica. 2017;102:1810–22.

Malard F, Labopin M, Stuhler G, et al. Sequential intensified conditioning regimen allogeneic hematopoietic stem cell transplantation in adult patients with intermediate- or high-risk acute myeloid leukemia in complete remission: a study from the Acute Leukemia Working Party of the European Group for Blood and Marrow Transplantation. Biol Blood Marrow Transplant. 2017;23:278–84.

McSweeney PA, Niederwieser D, Shizuru JA, et al. Hematopoietic cell transplantation in older patients with hematologic malignancies: replacing high-dose cytotoxic therapy with graft-versus-tumor effects. Blood. 2001;97:3390–400.

Mills W, Chopra R, McMillan A, et al. BEAM chemotherapy and autologous bone marrow transplantation for patients with relapsed or refractory non-Hodgkin's lymphoma. J Clin Oncol. 1995;13:588–95.

Mohty M, Labopin M, Volin L, et al. Reduced-intensity versus conventional myeloablative conditioning allogeneic stem cell transplantation for patients with acute lymphoblastic leukemia: a retrospective study from the European Group for Blood and Marrow Transplantation. Blood. 2010;116:4439–43.

Nagler A, Rocha V, Labopin M, et al. Allogeneic hematopoietic stem-cell transplantation for acute myeloid leukemia in remission: comparison of intravenous busulfan plus cyclophosphamide (Cy) versus total-body irradiation plus Cy as conditioning regimen—a report from the acute leukemia working party of the European group for blood and marrow transplantation. J Clin Oncol. 2013;31:3549–56.

Nagler A, Labopin M, Berger R, et al. Allogeneic hematopoietic SCT for adults AML using i.v. BU in the conditioning regimen: outcomes and risk factors for the occurrence of hepatic sinusoidal obstructive syndrome. Bone Marrow Transplant. 2014;49:628–33.

Nagler A, Labopin M, Beelen D, et al. Long-term outcome after a treosulfan-based conditioning regimen for patients with acute myeloid leukemia: a report from the Acute Leukemia Working Party of the European Society for Blood and Marrow Transplantation. Cancer. 2017;123:2671–9.

Pascal L, Mohty M, Ruggeri A, et al. Impact of rabbit ATG-containing myeloablative conditioning regimens on the outcome of patients undergoing unrelated single-unit cord blood transplantation for hematological malignancies. Bone Marrow Transplant. 2015;50:45–50.

Poiré X, Labopin M, Cornelissen JJ, et al. Outcome of conditioning intensity in acute myeloid leukemia with monosomal karyotype in patients over 45 year-old: a study from the acute leukemia working party (ALWP) of the European Group of Blood and Marrow Transplantation (EBMT). Am J Hematol. 2015;90:719–24.

Rambaldi A, Grassi A, Masciulli A, et al. Busulfan plus cyclophosphamide versus busulfan plus fludarabine as a preparative regimen for allogeneic haemopoietic stem-cell transplantation in patients with acute myeloid leukaemia: an open-label, multicentre, randomised, phase 3 trial. Lancet Oncol. 2015;16:1525–36.

Rubio MT, Savani BN, Labopin M, et al. Impact of conditioning intensity in T-replete haplo-identical stem cell transplantation for acute leukemia: a report from the acute leukemia working party of the EBMT. J Hematol Oncol. 2016;9:25.

Ruggeri A, Sanz G, Bittencourt H, et al. Comparison of outcomes after single or double cord blood transplantation in adults with acute leukemia using different types of myeloablative conditioning regimen, a retrospective study on behalf of Eurocord and the Acute Leukemia Working Party of EBMT. Leukemia. 2014;28:779–86.

Ruggeri A, Labopin M, Bacigalupo A, et al. Post-transplant cyclophosphamide for graft-versus-host disease prophylaxis in HLA matched sibling or matched unrelated donor transplant for patients with acute leukemia, on behalf of ALWP-EBMT. J Hematol Oncol. 2018;11:40.

Saraceni F, Labopin M, Hamladji RM, et al. Thiotepa-busulfan-fludarabine compared to busulfan-fludarabine for sibling and unrelated donor transplant in acute myeloid leukemia in first remission. Oncotarget. 2017;9:3379–93.

Savani BN, Labopin M, Kröger N, et al. Expanding transplant options to patients over 50 years. Improved outcome after reduced intensity conditioning mismatched-unrelated donor transplantation for patients with acute myeloid leukemia: a report from the Acute Leukemia Working Party of the EBMT. Haematologica. 2016;101:773–80.

Scott BL, Pasquini MC, Logan BR, et al. Myeloablative versus reduced-intensity hematopoietic cell transplantation for acute myeloid leukemia and myelodysplastic syndromes. J Clin Oncol. 2017;35:1154–61.

Shimoni A, Hardan I, Shem-Tov N, et al. Comparison between two fludarabine-based reduced-intensity conditioning regimens before allogeneic hematopoietic stem-cell transplantation: fludarabine/melphalan is associated with higher incidence of acute graft-versus-host disease and non-relapse mortality and lower incidence of relapse than fludarabine/busulfan. Leukemia. 2007;21:2109–16.

Shimoni A, Labopin M, Savani B, et al. Long-term survival and late events after allogeneic stem cell transplantation from HLA-matched siblings for acute myeloid leukemia with myeloablative compared to reduced-intensity conditioning: a report on behalf of the acute leukemia working party of European group for blood and marrow transplantation. J Hematol Oncol. 2016;9:118.

Shimoni A, Labopin M, Savani B, et al. Intravenous busulfan compared with treosulfan-based conditioning for allogeneic stem cell transplantation in acute myeloid leukemia: a study on behalf of the Acute Leukemia Working Party of European Society for Blood and Marrow Transplantation. Biol Blood Marrow Transplant. 2018;24:751–7.

Slavin S, Nagler A, Naparstek E, et al. Nonmyeloablative stem cell transplantation and cell therapy as an alternative to conventional bone marrow transplantation with lethal cytoreduction for the treatment of malignant and nonmalignant hematologic diseases. Blood. 1998;91:756–63.

Thomas ED, Clift RA, Hersman J, et al. Marrow transplantation for acute nonlymphoblastic leukemic in first remission using fractionated or single-dose irradiation. Int J Radiat Oncol Biol Phys. 1982;8:817–21.

Tutschka PJ, Copelan EA, Klein JP. Bone marrow transplantation for leukemia following a new busulfan and cyclophosphamide regimen. Blood. 1987;70:1382–8.

Vey N, De Prijck B, Faucher C, et al. A pilot study of busulfan and melphalan as preparatory regimen prior to allogeneic bone marrow transplantation in refractory or relapsed hematological malignancies. Bone Marrow Transplant. 1996;18:495–9.

Vose JM, Carter S, Burns LJ, et al. Phase III randomized study of rituximab/carmustine, etoposide, cytarabine, and melphalan (BEAM) compared with iodine-131 tositumomab/BEAM with autologous hematopoietic cell transplantation for relapsed diffuse large B-cell lymphoma: results from the BMT CTN 0401 trial. J Clin Oncol. 2013;31:1662–8.

Bone Marrow Harvesting for HSCT

Norbert Claude Gorin

14.1 Introduction

Historically, the bone marrow (BM) has been the first source of stem cells considered since the early 1960s for HSCT (Santos 1990; Thomas et al. 1979; Mathe 1964; Gorin et al. 1990). Parallel attempts at using fetal liver cells at that time have remained unsuccessful. In 1986 the first success of an unrelated cord blood (UCB) transplantation in a child promoted UCB (Gluckman et al. 1997) as an alternative source in certain settings.

Since 1994 and the initial demonstration that PBSC mobilized by cytokines (G-CSF first and more recently when needed plerixafor) could be used as well as BM, the proportion of PB transplants has considerably increased to reach about 70–95% of all stem cell transplants (Passweg et al. 2012, 2016), so that nowadays BM transplantation accounts for a minority of transplants.

There remain however several situations where and when a marrow harvest can still be of interest or even is highly recommended.

This chapter indicates the principal indications of BM transplantation, compares schematically the advantages of BM versus PB, and details the technique of BM harvesting.

14.2 Indications for Considering and Possibly Selecting BM as a Preferred Source of HSC

It is not the purpose of this chapter to review the benefit/risk ratio of BM versus peripheral mobilized blood as sources of HSC. Several studies, including prospective randomized studies, have shown in general with BM when compared to PB slower engraftment but lower incidence and lower severity of acute and chronic GVHD with in the end similar disease free and overall survivals (Schmitz et al. 2005). However, some retrospective studies for both auto- and allo-HSCT have shown better survival with rich BM collections (Gorin et al. 2003) or BM versus PB (Gorin et al. 2009, 2010). Also, the quality of life has not been carefully analyzed (Sun et al. 2010), and further studies may be in favor of BM (Ruggeri et al. 2018; Lee et al. 2016).

Time and cost constraints have however in general favored leukaphereses and PB transplants which represent about 95% of all auto-HSCT and 70% of allo-HSCT (Passweg et al. 2016). Table 14.1 lists the situations when nowadays marrow may appear as a better choice.

For allo-HSCT, BM is preferred/mandatory whenever the wish to reduce toxicity, NRM, and most of all GVHD (particularly extensive chronic)

N. C. Gorin MD, PhD (✉)
Department of Hematology and Cell Therapy, EBMT Paris Office, Hôpital Saint Antoine APHP, Paris, France

Paris Sorbonne University, Paris, France
e-mail: norbert-claude.gorin@aphp.fr

Table 14.1 Preferences for BM as source of stem cells in ALLO-HSCT

Allo-HSCT	Rationale	Justification 1	Justification 2	Reference
Children donors and/or recipients	Administration of GCSF to and leukapheresis of the donor more difficult to set	More cGVHD and NRM after PB compared with BM	In some countries, the use of GCSF (and plerixafor) is not allowed in children	Simonin et al. (2017)
Aplastic anemia	BM mandatory, associated with better results	Higher risk of GVHD with PB	Included in EBMT and CIBMTR guidelines	Bhella et al. (2018), Schrezenmeier et al. (2007), Bacigalupo et al. (2012), Eapen et al. (2011), and Barone et al. (2015)
MAC with a MUD and no ATG	BM associated with better results and less cGVH	Randomized trial with no ATG showing less cGVH and better QOL with BM	If a suitable BM donor is available. Otherwise PB with ATG	Anasetti et al. (2012), Lee et al. (2016), Eapen et al. (2007), and Walker et al. (2016)
Haploidentical transplantation	BM or combination of PB and BM favored by some teams	Team choice or clinical trial	High-dose CY for GVH prevention	Kasamon et al. (2017) and Luznik et al. (2010)

is considered as priority, such as for children with aplastic anemia and for some teams for haploidentical transplantation (see Table 14.1). The outcome considered to favor this choice is the GRFS (GVHD and relapse-free survival) as defined by EBMT (Ruggeri et al. 2016).

Conversely, PB can be a first choice in patients with hematological malignancies at high or very high risk of progression/relapse, such as AML FLT3ITD positive, lymphomas in progression after relapse from auto-HSCT, etc. for whom the risk of relapse is considered as first priority despite the risk of increasing NRM. Usually, this choice is made in parallel to the decision whether the conditioning regimen should be MAC or RIC (Gilleece et al. 2018).

For autologous HSCT (Table 14.2) the two major reasons for using BM are autologous transplantation for AML in remission and attempts at increasing the stem cell dose infused following poor marrow collections.

14.3 Mobilized or Primed Marrow

Following the discovery of cytokines, G-CSF in particular, the use of BM collected after 2–4 days of GCSF administration has been investigated in the year 2000–2005. G-CSF-primed marrow harvesting results in a graft with more mononuclear

cells collected and higher CD34(+) stem and progenitor cell doses s (Grupp et al. 2006). The clinical significance of different HSC sources (primed marrow, mobilized blood, and steady-state marrow) in auto- and allo-HSCT was reviewed in 2004 (Elfenbein and Sackstein 2004). Mobilized marrow speeds up engraftment for both auto- and allo-HSCT, with a possible (unproven) reduction of GVHD rate and severity. Its use nowadays is rare, but it is for some teams the preferred stem cell source or part of a combination of primed marrow + PB as stem cell source for haploidentical donor transplantation (Huang et al. 2009; Ly et al. 2015).

14.4 Technique of BM Collection and Impact of the Dose of Nucleated Cells Infused

Marrow is collected from the posterior superior iliac crests, usually under general anesthesia, although few teams have used sedation or locoregional anesthesia (Fig. 14.1).

Marrow is aspirated with bone needles with multiple holes all around, which makes collection easier and the procedure more rapid. However, to avoid large dilution with blood, it is recommended to limit each aspiration to a volume of less than 5 mL, before transferring the

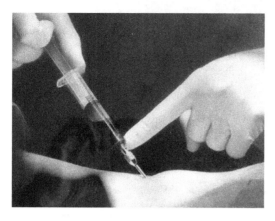

Fig. 14.1 Bone marrow harvest

aspirate through a three-way tap to the collection bag. The collection bag contains ACD anticoagulant solution and the syringes are rinsed with heparin (5.000 U/mL).

The goal is nowadays to obtain typically at least 3×10^8 nucleated cells/kg, although 2×10^8 nucleated cells/kg has long been in the past the usual target and remains acceptable. However, it should be kept in mind that old studies in the early development of BMT have indicated better results both in terms of engraftment but also decrease in NRM and RI and better outcome, with higher marrow doses (Gorin et al. 1999, 2003; Sierra et al. 1997):

- For Allo-HSCT with identical siblings, an early EBMT retrospective study evaluated the impact of the marrow cell dose infused: The median BM cell dose was 2.7×10^8/kg ($0.17–29 \times 10^8$/kg). In multivariate analyses, high-dose BM compared to PB was associated with lower NRM, better LFS, and better OS (RR = 0.64; 95% CI, 0.44–0.92; $P = 0.016$). Results in patients with AML receiving allografts in CR1 indicated a better outcome with BM as compared to PB, when the dose of BM infused was above the median value.
- For Allo-HSCT fully with matched unrelated donors (Sierra et al. 1997), transplantation of a marrow cell dose above the median value of 3.65×10^8/kg was associated with faster neutrophil and platelet engraftment and decreased

incidence of severe acute GVHD. Transplant in remission of acute leukemia with a high dose of marrow cells was associated with the best outcome in both children and adults.

If the targeted goal cannot be achieved, additional collection can be made from the anterior iliac crests, although it is time consuming and potentially more harmful for the patient or the donor, who must be turned over with all sterile fields to be reinstalled.

All things considered the maximum accepted volume collected should not go over 20 mL/kg donor body weight. Depending on the volume collected, three attitudes regarding transfusion during marrow collection may be followed: no transfusion and liquid replacement is the first option for many teams. Autotransfusion (to prepare beforehand in the 3 weeks preceding marrow collection, which adds some constraint) is the other recommended transfusional option. In rare circumstances allo-transfusion remains possible; usually two packs of concentrated red cells are enough.

Another option to consider to increase the stem cell dose to infuse when marrow collection has been insufficiently productive is the addition of PBSC. This however can be a complex decision which should take into account the disease and disease status, whether it concerns an autograft or an allograft or in this last situation whether a possible increase in the incidence and severity of GVHD associated with GVL/tumor is potentially beneficial or harmful. Two examples of this dilemma are summarized below:

1. In the context of auto-HSCT for leukemias or lymphomas, when analyzing patients receiving combinations of BM and PBSC (either because PBSC were collected to supplement poor BM or the reverse), outcomes are poor. One likely explanation is the existence of a bias since in most of these patients, poor collections (either BM or PBSC or both) are surrogate markers of multiple previous lines of chemotherapy for resistant/progressing diseases.
2. In contrast, for some teams, the combination of BM and PBSC has become the standard stem cell source for HSCT (see Table 14.1).

Table 14.2 Preferences for BM as source of stem cells in AUTO-HSCT

Auto-HSCT	Rationale	Justification	Comments
Poor PB collection	Increase the dose of HSC in the autograft	Ensure safer engraftment	However, poor mobilizers are likely to also produce poor marrow collection*
AML	Outcome better when compared to PB		Several EBMT retrospective studies

*Although there are biases, data from the EBMT registry indicate that poor mobilizers (often previously heavily treated with chemotherapy) have a poor outcome Shouval et al. (2018)

14.5 Complications of Bone Marrow Collections

One cannot ignore that on theoretical grounds two major hazards of marrow collection although very rare are death secondary to general anesthesia (<1/200,000) and major organ damage by mechanical mismanipulation of the bone needles that may sideslip if sufficient expertise and caution are not present.

The NMDP analyzed in 1993, 493 volunteers who donated unrelated marrow from October 1991 in 42 centers (Stroncek et al. 1993). The median volume of marrow collected was 1050 mL (range 180–2983 mL). Autologous red blood cells were transfused to 90% of donors, but only three donors received allogeneic blood. Apnea during anesthesia occurred in one donor. Other acute complications related to the collection procedure occurred in 6% of donors. Following marrow collection 75% experienced tiredness, 68% experienced pain at the marrow collection site, and 52% of the donors experienced low back pain. Mean recovery time was 16 days, but 42 donors felt that it took them at least 30 days to recover fully. The duration of the marrow collection procedure and duration of anesthesia both positively correlated with donor pain and/or fatigue following the collection. The recommendation of this study was the duration of the collection procedure and probably the duration of anesthesia, and therefore the volume of marrow collected should be kept to a minimum, but this conclusion is to be weighed against the wish to collect stem cell doses as high as possible to ensure fast engraftment and improve outcome.

14.6 Bone Marrow Cryopreservation

In the context of auto-HSCT, BM and PBSC are almost always cryopreserved and stored either in liquid nitrogen (-196 °C) or the gas phase of liquid nitrogen (-140 °C). The technique of freezing at -1 °C/min with dimethyl sulfoxide (DMSO) and the technique of rapid thawing are well established (Gorin 1986). Harmless long duration of storage has been reported up to 11 years (Aird et al. 1992). Recently some attempts at avoiding cryopreservation to replace it by storage at 4 °C in the refrigerator have produced interesting results, but using refrigerator storage is not presently validated and cannot be recommended by EBMT (Sarmiento et al. 2018).

Cryopreservation and storage of a marrow in view of an allo-HSCT is possible. However, it should be kept in mind that any cryopreservation procedure, would it seem perfect, results in some measurable (CFU-GM, BFU-E) and many less measurable (immune functions, etc.) damages. Therefore, it should be reserved to special situations when, for instance, the donor cannot be available at the very time of the transplantation procedure. As a rule, fresh marrow is preferable to frozen marrow.

14.7 Quality Control for BM Harvesting and Cryopreservation

The major indicator for successful BM collection is the dose collected, as discussed above, i.e., the number of nucleated cells expressed per kg of body weight for the recipient. It is very usual to have a blood count done at the mid time of the collection to ensure proper richness. With a goal of a minimum of 3×10^8 nucleated cells/kg, any richness above this value can be seen as a bonus. Harvest below this level, around 2×10^8 or even lower, however has been associated with correct engraftment.

CD34+ evaluation is not routinely performed for BM, while it is the rule for PB.

For cryopreserved marrow, some teams routinely cryopreserve small samples in minibags or ampoules, enabling viability testing before thawing the graft (usually an autograft). However, and importantly, a technical bias has been observed with ampoules since differences in cooling rates prevent ampoules from being a reliable index of HSC cryopreservation in large volumes (Douay et al. 1986a).

More pertinent testing consists in the evaluation of CFU-GM which represents in this setting the most reliable functional viability indicator (Douay et al. 1986b). Although there is no guideline, experience has shown that the results in CFUGM/kg are about 1–1.5 log below the expected or calculated results in CD34+ cells /kg (therefore expressed in 10^5/kg). CFU-GM evaluation is not a consensual prerequisite since it is an additional time-consuming effort, but it may bring important information in some cases, for instance, when dealing with marrow collections below 2×10^8/kg.

14.8   Conclusions

PB collections and transplantation nowadays represent 70–90% of all stem cell sources for transplants.

However, BM transplantation has not disappeared and is likely to persist in some limited situations and indications.

Further studies may revisit and increase the choice of marrow as stem cell source.

The Five Key Points of Marrow Collection

- Harvest with small (2–5 mL) aspirate volumes to avoid dilution with blood.
- The goal should be at least 3×10^8 nucleated cells per kg, but the more the better. The maximum volume collected should not go over 20 mL/kg donor body weight. Decision for no transfusion with liquid replacement (recommended) or autotransfusion (second best option) or in rare cases Allotransfusion during collection relies on the judgment of the local medical team.
- Cryopreservation is the rule for autoBMT, while it should be avoided and used only in rare specific conditions for allogeneic transplantation.
- BM is mandatory in children and patients with aplastic anemias. It is presently favored by some teams in the context of haploidentical transplantation.
- BM when compared with PBSC results in less NRM, less GVHD (in particular less chronic extensive GVHD), but less GVL/lymphoma/tumor effect.

References

Aird W, Labopin M, Gorin NC, Antin JH. Long-term cryopreservation of human stem cells. Bone Marrow Transplant. 1992;9:487–90.

Anasetti C, Logan BR, Lee SJ, et al. Peripheral-blood stem cells versus bone marrow from unrelated donors. N Engl J Med. 2012;367:1487–96.

Bacigalupo A, Socie G, Schrezenmeier H, et al. Bone marrow versus peripheral blood as the stem cell source for sibling transplants in acquired aplastic anemia: survival advantage for bone marrow in all age groups. Haematologica. 2012;97:1142–8.

Barone A, Lucarelli A, Onofrillo D, et al. Diagnosis and management of acquired aplastic anemia in childhood. Guidelines from the marrow failure study group of the pediatric haemato-oncology Italian association (AIEOP). Blood Cells Mol Dis. 2015;55:40–7.

Bhella S, Navneet S, Majhail NS, Betcher J, et al. Choosing wisely BMT: American society for blood and marrow transplantation and Canadian blood and marrow transplant group's list of 5 tests and treatments to question in blood and marrow transplantation. Biol Blood Marrow Transplant. 2018;24:909–13.

Douay L, Lopez M, Gorin NC. A technical bias: differences in cooling rates prevent ampoules from being a reliable index of stem cell cryopreservation in large volumes. Cryobiology. 1986a;23:296–301.

Douay L, Gorin NC, Mary JY, et al. Recovery of CFUGM from cryopreserved marrow and in vivo evaluation after autologous bone marrow transplantation are predictive of engraftment. Exp Hematol. 1986b;14:358–65.

Eapen M, Logan BR, Confer DL, et al. Peripheral blood grafts from unrelated donors are associated with increased acute and chronic graft-versus-host disease without improved survival. Biol Blood Marrow Transplant. 2007;13:1461–8.

Eapen M, Le Rademacher J, Antin JH, et al. Effect of stem cell source on outcomes after unrelated donor transplantation in severe aplastic anemia. Blood. 2011;118:2618–21.

Elfenbein GJ, Sackstein R. Primed marrow for autologous and allogeneic transplantation: a review comparing primed marrow to mobilized blood and steady-state marrow. Exp Hematol. 2004;32:327–39.

Gilleece M, Labopin M, Yakoub-Agha I, et al. Measurable residual disease, conditioning regimen intensity and age predict outcome of allogeneic hematopoietic cell transplantation for acute myeloid leukaemia in first remission: a registry analysis of 2292 patients by the acute leukemia working party European society of blood and marrow transplantation. Am J Hematol. 2018;93:1142–52.

Gluckman E, Rocha V, Boyer-Chammard A, et al. Outcome of cord-blood transplantation from related and unrelated donors. Eurocord transplant group and the European blood and marrow transplantation group. N Engl J Med. 1997;337:373–81.

Gorin NC. Collection, manipulation and freezing of haemopoietic stem cells. Clin Haematol. 1986;15:19–48.

Gorin NC, Aegerter P, Auvert B, et al. Autologous bone marrow transplantation for acute myelocytic leukemia in first remission: a European survey of the role of marrow purging. Blood. 1990;75:1606–14.

Gorin NC, Labopin M, Laporte JP, et al. Importance of marrow dose on posttransplant outcome in acute leukemia: models derived from patients autografted with mafosfamide-purged marrow at a single institution. Exp Hematol. 1999;27:1822–30.

Gorin NC, Labopin M, Rocha V, et al. Marrow versus peripheral blood for geno-identical allogeneic stem cell transplantation in acute myelocytic leukemia: influence of dose and stem cell source shows better outcome with rich marrow. Blood. 2003;102:3043–51.

Gorin NC, Labopin M, Blaise D, et al. Higher incidence of relapse with peripheral blood rather than marrow as a source of stem cells in adults with acute myelocytic leukemia autografted during the first remission. J Clin Oncol. 2009;27:3987–93.

Gorin NC, Labopin M, Reiffers J, et al. Higher incidence of relapse in patients with acute myelocytic leukemia infused with higher doses of CD34+ cells from leukapheresis products autografted during the first remission. Blood. 2010;116:3157–62.

Grupp SA, Frangoul H, Wall D, et al. Use of G-CSF in matched sibling donor pediatric allogeneic transplantation: a consensus statement from the Children's Oncology Group (COG) Transplant Discipline Committee and Pediatric Blood and Marrow Transplant Consortium (PBMTC) Executive Committee. Ped Blood Cancer. 2006;46:414–21.

Huang XJ, Liu DH, Liu KY, et al. Treatment of acute leukemia with unmanipulated HLA-mismatched/haploidentical blood and bone marrow transplantation. Biol Blood Marrow Transplant. 2009;15:257–65.

Kasamon YL, Ambinder RF, Fuchs EJ, et al. Prospective study of nonmyeloablative, HLA-mismatched unrelated BMT with high-dose posttransplantation cyclophosphamide. Blood Adv. 2017;1:288–92.

Lee SJ, Logan B, Westervelt P, et al. Comparison of patient-reported outcomes in 5-year survivors who received bone marrow vs peripheral blood unrelated donor transplantation: long-term follow-up of a randomized clinical trial. JAMA Oncol. 2016;2:1583–9.

Luznik L, Bolanos-Meade J, Zahurak M, et al. High-dose cyclophosphamide as single-agent, short-course prophylaxis of graft-versus-host disease. Blood. 2010;115:3224–30.

Ly M, Zhao XS, Hu Y, et al. Monocytic and promyelocytic myeloid-derived suppressor cells may contribute to G-CSF-induced immune tolerance in haplo-identical allogeneic hematopoietic stem cell transplantation. Am J Hematol. 2015;90:E9–E16.

Mathe G. Treatment of leukemia with allogenic bone marrow transplantation. Brux Med. 1964;44:559–62.

Passweg JR, Baldomero H, Gratwohl A, Bregni M, Cesaro S, Dreger P, et al. The EBMT activity survey: 1990–2010. Bone Marrow Transplant. 2012;47:906–23.

Passweg JR, Baldomero H, Bader P, et al. Hematopoietic stem cell transplantation in Europe 2014: more than 40 000 transplants annually. Bone Marrow Transplant. 2016;51:786–92.

Ruggeri A, Labopin M, Ciceri F, et al. Definition of GvHD-free, relapse-free survival for registry-based studies: an ALWP-EBMT analysis on patients with AML in remission. Bone Marrow Transplant. 2016;51:610–1.

Ruggeri A, Labopin M, Bacigalupo A, et al. Bone marrow versus mobilized peripheral blood stem cells in haploidentical transplants using posttransplantation cyclophosphamide. Cancer. 2018;124:1428–37.

Santos GW. Bone marrow transplantation in hematologic malignancies. Current status. Cancer. 1990;65(3 Suppl):786–91.

Sarmiento M, Ramirez P, Parody R, et al. Advantages of non-cryopreserved autologous hematopoietic stem cell transplantation against a cryopreserved strategy. Bone Marrow Transplant. 2018;53:960–6. https://doi.org/10.1038/s41409-018-0117-5.

Schmitz N, Beksac M, Bacigalupo A, et al. Filgrastim-mobilized peripheral blood progenitor cells versus bone marrow transplantation for treating leukemia: 3-year results from the EBMT randomized trial. Haematologica. 2005;90:643–8.

Schrezenmeier H, Passweg JR, Marsh JC, et al. Worse outcome and more chronic GVHD with peripheral blood progenitor cells than bone marrow in HLA-matched sibling donor transplants for young patients with severe acquired aplastic anemia. Blood. 2007;110:1397–400.

Shouval R, Labopin M, Bomze D, et al. Prediction of leukemia free survival following autologous stem cell transplantation in AML. A risk score developed by the ALWP of the EBMT. EHA 23rd annual meeting, Stockholm, 2018. Abstract.

Sierra J, Storer B, Hansen JA, et al. Transplantation of marrow cells from unrelated donors for treatment of high-risk acute leukemia: the effect of leukemic burden, donor HLA matching and marrow cell dose. Blood. 1997;89:4226–35.

Simonin M, Dalissier A, Labopin M, et al. More chronic GvHD and non-relapse mortality after peripheral blood stem cell compared with bone marrow in hematopoietic transplantation for paediatric acute lymphoblastic leukemia: a retrospective study on behalf of the EBMT Paediatric Diseases Working Party. Bone Marrow Transplant. 2017;52:1071–3.

Stroncek DF, Holland PV, Bartch G, et al. Experiences of the first 493 unrelated marrow donors in the National Marrow Donor Program. Blood. 1993;81:1940–6.

Sun CLFL, Kawashima T, Leisenring W, et al. Prevalence and predictors of chronic health conditions after hematopoietic cell transplantation: a report from the bone marrow transplant survivor study. Blood. 2010;116:3129–39.

Thomas ED, Buckner CD, Clift RA, et al. Marrow transplantation for acute non lymphoblastic leukemia in first remission. N Engl J Med. 1979;301:597–9.

Walker I, Panzarella T, Couban S, et al. Pretreatment with anti-thymocyte globulin versus no anti-thymocyte globulin in patients with haematological malignancies undergoing haemopoietic cell transplantation from unrelated donors: a randomised, controlled, open-label, phase 3, multicentre trial. Lancet Oncol. 2016;17:164–73.

Mobilization and Collection of HSC

Kai Hübel

15.1 Introduction

The intravenous infusion of patient's own HSC to restore BM damage is the basic principle of high-dose chemotherapy, since otherwise the patient would expect long-lasting aplasia with life-threatening infections. Therefore, a sufficient collection of HSC before application of high-dose therapy is mandatory. Since HSC expresses CD34 on their surface, the number of CD34+ cells in the transplant material is considered as an indicator of the HSC content.

In principle, there are two ways how to collect stem cell: by repeated aspiration of BM from the pelvic crest or by leukapheresis after mobilization of HSC into the PB. The latter one is favored and considered as standard because it is less stressful for the patient and leads to faster engraftment and hematologic reconstitution which may improve patient outcomes (Gertz 2010).

Usually, HSC circulates in a very small number in the PB. Therefore, mobilization of HSC from the BM to the PB is an essential part of auto-HSCT programs. Following sufficient mobilization, patient will need leukapheresis which is often performed by central lines to facilitate the procedure. Finally, HSC will be cryopreserved using dimethyl sulfoxide (DMSO) until transfusion.

15.2 Strategies of Mobilization

There are two different strategies to mobilize HSC from the BM to the PB: the so-called "steady-state" mobilization and the mobilization by chemotherapy.

15.2.1 Mobilization Without Chemotherapy ("Steady State")

Using this approach, HSC will be mobilized by the use of cytokines only. The only recommended cytokine for mobilization is G-CSF, since GM-CSF is no longer available in many countries after commercial failure and withdrawal. G-CSF induces myeloid hyperplasia and the release of CD34+ cells into the circulation through proteolytic cleavage of adhesion molecules (Lapidot and Petit 2002). Currently, the G-CSF cytokines filgrastim and lenograstim have market approval for mobilization of HSC in Europe.

The recommended doses are filgrastim 10 μg/kg/day SC for 5–7 consecutive days and lenograstim 10 μg/kg/day SC for 4–6 consecutive days. The use of biosimilar G-CSF has equivalent efficacy (Schmitt et al. 2016).

K. Hübel (✉)
University of Cologne, Department of Internal Medicine, Cologne, Germany
e-mail: kai.huebel@uni-koeln.de

Leukapheresis usually is performed on day 5 independent whether filgrastim or lenograstim was used for mobilization. The measurement of CD34+ cells in the PB before leukapheresis is not mandatory but could help to estimate the expected collection yield and the duration of leukapheresis. If the number of cells collected is inadequate, mobilization with G-CSF may be continued for 1–2 days. However, if the collection goal is not reached after the third leukapheresis, a successful mobilization is unlikely.

The major advantages of steady-state mobilization are the relatively low toxicity, the predictable time of leukapheresis, the outpatient administration, and the reduced costs compared to chemo-mobilization. The major disadvantages are variable mobilization failure rates and the lower CD34+ cell yields compared to chemo-mobilization. Mobilization with G-CSF only may be used in patients without further need of chemotherapy, e.g., in patients with a stable remission of the underlying disease.

15.2.2 Mobilization with Chemotherapy

The use of chemotherapy in combination with G-CSF is the preferred way of mobilization for all patients who will need further decrease of tumor burden and/or who have to collect a high number of HSC.

CY in a dose of 2–4 g/m^2 is widely used for HSC mobilization. It is also possible to mobilize HSC not by a separate chemotherapy but as part of the disease-specific chemotherapy, e.g., to mobilize HSC following salvage treatment with R-DHAP or R-ICE in lymphoma patients. The choice of a specific chemo-mobilization approach is based on patient's disease characteristics and local clinical practice guidelines.

Approved doses of G-CSF for HSC mobilization after myelosuppressive therapy are filgrastim 5 µg/kg/day SC and lenograstim 150 µg/m^2/day

SC. There are reports of the use of higher doses of G-CSF (Romeo et al. 2010), but there are no randomized trials and additional side effects are possible. Mobilization with G-CSF should start after completion of chemotherapy at the earliest and at the leukocyte nadir at the latest and should continue until the last leukapheresis. Most protocols recommend the initiation of G-CSF within 1–5 days after the end of chemotherapy.

The major advantage of adding chemotherapy to cytokines, besides the effect on the tumor, is the expected improvement of the collection yield with fewer apheresis sessions (Sung et al. 2013). The major disadvantages of chemo-mobilization are the therapy-related toxicity, the requirement of in-hospital treatment in most cases, the bone marrow damage by the chemotherapy which may impair future mobilizations, and higher mobilization costs. Furthermore, an exact prognosis of the CD34+ cell peak in the PB and the optimal start of leukapheresis are difficult and require daily monitoring of CD34+ cells in the PB. Table 15.1 summarizes a recommendation of timing of G-CSF following most used chemotherapy regimens and start of monitoring of CD34+ cells in the PB.

In several clinical trials, it was documented that relapse rate after auto-HSCT following mobilization with and without chemotherapy is comparable (Tuchman et al. 2015).

Table 15.1 Recommended start of G-CSF and start of CD34+ monitoring for most used mobilization chemotherapy regimens

Chemotherapy	Start G-CSF	Start CD34+ monitoring
CY 2 g/m^2	Day 5	Day 10
CAD	Day 9	Day 13
(R)CHOP/CHOEP	Day 6	Day 11
(R)DHAP	Day 9	Day 14
(R)ICE	Day 6	Day 12
(R)AraC/TT	Day 5	Day 10

Day 1: first day of chemotherapy application (without rituximab). Adapted from (Kriegsmann et al. 2018)

15.3 CD34+ Cell Count and Timing of Leukapheresis

Up to date, CD34+ cell count in mobilized peripheral blood product is the most important parameter of graft quality, as it is the only recognized predictor of stable hematopoietic engraftment after auto-HSCT (Saraceni et al. 2015). Monitoring of CD34+ cells in the PB is optional in steady-state mobilization but an essential part of chemo-mobilization. Following chemotherapy, the daily measurement of leukocytes and thrombocytes is recommended. If not otherwise specified by the protocol, CD34 monitoring should be initiated at the latest if leukocytes increase up to 1000/µL during recovering from aplasia. This increase of leukocytes is mostly accompanied with an increase of thrombocytes. A prompt start of leukapheresis is required of CD34+ cell count of $\geq 20/\mu L$ (Mohty et al. 2014); for more details, please see Sect. 15.6.

15.4 Target HSC Collection Count

The target quantity of HSC to be collected is dependent on the underlying disease. Most patients with NHL or HL (expect for rare case of patients with HL who require double auto-HSCT) will need one autograft. The generally accepted minimum CD34+ cell yield to proceed to transplantation is 2×10^6 cells/kg (Mohty et al. 2014); however, higher yields of $4–5 \times 10^6$ CD34+ cells/kg are aimed for at many centers since they have been associated with faster neutrophil and platelet recovery, reduced hospitalization, blood transfusions, and antibiotic therapy (Stiff et al. 2011; Giralt et al. 2014). Patients mobilizing $>8–10 \times 10^6$ cells/kg are called "super mobilizer"; however, the reported positive effect after infusion of such a high number of HSC on the outcome and prognosis of the patient is highly speculative. For patients with a chance of two or even more transplantations (mainly patients with MM), it is essential to collect the required number of HSC before the first high-dose therapy since mobilization after high-dose therapy has an increased risk of failure. For tandem transplantation, the required cell dose for one transplantation is also at least 2×10^6 CD34+ cells/kg.

15.5 Leukapheresis

Collection of peripheral HSC for auto-HSCT is a well-established process. The duration of one leukapheresis session should not exceed 5 h, and the total number of leukapheresis session should not exceed four procedures since more sessions are useless in most cases and will stress the patient. CD34+ cell collection has been shown to be more effective with larger apheresis volume (4.0–5.3 times the patient's total blood volume), and no difference in CD34+ cell viability was observed compared with normal-volume apheresis (2.7–3.5 times the patient's total blood volume) (Abrahamsen et al. 2005). Enhanced volumes are especially recommended for patients with a high risk of mobilization failure or for patients with a high individual CD34+ cell collection goal. However, not all patients are eligible for enhanced volume strategies. Larger transfusion volumes and related higher DMSO contents have been associated with increased risk of cardiac side effects (Donmez et al. 2007).

15.6 Poor Mobilizer

Despite widespread and established practice, current mobilization strategies vary between centers and differ in terms of feasibility and outcome. Although the majority of patients are able to mobilize sufficient CD34+ cells for at least a single auto-HSCT, approximately 15% fail to do so (Wuchter et al. 2010).

Poor mobilizers are usually defined as patients with less than 2×10^6 CD34+ cells/kg collected or patients mobilizing less than 10–20 CD34+ cells/μl into the PB. In general, there are two groups of poor mobilizers: predicted poor mobilizers and proven poor mobilizers (Olivieri et al. 2012). Proven poor mobilizers have low CD34+ peripheral counts circulating or do not achieve adequate HSC on day 1 of apheresis. Based on CD34+ cells, it is possible to identify the following subgroups: "borderline poor mobilizer" (11–19 CD34+ cells/μL), "relative poor mobilizer" (6–10 CD34+ cells/μL), and "absolute poor mobilizer" (0–5 CD34+ cells/μL) (Wuchter et al. 2010). If a patient has ≥20 CD34+ cells/μL at time of apheresis, the collection process should start. Between 15 and 20 CD34+ cells/μL, collection might be sufficient if not more than two

transplantations are planned and the patient has no risk factors for poor mobilization (see below).

Otherwise, the use of plerixafor (recommended dose 0.24 mg/kg/day SC) should be considered. If a patient has 10–15 CD34+ cells/μL, plerixafor application should be discussed. Below 10 CD34+ cells/μl, the use of plerixafor is clearly indicated to avoid mobilization failure. That means that there is a "gray area" between 10 and 20 CD34+ cells/μL, and the decision to use plerixafor in this situation is based on disease characteristics and treatment history (Fig. 15.1). Furthermore, if it is not possible to collect at least one third of the collection goal with the first apheresis, plerixafor should be applied because of high risk of mobilization failure (Mohty et al. 2014; Cheng et al. 2015).

Predicted poor mobilizers are defined by baseline patient or disease characteristics which are

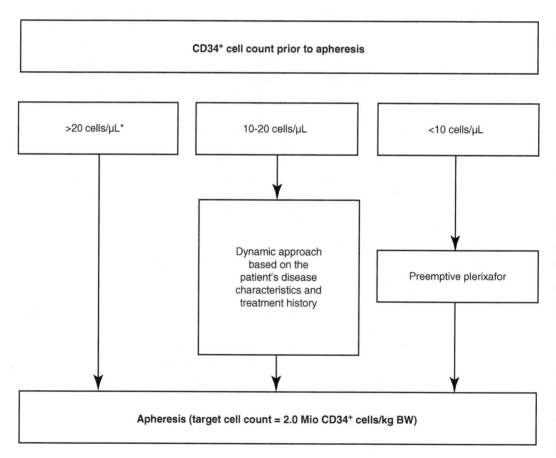

Fig. 15.1 Proactive intervention to rescue mobilization failure (Adapted from Mohty et al. 2014). *No active intervention required

Table 15.2 Factors described as predictive of poor mobilization or mobilization failure

Risk factors for poor mobilization
Age >60 years
Advanced stage of underlying disease
High number of prior treatment lines
Therapy with fludarabine, melphalan, and lenalidomide *(controversial)*
Low CD34+ cell count before apheresis
Low platelet count before mobilization *(controversial)*

Adapted from (Mohty et al. 2014)

associated with poor mobilization. These factors are listed in Table 15.2. In patients with one or more of these risk factors, the preemptive use of plerixafor should be considered. It is generally accepted that the most robust predictive factor for poor mobilization is the CD34+ cell count in PB before apheresis.

The use of plerixafor is not only valuable to avoid a failed mobilization in the described risk groups, bit it has also a documented effect on the resources of the centers. With the use of plerixafor, patients spend less time on apheresis with less blood volume processed and collect more CD34+ cells with the first apheresis, leading to a decreased number of apheresis sessions needed (Mohty et al. 2018). This has a direct effect on reducing mobilization costs. In case of a failed first mobilization attempt, the use of plerixafor for remobilization is clearly indicated (Hubel et al. 2011).

15.7 Future Directions

At this time, the number of CD34+ cells in the graft is the major and most important indicator for graft quality. A sufficient number of CD34+ cells are essential to overcome the toxicity of high-dose chemotherapy and to facilitate hematopoietic recovery. However, there is an increasing understanding that other graft subsets, e.g., CD34+ subpopulations or immune cell subsets (B cells, T cells, NK cells, dendritic cells), influence immune recovery. There are also reports that the mobilization regimen has a major impact on graft immune composition and patient's outcome (Saraceni et al. 2015). Therefore, stem cell

mobilization could not only be an important part of high-dose therapies but could also be part of an effective immunotherapy. The delineation of this approach has just been started.

Key Points
- Mobilization with chemotherapy plus G-CSF is the preferred method for patients who will need decrease of tumor burden or who have to collect a high number of HSC.
- Up to date, CD34+ cell count in the PB is the most important parameter of graft quality.
- The required HSC dose for one transplantation is at least 2×10^6 CD34+ cells/kg.
- The indication for the use of plerixafor depends on the CD34+ cell count in the PB, the collection goal, the collection yield with the first apheresis, and/or the presence of risk factors.

References

Abrahamsen JF, Stamnesfet S, Liseth K, et al. Large-volume leukapheresis yields more viable CD34+ cells and colony-forming units than normal-volume leukapheresis, especially in patients who mobilize low numbers of CD34+ cells. Transfusion. 2005;45:248–53.

Cheng J, Schmitt M, Wuchter P, et al. Plerixafor is effective given either preemptively or as a rescue strategy in poor stem cell mobilizing patients with multiple myeloma. Transfusion. 2015;55:275–83.

Donmez A, Tombuloglu M, Gungor A, et al. Clinical side effects during peripheral blood progenitor cell infusion. Transfus Apher Sci. 2007;36:95–101.

Gertz MA. Current status of stem cell mobilization. Br J Haematol. 2010;150:647–62.

Giralt S, Costa L, Schriber J, et al. Optimizing autologous stem cell mobilization strategies to improve patient outcomes: consensus guidelines and recommendations. Biol Blood Marrow Transplant. 2014;20:295–308.

Hubel K, Fresen MM, Salwender H, et al. Plerixafor with and without chemotherapy in poor mobilizers: results from the German compassionate use program. Bone Marrow Transplant. 2011;46:1045–52.

Kriegsmann K, Schmitt A, Kriegsmann M, et al. Orchestration of chemomobilization and G-CSF administration for successful hematopoietic stem cell collection. Biol Blood Marrow Transplant. 2018;24:1281–8.

Lapidot T, Petit I. Current understanding of stem cell mobilization: the roles of chemokines, proteolytic enzymes, adhesion molecules, cytokines, and stromal cells. Exp Hematol. 2002;30:973–81.

Mohty M, Azar N, Chabannon C, et al. Plerixafor in poor mobilizers with non-Hodgkin's lymphoma: a multicenter time-motion analysis. Bone Marrow Transplant. 2018;53:246–54.

Mohty M, Hubel K, Kroger N, et al. Autologous haematopoietic stem cell mobilisation in multiple myeloma and lymphoma patients: a position statement from the European group for blood and marrow transplantation. Bone Marrow Transplant. 2014;49:865–72.

Olivieri A, Marchetti M, Lemoli R, et al. Proposed definition of 'poor mobilizer' in lymphoma and multiple myeloma: an analytic hierarchy process by ad hoc working group Gruppo Italiano Trapianto di Midollo Osseo. Bone Marrow Transplant. 2012;47:342–51.

Romeo A, Chierichini A, Spagnoli A, et al. Standard- versus high-dose lenograstim in adults with hematologic malignancies for peripheral blood progenitor cell mobilization. Transfusion. 2010;50:2432–46.

Saraceni F, Shem-Tov N, Olivieri A, Nagler A. Mobilized peripheral blood grafts include more than hematopoi-etic stem cells: the immunological perspective. Bone Marrow Transplant. 2015;50:886–91.

Schmitt M, Hoffmann JM, Lorenz K, et al. Mobilization of autologous and allogeneic peripheral blood stem cells for transplantation in haematological malignancies using biosimilar G-CSF. Vox Sang. 2016;111:178–86.

Stiff PJ, Micallef I, Nademanee AP, et al. Transplanted CD34(+) cell dose is associated with long-term platelet count recovery following autologous peripheral blood stem cell transplant in patients with non-Hodgkin lymphoma or multiple myeloma. Biol Blood Marrow Transplant. 2011;17:1146–53.

Sung AD, Grima DT, Bernard LM, et al. Outcomes and costs of autologous stem cell mobilization with chemotherapy plus G-CSF vs G-CSF alone. Bone Marrow Transplant. 2013;48:1444–9.

Tuchman SA, Bacon WA, Huang LW, et al. Cyclophosphamide-based hematopoietic stem cell mobilization before autologous stem cell transplantation in newly diagnosed multiple myeloma. J Clin Apher. 2015;30:176–82.

Wuchter P, Ran D, Bruckner T, et al. Poor mobilization of hematopoietic stem cells-definitions, incidence, risk factors, and impact on outcome of autologous transplantation. Biol Blood Marrow Transplant. 2010;16:490–9.

Collection of HSC in Children

Volker Witt and Christina Peters

16.1 Introduction

Collecting or harvesting HSCs from children is a challenge, not only because children have different physiological and therefore anatomical situations but also because psychological, legal and ethical concerns in minors are sometimes more difficult compared to adult donors. In addition, parents and/or legal guardians have to be addressed in all issues. This chapter will focus on the technical, physiological, and ethical problems in the field of HSC collection from children rather than indications.

The main difference to the adult setting is the small bodyweight; the difficulties in accessing venous access, especially in the leukapheresis setting; and the need for blood cell substitution in case of BM harvest. In children the indications for autologous HSC harvesting is well-established (Passweg et al. 2014). Using children in the allogeneic setting as donors is a complete different issue (Bitan et al. 2016). Children should not donate HSCs if a comparable compatible adult volunteer HSC donor is available, if the indica-

tion for the stem cell therapy is not first line, or if the therapy is experimental (Sheldon 2004 Zinner 2004).

The main resources to harvest HSCs are BM and PBSCs. The basic techniques are quite similar to the techniques used in adults. For BM collection punctures of the iliac crests or in very small children, the tibia is used. For harvesting HSCs from the PB, leukapheresis is used with the same apheresis systems as in adults.

To perform these procedures in children, physicians and nursing practitioners must have working knowledge about the normal age-dependent physiological parameters, like vital signs, growth, and psychological and motorical development, and should be trained in the communication with children, parents, and/or their legal guardians (Anthias et al. 2016).

16.2 Bone Marrow Harvest (See Chap. 14)

The collection of HSCs from the BM is the historical oldest technique. Multiple punctures of the iliac crest are performed in general anesthesia by experienced physicians and practitioners. The bone marrow is harvested by aspirations through adequately dimensioned needles. In very small children and if the iliac crest is anatomically not suitable for punctures, the aspirations could also be performed by punctures of the proximal tibia.

V. Witt
Department of Pediatric Hematology and Oncology, St. Anna Kinderspital, Medical University Vienna, Vienna, Austria

C. Peters (✉)
Stem Cell Transplantation Unit, St. Anna Children's Hospital, Vienna, Austria
e-mail: christina.peters@stanna.at

For successful HSCT, it is necessary to obtain enough progenitor cells during the BM harvesting procedure. Most centers are using multiple aspirations of maximum 2 mL BM, while other centers are using few larger amount aspirations for BM harvesting (20–100–250 mL). It could be shown that the latter methods result in comparable grafts for transplantation (Witt et al. 2016). For some young donors with anatomically tiny situations or in diseases where a suitable donor should be used for more than one recipient a minimal harming procedure is warranted for the bone marrow harvest (Biral et al. 2008; Furey et al. 2018).

More recently, adult donors have received G-CSF because stimulated BM is richer in HSCs and therefore results in quicker engraftment (Ji et al. 2002). Experience with G-CSF-mobilized BM in pediatrics is limited. Recent data showed that a dose of 3–5 × 10⁶ CD34+ HPC/kg of recipient bodyweight is the optimal CD34+ cell dose infused to attain GVHD relapse-free survival in children with an HLA-matched sibling donor. A higher CD34+ cell dose did not impact clinical outcome. G-CSF-primed BM harvest might have a better impact on smaller amount of BM harvest volume needed for a sufficient stem cell graft, but the study was underpowered to give an answer on this urgent question (Frangoul et al. 2007; Furey et al. 2018).

16.3 Peripheral Blood Stem Cell Harvest

PBSCs are harvested by leukapheresis in very small children even below 6 kg bodyweight and are described since the 1990s of the last century (Kanold et al. 1994; Klingebiel et al. 1995; Diaz et al. 1996; Moon et al. 2013). Special experience and techniques are required to perform safe leukapheresis procedures in pediatric patients using apheresis systems who are constructed for the use in adults. Due to the large extracorporeal volume of the apheresis systems available on the market (ca. 160–220 mL), there is a need to calculate the expected blood loss in the set during procedure (Witt et al. 2007). This has to be done in each procedure to decide whether a priming of the set is needed with blood (Moon et al. 2013). In most of

the newest versions of the apheresis systems, an algorithm guides the user through this pediatric priming procedure. For priming only irradiated and leukodepleted packed RBCs should be used. In order to gain enough flow for the apheresis systems in very small children, a central venous catheter is needed, but also alternative line management with arterial lines is possible (Goldstein 2012; Even-Or et al. 2013; Hunt et al. 2013). It is important to know that in reports from registries, up to 50% of vascular access lines were peripheral venous access lines only in pediatric patients (Witt et al. 2008). For anticoagulation, citrate is used even in very small children. To avoid side effect, a calcium substitution is recommended (Kreuzer et al. 2011; Maitta et al. 2014).

For mobilization of the HPC into the PB, the longest experience exists with G-CSF in combination with chemotherapy in the autologous setting, but also plerixafor is reported in case series as suitable and safe in the use in children (Chambon et al. 2013). As in adults, a leukapheresis should be performed if a meaningful number of CD34+ HPCs are mobilized in the peripheral blood, to achieve the harvest of 2–5 × 10⁶/kg recipient with a minimum number of procedures (Fritsch et al. 2010).

16.4 Risk Analysis BM Versus PBMNC

A study from the EBMT Pediatric Diseases Working Party describes which factors influenced the safety of HSC collection. In this prospective evaluation, 453 pediatric donors were included. The children donated either BM or PBSCs according to center policy. A large variability in approach to donor issues was observed between the participating centers. Significant differences were observed between BM and PBSC donors regarding pain, need for blood allotransfusion, duration of hospital stay, and iron supplementation; however, differences between the groups undergoing BM vs PBSC donation preclude direct risk comparisons between the two procedures. The most common adverse event was pain, reported mainly by older children after BM harvest but also observed after CVC placement for PBSC collection. With regard to severe adverse events, one patient developed a pneumothorax with hydrothorax after CVC placement for PBSC collection. The risk of allo-transfusion after BM harvest was associated with a donor age of <4 years and a BM harvest volume of >20 mL/kg. Children <4 years were at higher risk than older children for allo-transfusion after BM harvest, and there was a higher risk of complications from CVC placement before apheresis. It was concluded that PBSC and BM collection are both safe procedures in children (Styczynski et al. 2012).

16.5 Pediatrics as Allogeneic Donors

Pediatric-aged donors vary widely in their ability to assent or consent to the risks of a donation procedure. There are key regulations and ethical imperatives, which must be addressed in deciding which donation procedure is appropriate for minors (van Walraven et al. 2013). In order to have general guidance, the American Academy of Pediatrics published in 2010 a recommendation on this issue. The authors strongly recommend the inclusion of the potential child donor in all decision-making process to the extent that they are capable. A minor's advocate should be an independent person who will help to prevent the delay of the donation procedure (Chan and Tipoe 2013).

The decision to take a minor family donor especially in inherited diseases is complicated to the fact that phenotypically healthy or minor symptomatic siblings with mild carrier status might be eligible for the severely ill recipient. One simple example is a sibling with thalassemia minor for a recipient with a thalassemia major (Biral et al. 2008). There are many other major diseases, including primary immunodeficiencies, chronic granulomatous disease, or sickle cell disease, where carriers are used as HSC donors. Potential family sibling donors with medical or psychological reasons not to donate should not be HLA typed (Bitan et al. 2016).

Key Points
- Pediatric donors can safely donate HSCs if an experienced team is performing the harvest procedure.
- Donors below 4 years of age have a higher risk for harvest-associated complications: With BM harvest, they have a higher need for Allo-transfusions, and there is a higher risk of complications from CVC placement before apheresis.
- Minors should only be recruited as HSC donors if no medically equivalent histocompatible adult person is available for donation and if there is a reasonable likelihood that the recipient will benefit.
- An informed consent (child assent) for the HSC donation has to be obtained by the legal guardians and from the pediatric donor. A donor advocate with expertise in pediatric development should be appointed for all individuals who have not reached the age of majority and who are considered as potential HSC donor.
- Long-term follow-up data should be collected to help determine the actual medical and psychological benefits and risks of child donors.

References

Anthias C, O'Donnell PV, Kiefer DM, et al. European group for blood and marrow transplantation centers with FACT-JACIE accreditation have significantly better compliance with related donor care standards. Biol Blood Marrow Transplant. 2016;22:514–9.

Biral E, Chiesa R, Cappelli B, et al. Multiple BM harvests in pediatric donors for thalassemic siblings: safety, efficacy and ethical issues. Bone Marrow Transplant. 2008;42:379–84.

Bitan M, van Walraven SM, Worel N, et al. Determination of eligibility in related pediatric hematopoietic cell donors: ethical and clinical considerations. Recommendations from a working group of the Worldwide Network for Blood and Marrow Transplantation Association. Biol Blood Marrow Transplant. 2016;22:96–103.

Chambon F, Merlin E, Rochette E, et al. Mobilization of hematopoietic stem cells by plerixafor alone in children: a sequential Bayesian trial. Transfus Apher Sci. 2013;49:453–8.

Chan TK, Tipoe GL. The policy statement of the American Academy of Pediatrics–children as hematopoietic stem cell donors–a proposal of modifications for application in the UK. BMC Med Ethics. 2013;14:43.

Diaz MA, Villa M, Alegre A, et al. Collection and transplantation of peripheral blood progenitor cells mobilized by G-CSF alone in children with malignancies. Br J Haematol. 1996;94:148–54.

Even-Or E, Grunspan A, Swerdlow Y, et al. Peripheral blood stem-cell harvest using percutaneous arterial lines in children. Pediatr Blood Cancer. 2013;60:946–8.

Frangoul H, Nemecek ER, Billheimer D, et al. A prospective study of G-CSF primed bone marrow as a stem-cell source for allogeneic bone marrow transplantation in children: a Pediatric Blood and Marrow Transplant Consortium (PBMTC) study. Blood. 2007;110:4584–7.

Fritsch P, Schwinger W, Schwantzer G, et al. Peripheral blood stem cell mobilization with pegfilgrastim compared to filgrastim in children and young adults with malignancies. Pediatr Blood Cancer. 2010;54:134–7.

Furey A, Rastogi S, Prince R, et al. Bone marrow harvest in pediatric sibling donors: role of granulocyte colony-stimulating factor priming and CD34(+) cell dose. Biol Blood Marrow Transplant. 2018;24:324–9.

Goldstein SL. Therapeutic apheresis in children: special considerations. Semin Dial. 2012;25:165–70.

Hunt EA, Jain NG, Somers MJ. Apheresis therapy in children: an overview of key technical aspects and a review of experience in pediatric renal disease. J Clin Apher. 2013;28:36–47.

Ji SQ, Chen HR, Wang HX, et al. Comparison of outcome of allogeneic bone marrow transplantation with and without granulocyte colony-stimulating factor (lenograstim) donor-marrow priming in patients with chronic myelogenous leukemia. Biol Blood Marrow Transplant. 2002;8:261–7.

Kanold J, Rapatel C, Berger M, et al. Use of G-CSF alone to mobilize peripheral blood stem cells for collection from children. Br J Haematol. 1994;88:633–5.

Klingebiel T, Handgretinger R, Herter M, et al. Autologous transplantation with peripheral blood stem cells in children and young adults after myeloab-

lative treatment: nonrandomized comparison between GM-CSF and G-CSF for mobilization. J Hematother. 1995;4:307–14.

Kreuzer M, Ahlenstiel T, Kanzelmeyer N, et al. Regional citrate anticoagulation—a safe and effective procedure in pediatric apheresis therapy. Pediatr Nephrol. 2011;26:127–32.

Maitta RW, Vasovic LV, Mohandas K, et al. A safe therapeutic apheresis protocol in paediatric patients weighing 11 to 25 kg. Vox Sang. 2014;107:375–80.

Moon JH, Kim MJ, Song SY. Safety and efficacy of G-CSF mobilization and collection of autologous peripheral blood stem cells in children with cerebral palsy. Transfus Apher Sci. 2013;49:516–21.

Passweg JR, Baldomero H, Peters C. Hematopoietic SCT in Europe: data and trends in 2012 with special consideration of pediatric transplantation. Bone Marrow Transplant. 2014;49:744–50.

Sheldon M. Children as organ donors: a persistent ethical issue. Camb Q Healthc Ethics. 2004;13:119–22.

Styczynski J, Balduzzi A, Gil L, et al. Risk of complications during hematopoietic stem cell collection in pediatric sibling donors: a prospective European Group for Blood and Marrow Transplantation Pediatric Diseases Working Party study. Blood. 2012;119:2935–42.

van Walraven SM, Straathof LM, Switzer GE, et al. Immediate and long-term somatic effects, and health-related quality of life of BM donation during early childhood. A single-center report in 210 pediatric donors. Bone Marrow Transplant. 2013;48:40–5.

Witt V, Beiglbock E, Ritter R, et al. Performance of a new separator system for routine autologous hematopoietic progenitor cell collection in small children. J Clin Apher. 2007;22:306–13.

Witt V, Pichler H, Fritsch G, Peters C. Multiple small versus few large amount aspirations for bone marrow harvesting in autologous and allogeneic bone marrow transplantation. Transfus Apher Sci. 2016;55:221–4.

Witt V, Stegmayr B, Ptak J, et al. World apheresis registry data from 2003 to 2007, the pediatric and adolescent side of the registry. Transfus Apher Sci. 2008;39:255–60.

Zinner S. Cognitive development and pediatric consent to organ donation. Camb Q Healthc Ethics. 2004;13:125–32.

Processing, Cryopreserving and Controlling the Quality of HSCs

Patrick Wuchter

17.1 Assessment of HSCs by Measuring CD34 and the Presence of Other Cell Subsets

The efficiency of an autologous, as well as an allogeneic, HSCs graft is mainly determined by the number of CD34+ cells present. The dose of transplanted CD34+ cells per kg body weight (BW) determines the kinetics of the neutrophil and platelet engraftment after auto-HSCT (Weaver et al. 1995). The measurement of CD34+ cells by flow cytometry is, therefore, an important method to assess the graft quantity.

The minimal number of CD34+ cells for an autologous transplant is ≥2.0 × 10⁶ CD34+ cells/ kg BW. Transplants below this threshold should only be used in cases where no additional stem cell collection is feasible and there is a vital indication for the autologous stem cell transplantation. Most transplant centres regard a cell dose of 2.5–6 × 10⁶ CD34+ cells/kg BW as optimal, based on published clinical data (Duong et al. 2014; Perez-Simon et al. 1999; Giralt et al. 2014; Lisenko et al. 2017b; Mohty et al. 2014). For an allo-HSCT, a cell dose of ≥4.0 × 10⁶ CD34+ cells/ kg BW is regarded as adequate.

P. Wuchter (✉)
Institute of Transfusion Medicine and Immunology, German Red Cross Blood Service Baden-Württemberg – Hessen, Medical Faculty Mannheim, Heidelberg University, Mannheim, Germany
e-mail: Patrick.Wuchter@medma.uni-heidelberg.de

In the autologous setting, it has been specu lated that the quality of CD34+ cells from poor mobilizers may be inferior. However, studies have found that the proportions of primitive and quiescent CD34+ subsets were comparable across mobilization groups (Jiang et al. 2012), and leu kocyte and platelet recovery after transplantation was not different (Wuchter et al. 2010).

The application of plerixafor in order to over come insufficient HSCs mobilization not only increases the number of CD34+ cells but also the proportion of more primitive HSCs subsets, the absolute lymphocyte count and the numbers of lymphocytes in various subsets (CD19+ cells, CD3 cells, T-cells and NK-cells) in the autograft (Fruehauf et al. 2009; Taubert et al. 2011; Varmavuo et al. 2013). However, these variances do not trans late into relevant clinical differences regarding hae matopoietic recovery. Taken together, the graft quality from poor mobilizers can be regarded equivalent compared to that from good mobilizers, regardless of the use of plerixafor.

It was further speculated that the composition of cellular subsets in the transplant may have an influence on the haematopoietic reconstitution. However, based on the currently published data, no final conclusion can be drawn, and further investigations are warranted to determine the potential effects of autograft cell subsets on the patients' clinical outcomes. As delineated in an EBMT position statement from 2014, determina tion of cell subsets other than CD34+ cells is not routinely performed in clinical practice but only in clinical trials (Mohty et al. 2014). Accordingly, assessment of tumour cell contamination is usually not part of the clinical routine but can be of interest in clinical trials.

17.2   HSCs Cryopreservation

HSCs should be processed and stored in accordance with the respective Medical Council, responsible local and overarching authorities as well as scientific society's guidelines (e.g. EU: Guideline   2004/23/EG   and   2006/17/EG, EU-GMP-Guideline).

If necessary, collected cells can be stored for a maximum of up to 72 h at 2–6 °C before cryopreservation. However, cryopreservation within 48 h or less is recommended to maintain an optimal viability of the cells. In the case of storage for >24 h prior to cryopreservation, the maximum nucleated cell (NC) concentration should not exceed 2×10^8/mL.

For cryopreservation, a number of different protocols are used worldwide. Usually, the maximum accepted NC concentration is $\leq 4 \times 10^8$/mL. If necessary, PBSC products can be diluted with autologous plasma or commercial resuspension medium. Increasing the cell concentration by volume depletion minimizes the number of cryostored bags needed, but the upper limit of the NC concentration needs to be considered. The final product includes 5–10% dimethyl sulfoxide (DMSO) as a cryoprotectant and 0.05–0.25 mL of ACD-A stabilizer solution per ml of transplant. Freezing at a controlled rate of 1–2 °C per minute is recommended. Cells need to be stored in vapour phase nitrogen at a temperature of ≤ -140 °C. Cross-contamination while preparing and storing the cells must be prevented by taking appropriate measures.

At the time of auto-HSCT, cryopreserved bags must be thawed at the site of transplantation, and PBSCs should be reinfused within a maximum time span of 10–20 min of thawing using standard transfusion filters in order to minimize the detrimental effect of DMSO upon HSCs. Previous washing for purposes of DMSO depletion is not routinely performed, as the loss and damage of HSCs are regarded as too high.

Several studies demonstrated that under these storage conditions, CD34[+] HSCs remained viable for up to 19 years (Fernyhough et al. 2013; McCullough et al. 2010; Spurr et al. 2002). In addition, a recent study demonstrated that the duration of cryostorage of the transplant had no impact on the haematologic reconstitution after transplantation (Lisenko et al. 2017a).

17.3   HSCs Quality Assessment

HSCs product quality assessment needs to be performed at several time points during cell processing and storage. Volume measurement, enumeration of NC and red blood cells and flow cytometry-based CD34[+] cell quantification should be performed directly after PBSC collection in accordance with the Stem Cell Enumeration Committee Guidelines of the International Society of Hematotherapy and Graft Engineering (ISHAGE) (Sutherland et al. 1996). A validated protocol and external quality control (e.g. the round robin test) is strongly recommended (Whitby et al. 2012).

Shortly before freezing, microbiological culture samples must be obtained. NC enumeration and NC viability measurement (e.g. by staining with trypan blue, 7-aminoactinomycin D [7-AAD] or propidium iodide) should be performed from aliquots of the final cell product after freezing and thawing. This viability testing is only valid for a defined and limited time span, often 2–5 years based on local guidelines, before it needs to be repeated prior to transplantation. As a result, a sufficient number of reference samples should be prepared for each HSCs product (the recommended minimum number is 3).

Target values need to be defined for the final product, mostly in accordance with local authorities. In most transplant centres in Europe, the following criteria are mandatory (together with additional criteria) for the release of an autologous transplant: NC concentration $\leq 4 \times 10^8$/mL, CD34[+] cell number $\geq 2 \times 10^6$/kg BW, red blood concentration ≤ 0.1 mL per mL of transplant, no microbial growth and minimum NC viability of >50% after freezing and thawing.

17.4 Collection of Reference (Retention) Samples for Quality Control

Reference samples for quality control must be taken and stored from the cell product. These samples allow the proof of quality and potency of the transplant in terms of sterility, purity and viability of the cells. In the case of an allo-HSCT, reference samples may also need to be collected from the donor, depending on the respective local legal situation, to allow for a retrospective analysis in terms of serological testing.

Reference samples are prepared in parallel with the cell product and stored under the same cryoconditions until they are analysed. As a release criterion for an autologous stem cell transplant, a reference sample should be cryopreserved for >24 h under the identical conditions as the cell product before the viability of $CD34^+$/$CD45^+$ cells is analysed. Performing a clonogenic assay (e.g. colony-forming assay) from the reference samples can assess the haematopoietic potency of the cells. However, this is not regarded as a release criterion but should be performed for process validation or in the case of prolonged cryostorage of a transplant (>2–5 years).

The final cell product must be labelled in accordance with respective legal requirements. In order to transport cryopreserved HSCs products, a validated shipping container is required, preferably with continuous temperature monitoring. The treating physician is responsible for application of the HSCs transplant after evaluating its integrity and the accompanying documents.

Key Points

- Minimal number of $CD34^+$ cells is $\geq 2.0 \times 10^6$/kg BW for an auto-HSCT and $\geq 4.0 \times 10^6$/kg BW for an Allo-HSCT.
- Determination of cell subsets other than $CD34^+$ is not routinely required.
- Cryopreservation needs to be performed within 72 h, preferably <48 h.

- The maximum NC concentration in the cryostored transplant should be $\leq 4 \times 10^8$/mL.
- The final product includes 5–10% DMSO as a cryoprotectant and 0.05–0.25 mL of ACD-A stabilizer solution per ml of transplant.
- Freezing at a controlled rate of 1–2 °C per minute is recommended, and cells need to be stored in vapour phase nitrogen at a temperature of ≤ -140 °C.
- NC viability should be >50% after freezing and thawing.
- At the time of ABSCT, cryopreserved bags must be thawed and reinfused within a maximum of 10–20 min of thawing.
- Reference samples for quality control must be prepared and cryostored in parallel and under identical conditions as the cell product.

References

Duong HK, Savani BN, Copelan E, et al. Peripheral blood progenitor cell mobilization for autologous and allogeneic hematopoietic cell transplantation: guidelines from the American Society for Blood and Marrow Transplantation. Biol Blood Marrow Transplant. 2014;20:1262–73.

Fernyhough LJ, Buchan VA, McArthur LT, Hock BD. Relative recovery of haematopoietic stem cell products after cryogenic storage of up to 19 years. Bone Marrow Transplant. 2013;48:32–5.

Fruehauf S, Veldwijk MR, Seeger T, et al. A combination of granulocyte-colony-stimulating factor (G-CSF) and plerixafor mobilizes more primitive peripheral blood progenitor cells than G-CSF alone: results of a European phase II study. Cytotherapy. 2009;11:992–1001.

Giralt S, Costa L, Schriber J, et al. Optimizing autologous stem cell mobilization strategies to improve patient outcomes: consensus guidelines and recommendations. Biol Blood Marrow Transplant. 2014;20:295–308.

Guidelines 2004/23/EG des Europäischen Parlaments und des Rates vom 31. März 2004 zur Festlegung von Qualitäts- und Sicherheitsstandards für die Spende, Beschaffung, Testung, Verarbeitung, Konservierung, Lagerung und Verteilung von menschlichen Geweben und Zellen. Amtsblatt der Europäischen Union.

Guidelines 2006/17/EG der Kommission vom 8. Februar 2006 zur Durchführung der Richtlinie 2004/23/EG des Europäischen Parlaments und des Rates hinsichtlich technischer Vorschriften für die Spende, Beschaffung und Testung von menschlichen Geweben und Zellen. Amtsblatt der Europäischen Union.

Guidelines EU-Leitfaden der Guten Herstellungspraxis – Humanarzneimittel und Tierarzneimittel (EU-GMP). Europäische Kommission: EudraLex;4.

Jiang L, Malik S, Litzow M, et al. Hematopoietic stem cells from poor and good mobilizers are qualitatively equivalent. Transfusion. 2012;52:542–8.

Lisenko K, Pavel P, Kriegsmann M, et al. Storage duration of autologous stem cell preparations has no impact on hematopoietic recovery after transplantation. Biol Blood Marrow Transplant. 2017a;23:684–90.

Lisenko K, Wuchter P, Hansberg M, et al. Comparison of different stem cell mobilization regimen in AL amyloidosis patients. Biol Blood Marrow Transplant. 2017b;23:1870–8.

McCullough J, Haley R, Clay M, et al. Long-term storage of peripheral blood stem cells frozen and stored with a conventional liquid nitrogen technique compared with cells frozen and stored in a mechanical freezer. Transfusion. 2010;50:808–19.

Mohty M, Hubel K, Kroger N, et al. Autologous haematopoietic stem cell mobilisation in multiple myeloma and lymphoma patients: a position statement from the European Group for Blood and Marrow Transplantation. Bone Marrow Transplant. 2014;49:865–72.

Perez-Simon JA, Martin A, Caballero D, et al. Clinical significance of CD34+ cell dose in long-term engraftment following autologous peripheral blood stem cell transplantation. Bone Marrow Transplant. 1999;24:1279–83.

Spurr EE, Wiggins NE, Marsden KA, et al. Cryopreserved human haematopoietic stem cells retain engraftment potential after extended (5–14 years) cryostorage. Cryobiology. 2002;44:210–7.

Sutherland DR, Anderson L, Keeney M, Nayar R, Chin-Yee I. The ISHAGE guidelines for CD34+ cell determination by flow cytometry. International Society of Hematotherapy and Graft Engineering. J Hematother. 1996;5:213–26.

Taubert I, Saffrich R, Zepeda-Moreno A, et al. Characterization of hematopoietic stem cell subsets from patients with multiple myeloma after mobilization with plerixafor. Cytotherapy. 2011;13:459–66.

Varmavuo V, Mantymaa P, Silvennoinen R, et al. CD34+ cell subclasses and lymphocyte subsets in blood grafts collected after various mobilization methods in myeloma patients. Transfusion. 2013;53:1024–32.

Weaver CH, Hazelton B, Birch R, et al. An analysis of engraftment kinetics as a function of the CD34 content of peripheral blood progenitor cell collections in 692 patients after the administration of myeloablative chemotherapy. Blood. 1995;86:3961–9.

Whitby A, Whitby L, Fletcher M, et al. ISHAGE protocol: are we doing it correctly? Cytometry B Clin Cytom. 2012;82:9–17.

Wuchter P, Ran D, Bruckner T, et al. Poor mobilization of hematopoietic stem cells-definitions, incidence, risk factors, and impact on outcome of autologous transplantation. Biol Blood Marrow Transplant. 2010;16:490–9.

Procurement and Management of Cord Blood

Sergio Querol and Vanderson Rocha

18.1 Introduction

Umbilical cord blood (UCB) cells for allogeneic use are collected and frozen in more than 130 public CB banks worldwide. More than seven hundred and fifty thousands CB units (CBU) are available for transplantation. In this chapter we will describe some procedures for cord blood collection, processing, banking and recommendations on how to choose a single or double UCB unit for transplantation (Garcia 2010).

18.2 Collection

Donor recruitment usually starts during the antenatal period, with objective information given by woman's health-care provider. After consent, trained personnel need to determine donor eligibility to ensure that donation is safe for future patients. To assess donor eligibility, a donor medical history interview shall be conducted identifying risk factors for transmissible and genetic disease. In addition, infectious disease markers (IDM) performed to maternal blood samples will be obtained within

7 days before or after the collection of the UCB unit. These samples will be tested for evidence of infection of HIV-1, HIV-2, hepatitis B, hepatitis C, HTLV-I, HTLV-II, syphilis and any additional markers according to local regulations.

Collection must not interfere with normal delivery attention. A successful collection should have a high collection volume and a high total nucleated cell count, be non-contaminated and have the proper documentation. A UCB collection typically involves cord clamping (delayed clamping up to 1–2 min is still compatible with public donations) (Frändberg et al. 2016), disinfection, venipuncturing of umbilical vein and draining by gravity avoiding clotting. Collection bag should be appropriately labelled.

There are two main techniques to collect UCB from the cord vein: before the placenta is delivered (in utero) or after the placenta is delivered (ex utero). Both collection techniques have their own unique advantages and disadvantages, but both techniques require that the individuals performing the collections be adequately trained.

After collection, typically health-care provider will complete a report describing labour and completing variables that could be useful to release the unit like the presence of fever, complications, type of delivery, etc. In case of unexpected adverse reactions during collection they need to be communicated to the competent authority. After collection, it may be required a follow-up of the donor including health questionnaires. Additionally, if

S. Querol (✉)
Banc Sang i Teixits, Barcelona, Spain
e-mail: squerol@bst.cat

V. Rocha
University of São Paulo, São Paulo, Brazil

University of Oxford, Oxford, UK

any abnormal result is detected during testing, a counseling process should be in place.

UCB units shall be transported to the processing facility, and sometimes, these facilities could be far away from the collection sites. A validated procedure for transportation between these two facilities is needed to demonstrate a reliable method. Standard procedures shall be in place to describe time and temperature of storage and transportation methods. All transportation records shall allow tracking back from the collection site to the UCB bank, and any deviation should be recorded.

18.3 Processing and Banking

18.3.1 UCB Cell Processing

Unrelated UCB unit must arrive at the processing laboratory in time to allow initiation of cryopreservation within 48 h of collection (this time is extended to 72 h for related or directed UCB donations). The decision as to whether a collected UCB unit will be acceptable for processing and banking will be made based on the acceptance criteria specified by the UCB bank. Many banks have further refined their acceptance criteria based on economics and the desire to build an international inventory of UCB units with very high TNC or percentage of ethnic minorities. Many UCB banks are now committed to processing and storing only those UCB units with high TNC (e.g. >20 × 10^7 TNC or higher), based on the greater likelihood of these units being used (Saccardi et al. 2016).

Volume reduction of UCB is considered essential to the provision of a high-quality product and cost-effective UCB banking. Reducing the volume of the final product allows for storage efficiency in terms of space and cost and, most importantly, reduces the risk of ABO incompatibility and DMSO toxicity to the potential recipient. Despite some loss of cells, volume reduction has additional practical and clinical benefits; the process yields RBC and plasma components as waste products that can be used for immediate or future testing, thereby minimizing the loss of the actual stem cell product for testing purposes.

Different methods for volume reduction are available (Hough et al. 2016).

The selection of a suitable protocol for cryopreservation of UCB for use in transplantation is critical to optimize the recovery of functionally viable progenitor cells, most of which lie within the CD34$^+$ compartment. Some important considerations that are potential sources of cell damage include the type and concentration of cryoprotectant, the cell concentration and the cooling and warming rates. UCB units must be stored in freezing bags designed and approved for the cryopreservation of human cells and placed into metal canisters to afford protection during freezing, storage, transportation and shipping. It is important that after filling, each freezing bag is visually examined for possible leaking and breakage of seals.

UCB units should be cryopreserved using a controlled rate freezer with a validated freezing programme. Liquid nitrogen-based controlled rate freezers have been used to ensure long-term maintenance. Minimizing transient-warming events is very important for that. Stability programmes should be designed in order to establish the expiration time of the UCB stored.

18.3.2 Testing and Quality Assessment

Table 18.1 shows release specification for UCB units. Quality assessment is written below:

Safety It is essential that UCB is screened for those infectious diseases which can be transmitted via blood (as described above). In addition, product should be free of microbial contamination (or with an appropriate antibiogram for related uses). Prior to release for administration, each UCB unit must have undergone hemoglobinopathy screening.

Identity At least, HLA-A, HLA-B, HLA-C and DRB1 loci must be determined using DNA-based methods and result included when listing a UCB unit on the search registries. It is recommended that HLA typing is performed in an accredited laboratory. ABO blood group and Rh type must be reported prior to listing a UCB

Table 18.1 Lists the specification requirements for CBU stored for clinical application, according to the sixth edition NetCord-FACT International Standards for Cord Blood Collection, Banking, and Release for Administration (www.factwebsite.org)

Specification requirements for cord blood units stored for clinical administration				
	Unrelated specification		Related specification	
Test	Fresh post-processing sample	Post-thaw attached segment or representative sample prior to release	Fresh post-processing sample	Post-thaw attached segment or representative sample prior to release
Total nucleated cell count	$\geq 5.0 \times 10^8$		Enumerated	
Total nucleated cell recovery	Should be $\geq 60\%$		Should be $\geq 60\%$	
Total viability	$\geq 85\%$		$\geq 70\%$	
Viable CD34 count	$\geq 1.25 \times 10^6$			
Viability of CD34 cells	$\geq 85\%$	$\geq 70\%$	$\geq 85\%$	$\geq 70\%$
Viability of CD45 cells		$\geq 40\%$		$\geq 40\%$
CFU (or other validated potency assay)[a]		Growth (or positive result for potency)		Growth (or positive result for potency)
Sterility	Negative for aerobes, anaerobes, fungus		Negative for aerobic and anaerobic bacteria and fungi—OR—identify and provide results of antibiotic sensitivities	
Donor screening and testing	Acceptable as defined by Applicable Law and NetCord-FACT standards		Acceptable as defined by Applicable Law and NetCord-FACT standards	
Identity		Verified		Verified

[a]There should be evidence of potency by CFU or other validated potency assay on a fresh post-processing sample

unit for search. Prior to release of a UCB unit for administration, it is imperative that HLA identity is confirmed. Ideally, confirmatory typing will be performed on a sample taken from a contiguous segment. HLA typing on maternal blood may also be performed prior to release of a UCB unit. Haplotype matching between maternal donor and infant donor confirms linkage between the two and serves as a secondary confirmation of identity.

Purity UCB unit specifications report total nucleated cells, total nucleated RBC count and CD34+ cells, and a cell blood count with differential should be performed, with parameters for neutrophils, lymphocytes, monocytes and platelets defined.

Potency Potency testing to determine the growth potential and viability of progenitor cells in a UCB unit should be performed post-processing (prior to cryopreservation), in addition to being performed on a representative thawed sample prior to release for administration.

18.4 Selecting CBU for Transplantation

The success of the UCB transplantation (UCBT) will depend on the characteristics of the CBU. Tables 18.2 and 18.3 list the recommendation of choosing single and double cord blood units, respectively, for transplantation.

Table 18.2 Recommendations for unrelated CBU selection and transplantation[a]

Initial selection of single CBU should be based upon

(a) HLA matching of the recipient and CBU

(b) CBU collected cell dose (TNC ± CD34$^+$)

(c) Patient's diagnosis (malignant versus non-malignant)

(d) Avoiding CBU containing Ag that match the specificity of any pre-transplant donor-specific anti-HLA Ab in the recipient

HLA matching

• *Malignant disorders* (Eapen et al. 2014)

HLA matching should be based upon allelic typing for HLA-A, HLA-B, HLA-C and HLA-DRB1 for single CBT

1. Select an HLA-matched (8/8) CBU. TNC dose should be >3 × 10^7/kg

2. If an HLA-matched (8/8) CBU is unavailable, select a CBU matched at 7/8 HLA loci. HLA-A or HLA-B mismatches are preferable to HLA-DRB1 mismatches. TNC dose should be >5 × 10^7/kg for 5–7/8 matched units

3. If a CBU matched at 8/8 or 7/8 HLA loci is unavailable, consider a CBU matched at 5 or 6/8 HLA loci. Avoid mismatches in HLA-DRB1

4. If CBU 4/8 matched, CBU may rarely be considered as a single CB graft if no other option is available. TNC dose should be >5 × 10^7/kg for 4/8 matched units

5. CBU 3/8 HLA-matched CBU are not recommended

• *Non-malignant disorders* (Eapen et al. 2017)

1. CBU with HLA 8/8 or 7/8 give same survival results

2. CBU with HLA 6/8 and 5/8 give inferior survival rates and are alternative options

3. We do not recommend selecting cord blood units with more HLA disparities

TNC and CD34$^+$ cell dose

• *Malignant disorders*

Nucleated cell dose[b]	At freezing, minimum TNC dose 3.0 × 10^7/kg, or
	After thawing, minimum TNC of 2.0–2.5 × 10^7/kg
CD34$^+$ cell dose[c]	At freezing, 1.0–1.7 × 10^5/kg, or
	After thawing, around 1.0–1.2 × 10^5/kg

• *Non-malignant disorders*[d]

Nucleated cell dose	At freezing, minimum cell dose 3.5 × 10^7/kg, or
	After thawing, minimum cell dose 3.0 × 10^7/kg
CD34$^+$ cell dose	At freezing or after thawing, >1.7 × 10^5/kg

Colony-forming unit assay: This assay is important to evaluate the functional capacity of HPCs after thawing an aliquot or after thawing the product; however it is difficult to establish a generalized CFU-GM dose due to variations of colony setup and counting between centres

Other considerations when selecting single CB units

If many CBU meeting the criteria above are available, the following factors should also be considered

• *Use accredited cord blood banks.* For safety, only accredited banks recognized by national and international organizations should be used

• *ABO compatibility:* ABO compatibility may be associated with improved outcomes, although the data are conflicting

• *NIMA:* If the cord banks have the mother's HLA typing, the potential effect of NIMA should be noted in context of clinical trials

• *KIR ligand:* Due to conflicting data, KIR ligand matching should not be used in the selection of CBUs

• *Sex matching:* Sex matching between CBUs and patients in single or double UCBT is not necessary

[a]Based on Eurocord and British Society of Blood and Marrow Transplantation recommendations (Hough et al. 2016, modified)

[b]If the infused TNC dose is 1.0–2.0 × 10^7/kg, the number of CD34$^+$ cells or CFU-GM should be taken into consideration to predict the probability of neutrophil recovery and to discuss the possibility of a second transplant. If both cell doses are lower than recommended, a BM aspirate and chimerism analysis should be performed between days +20–28. The absence of engraftment indicates the need for a second transplant; preliminary data shows that haploidentical or double CBT should be considered

[c]Due to variation in counting CD34$^+$ cells, this recommendation should be taken with caution. However, if colonies are not growing, the transplant physicians should consider a second transplant after day +30

[d]For patients with BMF syndromes (aplastic anaemia or congenital bone marrow failure states) or haemoglobinopathies, the number of TNC at freezing should be greater than 5 × 10^7/kg

Table 18.3 Additional criteria for double CBU selection

– When a single CBU unit contains insufficient cells (as specified above), double UCBT is recommended for the treatment of malignant disorders	
– There are currently insufficient data to make recommendations for double UCBT in the treatment of non-malignant disorders	
HLA matching	
• The historical stringency of HLA matching for CBUs with the recipient for double UCBTs should be used, i.e. the minimum acceptable HLA matching between either CBU and the recipient is 4/6 using low/intermediate typing (antigen) for HLA-A and HLA-B and high- resolution typing (allelic) for HLA-DRB1	
• There is no requirement for inter-cord HLA matching	
• The role of high-resolution (allele) typing is not yet defined for double CBT	
Cell dose	
Nucleated cell dose	At freezing, the sum of both CBUs $>3.5 \times 10^7$/kg
	The minimum cell dose of each unit should be $>1.5 \times 10^7$/kg
CD34$^+$ cell dose	At freezing or after thawing, the sum of both CBUs $>1.8 \times 10^5$/kg
ABO matching	
Recently, a retrospective study of Eurocord of almost 1000 double UCBT recipients has shown an important association between ABO compatibility of 2 units with the patient on acute GVHD, NRM and OS. Thus, ABO compatibility between units and patients should be preferred over minor or major compatibility of one of the units between CB and patient (V Rocha on behalf of Eurocord, personal recommendation)	

Key Points

- Cord blood donation comprises the following steps: informative and consent process, revision of eligibility criteria, cord blood collection and finally fresh storage before a standardized transportation to the processing cell lab.
- Cell processing labs require coordination of production and quality control labs to transform the altruistically donated raw material in a medicinal product with predefined specifications that ensure its safety, identity, purity and potency.
- A public cord blood bank is a stem cell registry that provides ready-to-use banked medicinal products for any patient in need through international networking of stem cell donor organizations.
- Cord blood selection is based on sorting CB units using primary criteria (cell content and HLA matching) followed by ranking based in secondary criteria depending on disease status, conditioning, age and recipient's weight.

References

Eapen M, Klein JP, Ruggeri A, Spellman S, Lee SJ, Anasetti C, Arcese W, Barker JN, Baxter-Lowe LA, Brown M, Fernandez-Vina MA, Freeman J, He W, Iori AP, Horowitz MM, Locatelli F, Marino S, Maiers M, Michel G, Sanz GF, Gluckman E, Rocha V, Center for International Blood and Marrow Transplant Research, Netcord, Eurocord, and the European Group for Blood and Marrow Transplantation. Impact of allele-level HLA matching on outcomes after myeloablative single unit umbilical cord blood transplantation for hematologic malignancy. Blood. 2014;123: 133–40.

Eapen M, Wang T, Veys PA, Boelens JJ, St Martin A, Spellman S, Bonfim CS, Brady C, Cant AJ, Dalle JH, Davies SM, Freeman J, Hsu KC, Fleischhauer K, Kenzey C, Kurtzberg J, Michel G, Orchard PJ, Paviglianiti A, Rocha V, Veneris MR, Volt F, Wynn R, Lee SJ, Horowitz MM, Gluckman E, Ruggeri A. Allele-level HLA matching for umbilical cord blood transplantation for non-malignant diseases in children: a retrospective analysis. Lancet Haematol. 2017;4:e325–33.

Frändberg S, Waldner B, Konar J, Rydberg L, Fasth A, Holgersson J. High quality cord blood banking is feasible with delayed clamping practices. The eight-year experience and current status of the national Swedish Cord Blood Bank. Cell Tissue Bank. 2016;17(3):439–48.

Garcia J. Allogeneic unrelated cord blood banking worldwide: an update. Swedish bank reference delay clamping. Transfus Apher Sci. 2010;42:257–63.

Hough R, Danby R, Russell N, Marks D, Veys P, Shaw B, Wynn R, Vora A, Mackinnon S, Peggs KS, Crawley C, Craddock C, Pagliuca A, Cook G, Snowden JA, Clark A, Marsh J, Querol S, Parkes G, Braund H, Rocha V. Recommendations for a standard UK approach to incorporating umbilical cord blood into clinical transplantation practice: an update on cord blood unit selection, donor selection algorithms and conditioning protocols. Br J Haematol. 2016;172:360–70.

Saccardi R, Tucunduva L, Ruggeri A, Ionescu I, Koegler G, Querol S, Grazzini G, Lecchi L, Nanni Costa A, Navarrete C, Pouthiers F, Larghero J, Regan D, Freeman T, Bittencourt H, Kenzey C, Labopin M, Baudoux E, Rocha V, Gluckman E. Impact of cord blood banking technologies on clinical outcome: a Eurocord/Cord Blood Committee (CTIWP), European Society for Blood and Marrow Transplantation and NetCord retrospective analysis. Transfusion. 2016;56:2021–9.

Graft Manipulation

Michael Schumm, Peter Lang,
and Rupert Handgretinger

19.1 Introduction

Graft manipulation is performed to define and to optimize the volume and cellular composition of stem cell sources like apheresis products, bone marrow, or umbilical cord blood.

Basic manipulations comprise centrifugation procedures for depletion of erythrocytes and volume reduction and are required to cryopreserve grafts in the presence of cryoprotectants like DMSO (Dimethylsulfoxide) (Rowley 1992). These are standard procedures for BM and CB, while apheresis products usually can be cryopreserved without further manipulation.

More complex manipulations are used to optimize the cellular composition and to meet requirements of the individual transplant regimen. Selection of CD34+ or AC133+ progenitors from apheresis or BM has been used to produce concentrated stem cell grafts. In recent years, the selective depletion of unwanted cells like CD3+ T cells, TcRαβ+ T cells, and others provides a custom-tailored graft. For both enrichment and depletion, immunomagnetic cell sorting using

M. Schumm · P. Lang · R. Handgretinger (✉)
Department of Hematology/Oncology
and General Pediatrics, Children's University
Hospital, University of Tuebingen, Tuebingen,
Germany
e-mail: rupert.handgretinger@med.uni-tuebingen.de

monoclonal antibodies and paramagnetic microbeads in combination with semi- or fully automated devices has become the standard technique in most laboratories.

19.2 Graft Manipulation

19.2.1 Physical Manipulations

19.2.1.1 Volume Reduction
Volume reduction might be necessary in small children and is done by a simple centrifugation process and removal of the supernatant.

19.2.1.2 Washing to Reduce Plasma Antibodies or Anticoagulants
Washing might be necessary in case of unwanted isoagglutinins or to lower the heparin concentration and is also done by centrifugation in a bag or dedicated devices and by exchange of plasma with a suitable solution like 0.9% NaCl. Addition of anticoagulant is not necessary as coagulating agents are washed out by the treatment.

19.2.1.3 Depletion of Erythrocytes
Depletion of erythrocytes is necessary in case of blood group incompatibities and usually confined to bone marrow. Several procedures

are employed including centrifugation with an apheresis device or centrifugation in bags or tubes and subsequent harvest of the buffy coat. In special cases, a separation using density gradient centrifugation (e.g., Ficoll) might be useful with an even stronger depletion of erythrocytes.

19.2.2 Immunomagnetic Procedures

19.2.2.1 CD34 Enrichment

Enrichment of CD34+ stem cells was the first method which provided grafts with a very low number of T cells and therefore allowed to avoid GvHD highly effective even in haploidentical HSCT (Ringhoffer et al. 2004; Handgretinger et al. 2001).

The method has also been successfully used in MSD and MUD HSCT to minimize the rate of GvHD (Pasquini et al. 2012; Lang et al. 2003) and showed a clear advantage regarding combined cGVHD-free and relapse-free survival compared to unmanipulated grafts in myeloid diseases (Tamari et al. 2018).

Moreover, CD34 selection is used as a graft backbone to which other cell types (unmanipulated DLI, CD45RA depleted DLI, and others) can be added.

Enrichment can be performed with the Miltenyi Biotec CD34 reagent system which uses a mAb for the CD34 class 2 epitope and therefore has to be detected by an Ab to a different epitope (normally class 3). Stem cells after separation normally show a high purity with extremely low amounts of other contaminating cell types. In some cases various amounts of monocytes are found without detrimental effect on the graft. Due to the small size of the graft, absolute numbers of contaminating T cells remain low even if a significant percentage persists. B cells are passively depleted as well, whereas CD34+CD19+ B-cell precursors are retained: 1–3% in PB, up to 30% in BM preparations.

Recovery of CD34+ cells is in the range of 50–90% (Schumm et al. 1999).

19.2.2.2 CD133 Enrichment

CD133 detects a slightly smaller subpopulation of CD34+ cells and can also be used for enrichment of stem cells with similar results (Koehl et al. 2002; Lang et al. 2004).

19.2.2.3 T-Cell Depletion

Immunomagnetic TCD is technically more demanding than CD34+ enrichment as the processed grafts contain a much higher overall number of cells and even extremely low percentages of contaminating T cells can endanger the success of the manipulation. Moreover, the correct enumeration of T cells in a depleted graft is challenging and needs special protocols.

CD3 Depletion

Depletion of CD3+ T cells provides almost untouched grafts with potential antileukemic effectors (e.g., NK cells) enabling fast engraftment and reliable prevention of GvHD. Prospective phase I/II trials showed low TRM rates after haplo-HSCT in combination with toxicity- and intensity-reduced conditioning regimens in children and adults (Lang et al. 2014; Federmann et al. 2012).

Depletion can be done using the CliniMACS LS tubing set or the DTS tubing set. In both cases the depletion efficacy can be 0.5 log lower than in CD34+ selection. Since in haplo-HSCT residual T cells should not exceed 50×10^3/kg, it might be occasionally necessary to perform a CD34+ selection with parts of the apheresis to remain below the requested thresholds and to guarantee a sufficient number of progenitor cells (Lang et al. 2014; Federmann et al. 2012; Huenecke et al. 2016).

It should be ensured that during the incubation process, all cells come into contact with the CD3 reagent to avoid unstained T cells which can impair the result of the depletion significantly. This may happen when transferring stained cells into a second bag system leaving unstained cells in the tubing ends and crinkles of the bag behind. Even smallest amounts of 20–50 µL can contain more T cells than the whole graft should have.

Analysis of CD3 depleted grafts needs special protocols and has to take into account the rare number of T cells among the huge overall number of cells. Therefore, a multigating strategy should be implemented and validated, and T cells should be determined using several parameters. Exclusion of myeloid cells by CD33 could be helpful as well as the use of CD3 in a bright fluorochrome like APC. Gating can be facilitated by using a "spiked" probe with cells of the negative fraction and a small percentage of cells from the positive fraction added to set the gate for subsequent analysis of the negative fraction. For statistical reasons, a minimum of 1×10^6 events should be acquired. To prevent takeover of cells from a previous tube, special care should be taken like flushing the cannula with water before the actual acquisition or to clean the cannula on the outside (Schumm et al. 2013).

TcRαβ Depletion

This procedure removes αβ + T lymphocytes via a biotinylated anti-TcRαβ Ab followed by an anti-biotin Ab conjugated to magnetic microbeads while retaining both γδ + T lymphocytes and natural killer cells in the graft.

Depletion with the TcRab reagent has been shown to be associated with a high depletion efficacy (4.7 log), better than after CD3 depletion (4.0 log) and similar to CD34+ enrichment (4.6 log). Moreover, the results differ less than those after CD3 depletion, resulting in <50 × 10³/kg infused residual TCRαβ+ T cells, even in small children (Schumm et al. 2013).

Compared to CD34 selected grafts, a faster expansion was seen for CD3+ and for CD56+ in the early phase after haplo-HSCT, probably caused by expansion of co-transfused γδ T cells and NK cells (Lang et al. 2015). Moreover, clinical trials in children and adults demonstrated a very low incidence of acute and chronic GvHD as well as favorable engraftment and TRM rates (Locatelli et al. 2017; Kaynar et al. 2017). The method was successfully used to avoid GvHD also in MUD HSCT (Maschan et al. 2016).

Detection of TcRαβ+ T cells should be done with the same precaution used for CD3 depleted cells, with a minimum of 1×10^6 events and several parameters for the identification of the TcRαβ+ cells. Pregating on CD3-PE vs 7-AAD has been shown to be very helpful as well as gating on TcRαβ and TcRγδ cells in the consecutive dot plot (Schumm et al. 2013).

CD19 Depletion

Depletion of CD19+ B cells can be done together with CD3 or TcRαβ depletion and prevents effectively the occurrence of EBV-associated PTLD. Although the threshold dose of contaminating B cells is still not defined, no cases of PTLD were observed in two multicenter trials with 104 children and adults after infusion of median numbers of 28 and 7×10^3 CD20+ cells/kg BW, respectively (Lang et al. 2014; Federmann et al. 2012).

Alternatively, B-cell depletion can be done in vivo by infusion of therapeutic anti-CD20 mAbs (Locatelli et al. 2017).

Detection of CD19+ B cells needs special attention as the binding of fluorescence-labeled antibody is impaired when cells were preincubated with the CD19 reagent. Therefore, the detection has to be done with an antibody for CD20 which is co-expressed on B cells (Schumm et al. 2006).

Stem Cell Boosts

Poor graft function after HSCT is a relevant complication and is defined as at least bilinear severe cytopenia and/or transfusion requirement, which occurs in a situation of full donor chimerism.

Administration of stem cell boosts from the original donor offers a therapeutic option (Remberger et al. 1998).

To reduce the risk of GvHD, ex vivo TCD procedures as mentioned above are recommended (Olsson et al. 2013). Most experience exists with CD34 selected boosts. Response rates of 80% and a low risk of de novo GvHD between 6% and 22% were observed, even in the case of mismatched donors (Askaa et al. 2014; Mainardi et al. 2018).

19.2.3 DLI and T Cells

T cells may be added to a graft or administered post transplant to provide T cell immunity in various situations. The tolerable dose of T cells varies strongly depending on the HLA disparity, the T cell chimerism in the patient, and the time after transplantation. In MUD HSCT or in haploidentical HSCT, it can be helpful to cryopreserve a number of vials with a defined number of T cells (i.e., 100×10^3 CD3+/kg and 25×10^3 CD3+/kg, respectively) for easy access in case of increasing recipient chimerism.

19.2.3.1 CD45RA Depletion
DLI with CD45RA+-depleted T cells takes advantage of the CD45R0+ T cells which obviously exert little graft-versus-host reaction but can provide antileukemic and antiviral activity. Depletion can be done using the same equipment and reagents for depletion. Depletion is highly effective, and contaminating CD45RA+ cells cannot be found at all (Teschner et al. 2014).

19.2.3.2 DLI in Relapse
DLI has been first used in CML patients after relapse and was given as unmanipulated non-mobilized apheresis in the HLA-matched setting.

19.2.3.3 DLI in Mixed Chimerism
Repetitive DLI can be used to revert a mixed T cell chimerism. Depending on the type of the donor, various cell numbers are employed. In MSD or MUD HSCT, doses between 1×10^5 and 1×10^6/kg are usual, whereas after mismatched or haploidentical HSCT, starting doses of 25×10^3 CD3/kg are recommended (Haines et al. 2015) (and own experience).

19.2.3.4 Virus-Specific T Cells
Virus-specific T cells can be enriched from peripheral blood or an unstimulated apheresis of the original (seropositive) stem cell donor or—if not possible—alternatively from a partially matched third-party donor.

Donor-derived-specific T cells against ADV-, CMV-, or EBV-associated antigens have been already used in many patients suffering from life-threatening infections post transplant, and clinical or virological response rates between 70% and 86% were observed (Icheva et al. 2013; Feucht et al. 2015; Feuchtinger et al. 2010).

The most common technique in the field of graft manipulation is the cytokine capture system which employs the secretion of IFNg after stimulation with appropriate Ag or peptide mixtures for immunomagnetic selection of specific T cells. Simultaneous stimulation with several Ag is possible and generates multispecific T cells.

The selection procedure can be done with a CliniMACS Prodigy® from a maximum of 1×10^9 cells from a non-mobilized or a mobilized apheresis and yields 6–7 ml of cells, with $0.1–2 \times 10^6$ CD3+IFNg+ target cells.

Accompanying debris and dead cells require an accurate analysis. Moreover, the small amount of target cells limits the sample size available for analysis, and therefore a single platform procedure including cell count and viability in one measurement is recommended. The first step should be done without washing and includes a cell gate to exclude debris. CD45 and 7-AAD can be used for proper determination of cell viability. A second sample can be analyzed after washing for CD3+, CD4+, and CD8+ numbers and the percentage of IFNg+ cells in these subsets. Bystander cells like B cells, monocytes, and granulocytes can be found in low numbers (Feuchtinger et al. 2006).

19.3 Regulatory Issues

Graft manipulation is regarded as drug manufacturing in most countries and has to follow the requirements of the EU GMP guidelines, the European Pharmacopoeia, and several EU directives. Therefore clean room areas are required for the manufacturing and a manufacturing license, and a marketing authorization is mandatory for distribution of the product. A quality assurance system has to be implemented, and specifications have to be in place for both raw material and drug product. In most cases, volume, cell number, cell dose, viability, and composition are minimum parameters. Sterility in the form of microbiological examination of cell-based preparations according to Pharm. Eu. 2.6.27 has to be shown either before release of the product or, in the case of limited stability, after release.

Peripheral blood stem cells from both blood and bone marrow for hematopoietic reconstitution are regarded as non-ATMP.

Key Points

- CD34 enrichment yields stem cell preparations with low contaminating T and B cells
- CD3/CD19 depletion preserves large numbers of NK cells in the grafts
- TcR αβ/CD19 depletion provides large numbers of NK cells and γδ T cells with very low amounts of TcRαβ T cells
- DLI with CD45RA-depleted T cells might reduce the risk of GvHD
- Virus antigen-specific donor- or third-party-derived T cells can be utilized post transplant in patients with therapy-refractory viral infections

References

Askaa B, Fischer-Nielsen A, et al. Treatment of poor graft function after allogeneic hematopoietic cell transplantation with a booster of CD34-selected cells infused without conditioning. Bone Marrow Transplant. 2014;49:720–1.

Federmann B, Bornhauser M, Meisner C, et al. Haploidentical allogeneic hematopoietic cell transplantation in adults using CD3/CD19 depletion and reduced intensity conditioning: a phase II study. Haematologica. 2012;97:1523–31.

Feucht J, Opherk K, Lang P, et al. Adoptive T-cell therapy with hexon-specific Th1 cells as a treatment of refractory adenovirus infection after HSCT. Blood. 2015;125:1986–94.

Feuchtinger T, Matthes-Martin S, Richard C, et al. Safe adoptive transfer of virus-specific T-cell immunity for the treatment of systemic adenovirus infection after allogeneic stem cell transplantation. Br J Haematol. 2006;134:64–76.

Feuchtinger T, Opherk K, Bethge WA, et al. Adoptive transfer of pp65-specific T cells for the treatment of chemorefractory cytomegalovirus disease or reactivation after haploidentical and matched unrelated stem cell transplantation. Blood. 2010;116:4360–7.

Haines HL, Bleesing JJ, Davies SM, et al. Outcomes of donor lymphocyte infusion for treatment of mixed donor chimerism after a reduced-intensity preparative regimen for pediatric patients with nonmalignant diseases. Biol Blood Marrow Transplant. 2015;21:288–92.

Handgretinger R, Klingebiel T, Lang P, et al. Megadose transplantation of purified peripheral blood CD34(+) progenitor cells from HLA-mismatched parental donors in children. Bone Marrow Transplant. 2001;27:777–83.

Huenecke S, Bremm M, Cappel C, et al. Optimization of individualized graft composition: CD3/CD19 depletion combined with CD34 selection for haploidentical transplantation. Transfusion. 2016;56:2336–45.

Icheva V, Kayser S, Wolff D, et al. Adoptive transfer of Epstein-Barr virus (EBV) nuclear antigen 1-specific t cells as treatment for EBV reactivation and lymphoproliferative disorders after allogeneic stem-cell transplantation. J Clin Oncol. 2013;31:39–48.

Kaynar L, Demir K, Turak EE, et al. TcRalphabeta-depleted haploidentical transplantation results in adult acute leukemia patients. Hematology. 2017;22:136–44.

Koehl U, Zimmermann S, Esser R, et al. Autologous transplantation of CD133 selected hematopoietic progenitor cells in a pediatric patient with relapsed leukemia. Bone Marrow Transplant. 2002;29:927–30.

Lang P, Bader P, Schumm M, et al. Transplantation of a combination of CD133+ and CD34+ selected progenitor cells from alternative donors. Br J Haematol. 2004;124:72–9.

Lang P, Feuchtinger T, Teltschik HM, et al. Improved immune recovery after transplantation of TCRalphabeta/CD19-depleted allografts from haploidentical donors in pediatric patients. Bone Marrow Transplant. 2015;50(Suppl 2):S6–10.

Lang P, Handgretinger R, Niethammer D, et al. Transplantation of highly purified CD34+ progenitor cells from unrelated donors in pediatric leukemia. Blood. 2003;101:1630–6.

Lang P, Teltschik HM, Feuchtinger T, et al. Transplantation of CD3/CD19 depleted allografts from haploidentical family donors in paediatric leukaemia. Br J Haematol. 2014;165:688–98.

Locatelli F, Merli P, Pagliara D, et al. Outcome of children with acute leukemia given HLA-haploidentical HSCT after alphabeta T-cell and B-cell depletion. Blood. 2017;130:677–85.

Mainardi C, Ebinger M, Enkel S, et al. CD34(+) selected stem cell boosts can improve poor graft function after paediatric allogeneic stem cell transplantation. Br J Haematol. 2018;180:90–9.

Maschan M, Shelikhova L, Ilushina M, et al. TCR-alpha/beta and CD19 depletion and treosulfan-based conditioning regimen in unrelated and haploidentical transplantation in children with acute myeloid leukemia. Bone Marrow Transplant. 2016;51:668–74.

Olsson R, Remberger M, Schaffer M, et al. Graft failure in the modern era of allogeneic hematopoietic SCT. Bone Marrow Transplant. 2013;48:537–43.

Pasquini MC, Devine S, Mendizabal A, et al. Comparative outcomes of donor graft CD34+ selection and immune suppressive therapy as graft-versus-host disease prophylaxis for patients with acute myeloid leukemia in complete remission undergoing HLA-matched sibling allogeneic hematopoietic cell transplantation. J Clin Oncol. 2012;30:3194–201.

Remberger M, Ringden O, Ljungman P, et al. Booster marrow or blood cells for graft failure after allogeneic bone marrow transplantation. Bone Marrow Transplant. 1998;22:73–8.

Ringhoffer M, Wiesneth M, Harsdorf S, et al. CD34 cell selection of peripheral blood progenitor cells using the CliniMACS device for allogeneic transplantation: clinical results in 102 patients. Br J Haematol. 2004;126:527–35.

Rowley SD. Hematopoietic stem cell cryopreservation: a review of current techniques. J Hematother. 1992;1:233–50.

Schumm M, Handgretinger R, Pfeiffer M, et al. Determination of residual T- and B-cell content after immunomagnetic depletion: proposal for flow cytometric analysis and results from 103 separations. Cytotherapy. 2006;8:465–72.

Schumm M, Lang P, Bethge W, et al. Depletion of T-cell receptor alpha/beta and CD19 positive cells from apheresis products with the CliniMACS device. Cytotherapy. 2013;15:1253–8.

Schumm M, Lang P, Taylor G, et al. Isolation of highly purified autologous and allogeneic peripheral CD34+ cells using the CliniMACS device. J Hematother. 1999;8:209–18.

Tamari R, Oran B, Hilden P, et al. Allogeneic stem cell transplantation for advanced myelodysplastic syndrome: comparison of outcomes between CD34(+) selected and unmodified hematopoietic stem cell transplantation. Biol Blood Marrow Transplant. 2018;24:1079–87.

Teschner D, Distler E, Wehler D, et al. Depletion of naive T cells using clinical grade magnetic CD45RA beads: a new approach for GVHD prophylaxis. Bone Marrow Transplant. 2014;49:138–44.

Documentation of Engraftment and Chimerism After HSCT

Peter Bader

20.1 Introduction

It is of central interest to document that the newly developing hematopoiesis post-transplant is of donor or recipient origin. The investigations of the genotype origin of post-transplant hematopoiesis are called chimerism analysis. The term "chimerism" was first introduced into medicine in 1951. Andresen wrote that an organism with cells from two or more distinct zygote lineages is a "chimera." Since 1956 this term was used in field of transplantation (Ford et al. 1956). Chimera refers itself to the Greek mythology where Homer described a fire-spitting monster with the head of a lion, a tail of a serpent, and the body of a goat terrorizing Lycia, a region in Minor Asia.

For a long time, it was believed that complete donor hematopoiesis is necessary to maintain engraftment after allo-HSCT. A few decades ago, it became apparent that donor and recipient hematopoiesis may coexist. This state of coexistence of hematopoietic cells is called mixed chimerism (MC). If all cells are of donor origin, the patient is referred to as "complete chimera," and he shows a "complete chimerism."

It is important to note that the state of hematopoietic chimerism may underlay a certain dynamic. Patients with a complete chimerism may develop a "mixed chimerism" at a later time point or vice versa. In the later patients, the amount of autologous cells may "increase" or "decrease." The patients then develop an "increasing mixed chimerism" or a decreasing mixed chimerism. To avoid misunderstandings as to whether donor or recipient hematopoiesis changes, it is recommended to report "increasing mixed donor chimerism" or "increasing mixed recipient chimerism."

Nowadays, it has become possible to analyze hematopoietic chimerism also in single cell subpopulations. If a patient's hematopoiesis is mixed only in different cell lines, these patients are referred to have a "split chimerism." Finally the applied method for chimerism analysis has also an impact on the degree of chimerism. A patient could be complete chimera with a method detecting about 1% autologous cells, whereas recipient cells could have been detected with a more sensitive technique (Bader et al. 2005).

20.2 Methods for Chimerism Analysis

Different methods have been developed for the assessment of hematopoietic chimerism. All these methods followed the same principle using

P. Bader (✉)
Division for Stem Cell Transplantation and Immunology, University Hospital for Children and Adolescents, Goethe University Frankfurt am Main, Frankfurt, Germany
e-mail: peter.bader@kgu.de

differences in polymorphic genetic markers and their products. Historically restriction fragment length polymorphism (RFLP), cytogenetics, red cell phenotyping, and fluorescence in situ hybridization techniques were used for the assessment of hematopoietic chimerism. All of these techniques have been very time-consuming and did not always offer the possibility to be used in every patient-donor constellation.

Widespread and timely clinical applicability has become possible after polymerase-chain-reaction (PCR) techniques were developed. During the 1990s, these analyses were mainly performed by amplification of variable number of tandem repeats (VNTR). Later in the decade short tandem repeats (STR) were used. Fluorescent labeling of the primers and resolution of PCR products with capillary electrophoresis allowed immediate and accurate quantification of the degree of chimerism. Semiautomated PCR analysis using the appropriate hardware allowed moreover high sample throughput. This made it possible to study chimerism in all patients and in short time intervals already early after transplantation. Accurate monitoring of engraftment as well as surveillance of impending graft rejection in patients transplanted for nonmalignant disease has become possible (McCann and Lawler 1993; Alizadeh et al. 2002; Thiede et al. 2001).

Recently, real-time PCR (rPCR) approaches using single nucleotide polymorphism (SNP) have also become available for the detection of chimerism. SNPs are biallelic variants that differ from each other only at a single nucleotide and occur on average every 1.3 kb in the human genome. This rPCR has an even higher sensitivity compared to STR-PCR assays, but their quantitative accuracy with a variation coefficient of only 30–50% is lower compared to 1–5% of the STR systems.

The latest developments for the detection of chimerism are the analysis using digital PCR (dPCR) procedures. This technology allows accurate and absolute quantification of DNA. This dPCR system is based on deletion/insertion polymorphism (DIP/INDEL) analysis. Clinical studies using this technique, however, are not yet performed (Jacque et al. 2015; Clark et al. 2015).

Based on these issues, the STR-PCR with fluorescent-labeled primers and resolution of the fragments with capillary electrophoresis is currently still considered to be the gold standard for the assessment of post-transplant chimerism. It is important to stress that whatever method is employed to study chimerism, it is important that the procedure is standardized and the chimerism laboratory is accredited and is participating in quality control rounds (Lion et al. 2012).

20.3 Chimerism Investigation in the Clinical Setting

20.3.1 Chimerism in Nonmalignant Diseases

Allo-HSCT is the only curative treatment option for many patients with inherited or acquired nonmalignant diseases such as immunodeficiency, storage diseases, osteopetrosis, thalassemia, sickle cell disease, severe aplastic anemia, bone marrow failure syndromes, and many others.

The aim of the transplant procedure in these diseases is to achieve stable and durable engraftment to (1) improve the hematopoietic function, to (2) correct the immune competence, and/or to (3) increase or normalize the respective enzyme shortage. As a consequence, it is not always necessary to replace the recipient hematopoiesis completely. For many diseases, it is sufficient to implement a state of mixed hematopoietic chimerism to improve the patients' well-being. To minimize toxic side effects intensity of conditioning regimens in these diseases is often reduced and therefore less myeloablative. MC is more likely, and graft rejection or non-engraftment remained the major causes of treatment failures in these patients (Bader et al. 2005; Thiede et al. 2001).

It could be shown that rapid donor cell presence and maintenance of early complete donor chimerism in NK and T cells may play an important role in achieving sustained engraftment especially in patients who were treated with reduced intensity conditioning regimens. Analysis of chimerism in disease characterizing cell subpopulations in patients with nonmalignant disease, e.g., in patients with severe combined immune deficiencies (SCID) or in patients with storages disease, enables the documentation of success of the transplant procedures (Preuner et al. 2016).

20.3.1.1 Intervention to Influence the Evolution of Chimerism: Transfusion of DLI

In patients with nonmalignant diseases, MC occurs frequently. The question whether individual patients with MC are at risk to reject their graft depends on the diagnosis and on the conditioning regimens. Studies have clearly shown that MC can be influenced by DLI. MC can be stabilized or even converted to complete donor chimerism by DLI. However, in treating patients with MC and DLI, physicians have to bear in mind the potential risk to induce GVHD which should be avoided in patients with nonmalignant disease with all efforts.

Hemoglobinopathies

In *thalassemia patients*, large studies have been published already from the Pesaro group of Guido Lucarelli, evaluating the influence of MC and disease recurrence. In general it was found that patients whose recipient MC increased to >30% autologous cells were by far more likely to ultimately reject and be transfusion dependent. However, there are patients with persisting high level MC who remained transfusion independent. Retrospective studies have been performed evaluating the possibility of influencing MC by DLI. It could be shown that a state of MC may be sufficient to remain transfusion independent. It was also shown that DLI is capable to convert MC to CC. However, no general recommendation could be given at the time being (Fitzhugh et al. 2014; Karasu et al. 2012; Abraham et al. 2017).

In *sickle cell disease (SCD)*, the impact of MC has been studied intensively as more and more patients with SCD were transplanted from matched but also from mismatched donors. In the late 1990s, first studies concluded that 10% of donor cell engraftment and persistence were needed for effective treatment of SCD in patients who were treated with a homozygous healthy donor; however, if the patient was grafted with the stem cells of a heterozygous HbAS donor, 30–40% donor cells are required. The presence of MC in patients transplanted for sickle cell disease does not warrant DLI per se. In patients with less than 30% of donor chimerism, DLI might be considered. In a most recent study, Fitzhugh and colleagues developed a mathematical model by which they could show that a donor chimerism in the myeloid compartment of 20% is necessary to reverse the sickle cell phenotype and to prevent patients from disease recurrence (Fitzhugh et al. 2017).

20.3.2 Chimerism in Malignant Diseases

Chimerism detected by molecular methods allows the assessment of persisting or reappearing recipient cells after allo-HSCT. These cells might be a reflection of either survival of malignant cells or of survival or recurrence of recipient hematopoietic cells or a combination of both. It could be shown by prospective studies already in the early 1990s that a MC frequently occurs in the mononuclear cell fraction, weakens thereby the GvL effect, and facilitates recurrence of the underlying leukemia.

Chimerism analysis does provide information about the alloreactivity and/tolerance induction of the graft and thereby serves more likely a "prognostic factor" than as an indirect marker for MRD. It has become evident that the development of post-transplant chimerism is a dynamic process. Hence, if chimerism analyses are performed in the intention to detect impending relapse, investigations need to be performed in short time intervals (Bader et al. 2004b; Thiede et al. 2001; Kröger et al. 2010a, b).

Initially, many pediatric studies using serial analysis of chimerism could clearly demonstrate that patients who develop a MC Post transplant have an increased risk for future relapse of their leukemia. This could later also be confirmed by studies in adult patients.

Moreover these and subsequent studies undoubtedly showed that by immunotherapeutic interventions, e.g., withdrawal of IS or transfusion of DLI, MC could be converted to complete chimerism, GvL effect restored, and many patients prevented from developing overt hematological relapse (Platzbecker et al. 2012; Bader et al. 2004a).

Based on its limited sensitivity to detect minor cell population of about 1%, chimerism analysis in the whole blood is not suitable to serve as a MRD marker. For the assessment of MRD, other techniques should be used, if possible. In patients and diseases lacking a disease-specific marker, for example, regularly in patients with MDS and often in patients with AML, chimerism analysis could be performed in cell subpopulations. Thiede et al. could clearly demonstrate that by the characterization of chimerism in the CD34-positive cell fraction, leukemia relapse could be anticipated in advance in many patients with AML and MDS. In ALL patients, several studies have been performed investigating the impact of MC after enrichment of entity specific subpopulation, e.g., CD 10, CD19, and CD 34 for precursor B ALL and CD3, CD4, CD5, and CD8 for T-lineages. Remarkable correlation between MRD and chimerism in different subsets could be proven (Platzbecker et al. 2012; Bornhäuser et al. 2009; Rettinger et al. 2011).

Serial and quantitative analysis of chimerism allows the identification of patients at highest risk for relapse. Not all patients can be identified, and time interval between the onset of MS and relapse is often short. It is essential to perform the analysis frequently and ideally: chimerism should be combined with MRD analysis to optimize the predictive value. These investigations can form the basis for individual preemptive immunotherapy strategies to prevent recurrence of the underlying disease.

Key Points

- Documentation of engraftment is the important step on the way to successful HSCT
- Post-transplant patients are carrying two different genetic profiles and are called chimera
- Analysis of hematopoietic chimerism offers the possibility to realize impending graft rejection and may also serve as an indicator for the recurrence of the underlying disease
- Since several years, these investigations have become the basis for intervention strategies to:
  - Avoid graft rejection
  - Maintain engraftment
  - To treat imminent relapse by preemptive immunotherapy

References

Abraham A, Hsieh M, Eapen M, et al. Relationship between mixed donor-recipient chimerism and disease recurrence after hematopoietic cell transplantation for sickle cell disease. Biol Blood Marrow Transplant. 2017;23:2178–83.

Alizadeh M, Bernard M, Danic B, et al. Quantitative assessment of hematopoietic chimerism after bone marrow transplantation by real-time quantitative polymerase chain reaction. Blood. 2002;99:4618–25.

Bader P, Kreyenberg H, Hoelle W, et al. Increasing mixed chimerism is an important prognostic factor for unfavorable outcome in children with acute lymphoblastic leukemia after allogeneic stem-cell transplantation: possible role for immuno-therapy. J Clin Oncol. 2004a;22:1696–705.

Bader P, Kreyenberg H, Hoelle W, et al. Increasing mixed chimerism defines a high-risk group of childhood acute myelogenous leukemia patients after allogeneic stem cell transplantation where pre-emptive immunotherapy may be effective. Bone Marrow Transplant. 2004b;33:815–21.

Bader P, Niethammer D, Willasch A, et al. How and when should we monitor chimerism after allogeneic stem cell transplantation? Bone Marrow Transplant. 2005;35:107–19.

Bornhäuser M, Oelschlaegel U, Platzbecker U, et al. Monitoring of donor chimerism in sorted CD34+ peripheral blood cells allows the sensitive detection of imminent relapse after allogeneic stem cell transplantation. Haematologica. 2009;94:1613–7.

Clark JR, Scott SD, Jack AL, et al. Monitoring of chimerism following allogeneic haematopoietic stem cell transplantation (HSCT). Br J Haematol. 2015;168:26–37.

Fitzhugh CD, Abraham A, Hsieh MM. Alternative donor/unrelated donor transplants for the β-thalassemia and sickle cell disease. Adv Exp Med Biol. 2017;1013:123–53.

Fitzhugh CD, Abraham AA, Tisdale JF, et al. Hematopoietic stem cell transplantation for patients with sickle cell disease. Hematol Oncol Clin North Am. 2014;28:1171–85.

Ford CE, Hamerton JL, Barnes DW, et al. Cytological identification of radiation-chimaeras. Nature. 1956;177:452–4.

Jacque N, Nguyen S, Golmard J-L, et al. Chimerism analysis in peripheral blood using indel quantitative real-time PCR is a useful tool to predict post-transplant relapse in acute leukemia. Bone Marrow Transplant. 2015;50:259–65.

Karasu GT, Yesilipek MA, Karauzum SB, et al. The value of donor lymphocyte infusions in thalassemia patients at imminent risk of graft rejection following stem cell transplantation. Pediatr Blood Cancer. 2012;58:453–8.

Kröger N, Bacher U, Bader P, et al. NCI first international workshop on the biology, prevention, and treatment of relapse after allogeneic hematopoietic stem cell transplantation. Biol Blood Marrow Transplant. 2010a;16:1325–46.

Kröger N, Bacher U, Bader P, et al. NCI first international workshop on the biology, prevention, and treatment of relapse after allogeneic hematopoietic stem cell transplantation. Biol Blood Marrow Transplant. 2010b;16:1187–211.

Lion T, Watzinger F, Preuner S, et al. The EuroChimerism concept for a standardized approach to chimerism analysis after allogeneic stem cell transplantation. Leukemia. 2012;26:1821–8.

McCann SR, Lawler M. Mixed chimaerism; detection and significance following BMT. Bone Marrow Transplant. 1993;11:91–4.

Platzbecker U, Wermke M, Radke J, et al. Azacitidine for treatment of imminent relapse in MDS or AML patients after allogeneic HSCT. Leukemia. 2012;26:381–9.

Preuner S, Peters C, Pötschger U, et al. Risk assessment of relapse by lineage-specific monitoring of chimerism in children undergoing allogeneic stem cell transplantation for acute lymphoblastic leukemia. Haematologica. 2016;101:741–6.

Rettinger E, Willasch AM, Kreyenberg H, et al. Preemptive immunotherapy in childhood acute myeloid leukemia for patients showing evidence of mixed chimerism after allogeneic stem cell transplantation. Blood. 2011;118:5681–8.

Thiede C, Bornhäuser M, Oelschlägel U, et al. Sequential monitoring of chimerism and detection of minimal residual disease after allogeneic blood stem cell transplantation (BSCT) using multiplex PCR amplification of short tandem repeat-markers. Leukemia. 2001;15:293–302.

Short- and Long-Term Controls After HSCT

Montserrat Rovira and Maria Suárez-Lledó

21.1 Introduction

Patients undergoing HSCT (mainly allo-HSCT) have a risk of developing complications related to pre-, peri-, and post-HSCT. The resulting morbidity of the HSCT process makes it necessary for patients to adopt a healthy lifestyle that promotes health and contemplate preventive measures for the detection and treatment of possible complications.

The short- and long-term controls allow for regular and systematic screening and at the same time are an opportunity to give advice on healthy lifestyle habits. Monitoring should be multidisciplinary with involvement of hematology, other medical specialties, physicians of primary care, nursing, and mental health professionals.

Early and late complications, as well as psychological problems, are discussed in Parts IV, V and VI of the Handbook.

After discharge, it is important that the patient has a summary of the treatment received and a long-term follow-up plan appropriate to the exposure and individual risk factors.

The recommendations related to screening and prevention post-HSCT can be consulted in several web pages (see references).

M. Rovira (✉) · M. Suárez-Lledó
HSCT Unit, Hematology Department, Hospital Clínic de Barcelona, University of Barcelona,
Barcelona, Catalunya, Spain
e-mail: mrovira@clinic.cat

21.2 Monitoring Depending on the Type of HSCT

21.2.1 Autologous HSCT

Timing	Monitoring
From discharge to day +100	Until full hematologic recovery, it is recommended to live near the hospital Recommended controls[a]: – Clinical evaluation and transfusions when necessary – Basic hematological and biochemical tests – Specific markers for different diseases
At +3 months	Evaluate the status of the primary disease Recommended controls[a]: – Hematological and biochemical tests, specific tumoral markers – MRD evaluation: Immunophenotype and molecular specific adapted to each disease – BM biopsy in case of NHL, HL, MPS, and solid neoplasms with previous marrow affectation, in the remaining disease BM smears (see specific chapters) – Imaging tests depending on primary disease
Long term	Visits every 6 months up to 2 years and then annually Recommended controls[a]: – Analytical and complementary explorations: See Table 21.1 – Baseline disease: Control of possible progression or relapse during at least 5 years – In patients treated with chemotherapy + radiotherapy, assess the risk of second malignancies or MDS after HSCT

[a]Variable frequency depending on the patient's condition

21.2.2 Allogeneic HSCT

Timing	Monitoring
From discharge to day +100	It is recommended that the patient resides near the transplant center during the first 3–6 months after HSCT Recommended controls[a]: – Weekly clinical evaluation, during the first month, every other week until 2 m, and then monthly up to 6–12 m, unless problems arise. It must include complete physical examination, with special emphasis on data of acute GvHD, infections, and pulmonary complications – Blood samples: Complete blood count, liver and kidney function, Mg, levels of IS agents, quantify CMV by PCR (and EBV if ATG); chimerism evaluation at 1 month – BM aspirate (or biopsy) in diseases with previous marrow affectation (usually within 1 month of HSCT)
At 3 months	Usually, this moment marks the turning point so that, if the patient does not have major problems, he/she can be monitored by the referring doctor. However, the patient should be periodically reevaluated at the transplant center (every 3–4 months during the first year, every 4–6 months during the second year, and annually after the third year) Recommended controls[a]: – Visit and complete physical exploration with special emphasis on the signs of acute and chronic GvHD (assessment by organs as indicated in Chaps. 43 and 44 and paragraph 21.3) – Blood test: Complete blood count, kidney function, liver function, clearance creatinine, IS levels; chimerism and sample for MRD follow-up. In patients aged <17 years, weight and height every 3 months
Long term	It depends on the complications that arise during follow-up. If there are no complications, it is recommended that a patient visits to the center every 6 months up to 3 years and annually thereafter Recommended controls: – Visit and complete physical examination including gynecological evaluation and endocrinological, if appropriate – Analytical and complementary explorations: See Sect. 21.3 – Specific controls: Specific MRD studies on diseases with markers (see corresponding chapters) – In patients treated with chemotherapy + radiotherapy, the risk of secondary neoplasms

[a]Variable frequency depending on the patient's condition

21.3 Organ-Specific Long-Term Monitoring

Table 21.1 analyzes organ by organ the long-term follow-up recommendations.

Table 21.1 Organ-specific monitoring[a]

Recommended screening[b]	6 months	1 year	An.	Comments
Ocular (see Chap. 48)				
– Clinical symptom evaluation	1	1	1	– Immediate exam if visual symptoms
– Visual acuity and fundus exam	+	1	+	– Special attention to *sicca* syndrome
Oral (Chap. 50)				
– Preventive oral health and dental maintenance	1	1	1	– Avoid smoking, sugar beverages, or oral piercing
– Clinical assessment	1	1	1	– If oral cGvHD, high-risk squamous cell cancer; evaluation every 6 months
– Dental assessment (+children)	+	1	1	
Respiratory (Chap. 52)				
– Clinical pulmonary assessment	1	1	1	* Active or passive
– Smoking tobacco avoidance*	1	1	1	– If cGVHD, spirometry test in each control (recommended for many authors)
– PFT (+chest Rx if symptoms)	+	+	+	
Cardiac and vascular[c] (Chap. 55)				
– CV risk factor assessment	+	1	1	– Counseling on heart healthy lifestyle – Active treatment of risk factors
Liver (Chaps. 38 and 49)				
– Liver function testing	1	1	1	– Monitor viral load by PCR if HCV or HBV
– Serum ferritin testing		1	+	– Additional testing if high ferritin levels (MRI/FerriScan®)
Kidney (Chap. 51)				
– Blood pressure screening	1	1	1	– Hypertension should be investigated and treated appropriately
– Urine protein screening	1	1	1	
– BUN/creatinine testing	1	1	1	– Avoid nephrotoxins
Muscle and connective (Chap. 54)				
– Physical activity counseling	1	1	1	– If risk of cGvHD, test joint mobility and touch skin to detect sclerotic changes
– Evaluation muscle weakness	2	2	2	– Treat cramps symptomatically
Skeletal (Chap. 54)				
– Bone density testing[d]		1	+	– Prevent bone loss and fractures with exercise, vitamin D, and calcium
Nervous system (Chap. 53)				
– Neurologic clinical evaluation	+	1	1	* Special attention of cognitive development in pediatric patients
– Cognitive development*		1	1	
Endocrine (Chap. 56)				
– Thyroid function testing		1	1	– Annual gynecological evaluation in women
– Growth speed in children		1	1	– Hormonal replacement if necessary
– Gonadal function assessment[e]	1	1	1	
– Gonadal function assessment[f]		1	+	
– Gonadal function assessment[g]		+	+	

Table 21.1 (continued)

Recommended screening[b]	6 months	1 year	An.	Comments
Mucocutaneous (Chap. 54)				
– Skin self-exam, sun counseling	1	1	1	– Avoid sunlight without adequate protection
– Gynecological exam in women		1	1	
Immunity				
– Encapsulated Microorg. Prophylaxis*	2	2	2	* If chronic GvHD and IS therapy, consider
– PJP prophylaxis (see Chap. 39)	1	2	2	endocarditis prophylaxis in high-risk patients
– Immunizations (see Chap. 29)	1	1	1	
Secondary neoplasia (Chap. 47)				
– Counseling and autoexamination		1	1	– Reduce UV skin exposure
– Same population screening		1	1	– Special attention to high-risk organs
				– If TBI, increase frequency mammography
Psychosocial and sexual				
– Psychosocial assessment (see Chap. 30)	1	1	1	– Add spousal/caregiver psychological
– QOL assessment (see Chap. 34)	1	1	1	adjustment and family functioning
– Evaluation of Sexual function	1	1	1	

An. annually, *1* recommended for all transplant recipients, *2* recommended for patients with ongoing chronic GvHD or IS, + reassessment recommended for abnormal testing in a previous time period or for new signs/symptoms
[a]Adapted from Majhail et al. (2012). Similar recommendations but focused in children have been elaborated by the Children's Oncology Group http://www.survivorshipguidelines.org
[b]In patients with chronic GVHD, these controls should be tightened, and their frequency increased
[c]Follow the American Heart Association for endocarditis prophylaxis in high-risk HSCT recipients
[d]Adult women, all allo-HSCT, and patients at high risk for bone loss
[e]Prepubertal men and women
[f]Postpubertal women
[g]Postpubertal men

21.4 Fertility (See Chap. 56)

21.5 Quality of Life (See Chap. 34)

- Monitoring should be multidisciplinary with involvement of hematology, other medical specialties, physicians of primary care, nursing, and mental health professionals

Key Points

- Patients auto- and mainly allo-HSCT have a risk of developing complications related to pre-, peri-, and post-HSCT
- The resulting morbidity of the HSCT process makes it necessary for patients to adopt a healthy lifestyle that promotes health and contemplate preventive measures for the detection and treatment of possible complications
- The short- and long-term controls allow for regular and systematic screening and at the same time are an opportunity to give advice on healthy lifestyle habits

Recommended References

DeFilipp Z, Duarte RF, Snowden JA, et al. Metabolic syndrome and cardiovascular disease after hematopoietic cell transplantation: screening and preventive practice recommendations from the CIBMTR and EBMT. Biol Blood Marrow Transplant. 2016;22:1493–503.

Dietz AC, Mehta PA, Vlachos A, et al. Current knowledge and priorities for future research in late effects after hematopoietic cell transplantation for inherited bone marrow failure syndromes: consensus statement from the Second Pediatric Blood and Marrow Transplant Consortium International Conference on Late Effects after Pediatric Hematopoietic Cell Transplantation. Biol Blood Marrow Transplant. 2017;23:726–35.

Dyer G, Gilroy N, Bradford J, et al. A survey of fertility and sexual health following allogeneic haematopoietic stem cell transplantation in New South Wales, Australia. Br J Haematol. 2016;172:592–601.

Elad S, Raber-Durlacher JE, Brennan MT, et al. Basic oral care for hematology-oncology patients and hematopoietic stem cell transplantation recipients: a position paper from the joint task force of the Multinational Association of Supportive Care in Cancer/International Society of Oral Oncology (MASCC/ISOO) and the EBMT. Support Care Cancer. 2015;23:223–36.

Fred Hutchinson Cancer Research Center/Seattle Cancer Care Alliance Version June 03, 2015. Long-Term Follow-Up After Hematopoietic Stem Cell Transplant General Guidelines For Referring Physicians.

Heimall J, Buckley RH, Puck J, et al. Recommendations for screening and management of late effects in patients with severe combined immunodeficiency after allogenic hematopoietic cell transplantation: a consensus statement from the Second Pediatric Blood and Marrow Transplant Consortium International Conference on Late Effects after Pediatric HCT. Biol Blood Marrow Transplant. 2017;23:1229–40.

Inamoto Y, Shah NN, Savani BN, et al. Secondary solid cancer screening following hematopoietic cell transplantation. Bone Marrow Transplant. 2015;50:1013–23.

Majhail NS, Rizzo JD, Lee SJ, et al. Recommended screening and preventive practices for long-term survivors after hematopoietic cell transplantation. Biol Blood Marrow Transplant. 2012;18:348–71.

National Marrow Donor Program Guidelines.: www.BeTheMatch.org/md-guidelines. For patients: www.BeTheMatch.org/Patient; For Pediatric patients: www.survivorshipguidelines.org.

Parsons SK, Tighiouart H, Terrin N. Assessment of health-related quality of life in pediatric hematopoietic stem cell transplant recipients: progress, challenges and future directions. Expert Rev Pharmacoecon Outcomes Res. 2013;13:217–25.

Persoon S, Kersten MJ, van der Weiden K, et al. Effects of exercise in patients treated with stem cell transplantation for a hematologic malignancy: a systematic review and meta-analysis. Cancer Treat Rev. 2013;39:682–90.

Shenoy S, Gaziev J, Angelucci E, et al. Late effects screening guidelines after Hematopoietic Cell Transplantation (HCT) for hemoglobinopathy: consensus statement from the Second Pediatric Blood and Marrow Transplant Consortium International Conference on Late Effects after Pediatric HCT. Biol Blood Marrow Transplant. 2018;24(7):1313–21.

Tichelli A, Rovó A. Survivorship after allogeneic transplantation-management recommendations for the primary care provider. Curr Hematol Malig Rep. 2015;10:35–44.

Part IV
General Management of the Patient

Topic leaders: Carlo Dufour, Silvia Montoto and John Murray

Vascular Access

Simone Cesaro and Federica Minniti

22.1 Introduction

The central venous catheter (CVC) is a key tool for patients undergoing a HSCT, and its introduction in the oncology setting has represented a clear improvement in the quality of patient health care. The use of a CVC requires correct maintenance to prevent malfunctioning due to partial or complete occlusion, dislodgement, kinking, rupture, thrombosis, or life-threatening complications such as catheter-related bloodstream infections (CRBSI).

CVCs are being designated by:

- Duration (e.g., temporary or short-term versus permanent or long-term)
- Site of insertion (e.g., subclavian vein, femoral vein, jugular vein, basilic vein)
- Number of lumens (single, double, or triple lumen)
- Characteristic of tip (open tip or closed tip)
- Materials to reduce complications (e.g., impregnation with heparin, antibiotics, or silver)

S. Cesaro (✉)
Pediatric Hematology Oncology, Azienda
Ospedaliera Universitaria Integrata, Verona, Italy
e-mail: simone.cesaro@aovr.veneto.it

F. Minniti
Mother and Child Department, Ospedale della Donna
e del Bambino, University of Verona, Verona, Italy

Table 22.1 shows the main maintenance actions for CVC (Cesaro et al. 2016).

Table 22.1 CVC maintenance: suggested main rules

1. Assessment of line functionality and dressing site daily for inpatients or every 2–3 days for outpatients
2. CVC care and maintenance as dictated by local policy or standard operating procedure[a]
3. Vigorous mechanical scrub for manual disinfection prior to each CVC access and allow it to dry. Acceptable disinfecting agents include 70% isopropyl alcohol, iodophors (i.e., povidone-iodine), or >0.5% chlorhexidine in alcohol solution
4. Change gauze dressing every 7 days or before in case of soiled, dampened, and loosened
5. Change the transfusion administration set and filter after the completion of each unit or every 4 h. If more than 1 unit can be infused in 4 h, the transfusion set can be used for a 4-h period
6. Change intermittent administration sets every 24 h
7. Replace administration sets for parenteral nutrition solutions at least every 24 h
8. Replace administration sets used for intravenous fat emulsions infused separately every 12 h
9. Change caps every 72 h (or 7 days if pressure-positive device is used)

[a]There may be a variability among EBMT centers regarding the practice of CVC care and maintenance such as the use of sterile gloves and mask by provider/assistant, the adoption of aseptic technique for all catheter entries, the use of prepackaged dressing change kit, the frequency of flushing, and the type of solution used for flushing CVC

22.2 Type of CVC Materials

Catheter materials should be biocompatible, kink resistant, inherently chemically resistant and neutral, biostable, soft, and deformable and should have a high tensile strength (Lim et al. 2018; Frasca et al. 2010). The most commonly used materials are polyurethane, polyethylene and polytetrafluoroethylene (Teflon), polyvinyl-chloride (PVC), silicone, and Vialon (Borretta et al. 2018). Silicone catheters are flexible, chemically stable, and well tolerated. Polyurethane catheters are preferred to those made of polyethylene or PVC because of their lower rate of CRBSI and their lower friability (Frasca et al. 2010). Polytetrafluoroethylene catheters are rigid and lose X-ray transparency when injected with opaque solutions. Polyurethane has a superior tensile strength.

Non-tunneled, semirigid catheters are usually made of polyurethane, while tunneled catheters are usually made of both silicone and polyurethane (Lim et al. 2018). The superiority of polyurethane catheters compared with silicone is debated. The two catheter types have no difference in surface degradation; however, silicone catheters are more prone to material failure as a result of the development of surface irregularities due to loss of barium sulfate molecules and thrombotic occlusion. Conversely, polyurethane catheters have a higher susceptibility for catheter-induced venous thrombosis and CRBSI (Blanco-Guzman 2018; Wildgruber et al. 2016).

22.3 Type of CVC

CVCs are classified in two main categories: *tunneled and non-tunneled*, according to whether or not they follow a subcutaneous route before accessing the central vein. Non-tunneled catheters are directly inserted into a peripheral or large central vein. Both tunneled and non-tunneled CVCs may have a single or multiple lumen. Tunnelization of CVCs was introduced to reduce the risk of infectious and mechanical (dislodgement) complications, and this type of CVC is ideal for long-term care (Cesaro et al. 2009).

Non-tunneled CVCs are usually inserted for a short to medium period (from 2–4 weeks to 1–3 months) (Lee and Ramaswamy 2018; Padmanabhan 2018). Tunneled CVCs are in turn classifiable in two subgroups: partially implanted and totally implanted. Partially implanted CVCs are characterized by an external part outside the patient's body whose extremity (hub) is used to draw blood sampling or to connect the infusion lines, a tunneled subcutaneous part with a Dacron cuff at a few centimeters from the skin entry point, and a final intravenous part with the tip positioned at the border between the superior vena cava and the right atrium (Padmanabhan 2018; Blanco-Guzman 2018). The Dacron cuff stimulates a fibrotic reaction of the subcutaneous tissues over 2–4 weeks ensuring stability and CVC securement. Both cuff and subcutaneous course are fundamental to prevent the CVC from becoming infected due to the migration of external microbes along the CVC. Broviac, Hickman, and Groshong CVCs belong to this group. Broviac-Hickman CVCs have an open tip and require the clamping of the external part of the CVC when they are not in use to avoid the backflow of the blood from the tip with breath or body movements. Groshong CVCs have a closed tip with lateral valves on their terminal part that open as fluid is withdrawn or infused, while they remain closed when the CVC is not in use. The CVC has to be clamped only if the catheter does not have a needle-free connector. The ideal situation to avoid backflow of blood is a neutral pressure needle-free connector with an open clamp (Padmanabhan 2018).

Totally implanted catheters (porth) consist of a reservoir (port) placed in a pocket in the subcutaneous tissue anteriorly on the chest wall, below the clavicle, that is connected to the catheter (Padmanabhan 2018; Blanco-Guzman 2018). This type of CVC has no part outside of the body, thus preserving the patient's body image and ensuring almost no limitations on sports activities, and body hygiene. The main drawback of this type of CVC is that its accessing needs a skin puncture with a special "non-coring" needle (Huber needle or gripper system). In case of frequently repeated port accesses, the procedure can be painful or discomforting for the patient, requiring the application of topical skin anesthetics for its prevention. Moreover, the needle does not permit the infusion or the extraction of high volumes making it less suitable for patients requiring high infusion or blood extraction rates. The recent introduction of port models with a modified reservoir chamber (vortex, tidal, power port) has allowed to obtain a higher flow rate suitable for leukapheresis, red blood cell exchange, extracorporeal photopheresis, and therapeutic plasma exchange (Blanco-Guzman 2018; Lim et al. 2018).

The *peripherally inserted central catheter (PICC)* is a CVC inserted into a vein of the arm, usually the basilic or cephalic veins; its tip is advanced through the axillary and subclavian veins up to the cavoatrial junction (Hashimoto et al. 2017; Cornillon et al. 2017). For more information on PICCs, see Chap. 32.

22.4   Venous Access

Central lines are usually inserted through the subclavian, the jugular, or, less frequently, the femoral vein. This last venous access is associated with a higher risk of infectious complications (O'Leary 2016), and it is more commonly used in critically ill patients admitted to intensive care units who require a non-tunneled CVC. Using the subclavian or jugular access, the tip of the catheter has to lie in the superior vena cava, just before the entrance of the right atrium, about 29–55 mm below the level of trachea carina (in adults). The incidence of pneumothorax after CVC insertion is about 1.5–3.1%, and it is higher with subclavian vein catheterization, whereas the risk of hemorrhage and bruise is slightly more common with the jugular venous line access.

In the positioning of a PICC, the incannulation of the basilic vein is preferred to that of the cephalic vein as it has low risk of complications. To minimize the risk of complications due to venous catheterizations, the routine use of ultrasound guidance to cannulate the vein is recommended instead of the classical (blind) technique (Cornillon et al. 2017; Crocoli et al. 2015).

A chest X-ray must be performed at the end of the CVC insertion procedure to confirm that the line is positioned inside the superior vena cava and, for the cannulation of subclavian or jugular veins, no pneumothorax was inadvertently caused. Recently, the use of intracavitary ECG (electrocardiographic method) has also been approved for clinical use to evaluate the correct position of the catheter tip (Borretta et al. 2018).

22.5   CVC Complications

Catheter-related complications may be classified into *infectious* (local or systemic) and *mechanical* (occlusion, rupture, dislodgement, accidental self-removal, and thrombosis) (Cesaro et al. 2009). As the catheter is itself a risk for developing complications, when there is no further need for a catheter, it should be removed. Removal of the catheter must also be considered in the event of catheter dysfunction; CRBSI by *Candida* spp., *Pseudomonas* spp., *Klebsiella* spp., and *Staphylococcus aureus*; persistent bacteria colonization or recurrent CRBSI; or contraindications against anticoagulant therapy.

22.5.1 Special Measures to Prevent Catheter-Related Infections

The key rules to prevent infections are proper handwashing by the performing provider, the use of aseptic technique over the patient at insertion time, thorough cleaning of the insertion site, and periodic review of the CVC exit site (Cesaro et al. 2016). Impregnation of the CVC with heparin may reduce the incidence of infectious and thrombotic complications. To prevent CRBSI and tunnel or exit-site infection, medication-impregnated dressings with different antimicrobial materials were developed to decrease the production of the biofilm by microorganisms and decrease the adhesion of them to the catheter walls. The most commonly used impregnating medications are chlorhexidine gluconate, silver sulfadiazine, rifampin, and minocycline (Frasca et al. 2010). Chlorhexidine gluconate impregnates the whole dressing or is applied using an impregnated sponge (e.g., Biopatch®) and covered by a transparent polyurethane semipermeable transparent dressing (Ullman 2015).

22.6 Catheters for Leukapheresis

The procedure of stem cell collection by apheresis is performed both for auto- and allo-HSCT to obtain PBSC (O'Leary 2016). As the procedure requires sustained high blood flow rates (50–100 mL/min), an adequate venous access is needed (O'Leary 2016). Peripheral access placed in the basilic, cephalic, brachial, median cubital and radial veins is recommended (Padmanabhan 2018; Lim et al. 2018; Hölig et al. 2012). Considering that the placement of a central CVC is associated with potentially life-threatening complications such as pneumothorax, bleeding, and embolism (Hölig et al. 2012), its use is not recommended for PBSC collection of a healthy volunteer donor. Conversely, in the case of auto-PBSC, if the patient has no adequate peripheral or central venous access, a temporary non-tunneled CVC may be placed in the internal jugular, subclavian, or femoral veins (Padmanabhan 2018; Lim et al. 2018; Vacca et al. 2014; Hölig et al. 2012; Cooling 2017a). Catheter removal is performed on donor laboratory values (PLT >50 × 10^9/L) or after the assessment of an adequate CD34+ dose and successful cryopreservation of the HPC product (O'Leary 2016; Vacca et al. 2014).

Partially implanted silicone CVCs are often used by pediatric oncologists-hematologists because they are most suitable for long-term complex treatment (Wildgruber et al. 2016). In the case of leukapheresis procedure, silicone CVCs are not ideal because they are more prone to collapse during automatic apheresis (Ridyard et al. 2017). On the other hand, the harvesting procedure of PBSC, which requires high blood flow rates and a large needle, may be difficult in children below 10 kg using a temporary peripheral venous access due to the small size of veins (Padmanabhan 2018; Cesaro et al. 2016). In this case, the placement of a short-term CVC made of

polyurethane may be needed (Cooling 2017a, b). However, in younger children, the rigidity of such material and the narrower lumens of the veins may represent a potential risk for thrombosis and infection (Ridyard et al. 2017; Cooling 2017b; Vacca et al. 2014).

Key Points

CVC indications and insertion

1. Type of CVC	Tunneled CVCs/Port/ PICCs	Long-term therapy (months, years) Port for intermittent use, tunneled CVC for continuous use Suitable for inpatient and outpatient
	Non-tunneled CVCs	Short-term therapy (2–4 weeks, 1–3 months) Suitable for inpatient
2. Number of lumens	Single lumen vs Double lumen	Double lumen in patients undergoing HSCT, critically ill patients, intensive intravenous therapy
3. Insertion	Percutaneous/ minimally invasive	Ultrasound guidance recommended Adequate training required
	Cutdown approach	Very limited indication (premature infants) Experienced operator
4. Material	Silicone	Tunneled CVC
	Polyurethane	Tunneled and non-tunneled CVC

References

Blanco-Guzman MO. Implanted vascular access device options: a focus review on safety and outcomes. Transfusion. 2018;58:558–68.

Borretta L, MacDonald T, Digout C, et al. Peripherally inserted central catheters in pediatric oncology patients: a 15-year population-based review from Maritimes, Canada. J Pediatr Hematol Oncol. 2018;40:e55–60.

Cesaro S, Cavaliere M, Pegoraro A, et al. A comprehensive approach to the prevention of central venous catheter complications: results of 10-year prospective surveillance in pediatric hematology-oncology patients. Ann Hematol. 2016;95:817–25.

Cesaro S, Tridello G, Cavaliere M, et al. Prospective, randomized trial of two different modalities of flushing central venous catheters in pediatric patients with cancer. J Clin Oncol. 2009;27:2059–65.

Cooling L. Performance and safety of femoral central venous catheters in pediatric autologous peripheral blood stem cell collection. J Clin Apher. 2017a;32:501–16.

Cooling L. Procedure-related complications and adverse events associated with pediatric autologous peripheral blood stem cell collection. J Clin Apher. 2017b;32:35–48.

Cornillon J, Martignoles JA, Tavernier-Tardy E, et al. Prospective evaluation of systematic use of peripherally inserted central catheters (PICC lines) for the home care after allogenic hematopoietic stem cells transplantation. Support Care Cancer. 2017;25:2843–7.

Crocoli A, Tornesello A, Pittiruti M,. et al. Central venous access devices in pediatric malignancies: a position paper of Italian Association of Pediatric Hematology and Oncology. J Vasc Access. 2015;16(2):130–6.

Frasca D, Dahyot-Fizelier C, Mimoz O. Prevention of central venous catheter-related infection in the intensive care unit. Crit Care. 2010;14:212.

Hashimoto Y, Fukuta T, Maruyama J, et al. Experience of peripherally inserted central venous catheter in patients with hematologic disease. Intern Med. 2017;56:389–93.

Hölig K, Blechschmidt M, Kramer M, et al. Peripheral blood stem cell collection in allogeneic donors: impact of venous access. Transfusion. 2012;52(12): 2600–5.

Lee K, Ramaswamy RS. Intravascular access devices from an interventional radiology perspective: indications, implantation techniques, and optimizing patency. Transfusion. 2018;58(Suppl 1):549–57.

Lim HS, Kim SM, Kang DW. Implantable vascular access devices–past, present and future. Transfusion. 2018;58:545–8.

O'Leary MF. Venous access for hematopoietic progenitor cell collection: an international survey by the ASFA HPC donor subcommittee. J Clin Apher. 2016;31(6):529–34.

Padmanabhan A. Cellular collection by apheresis. Transfusion. 2018;58:598–604.

Ridyard CH, Plumpton CO, Gilbert RE, Hughes DA. Cost effectiveness of pediatric central venous catheters in the UK: a secondary publication from the CATCH clinical trial. Front Pharmacol. 2017;8:644.

Ullman AJ, Cooke ML, Mitchell M, et al., Dressings and securement devices for central venous catheters (CVC). Cochrane Database Syst Rev. 2015;(9):CD010367.

Vacca M, Perseghin P, Accorsi P, et al. Central venous catheter insertion in peripheral blood hematopoietic stem cell sibling donors: the SIdEM (Italian Society of Hemapheresis and Cell Manipulation) point of view. Transfus Apher Sci. 2014;50:200–6.

Wildgruber M, Lueg C, Borgmeyer S, et al. Polyurethane versus silicone catheters for central venous port devices implanted at the forearm. Eur J Cancer. 2016;59:113–24.

Transfusion Support

Hubert Schrezenmeier, Sixten Körper,
Britta Höchsmann, and Christof Weinstock

23.1 General Aspects

Transfusions are an essential part of supportive care in the context of HSCT. RBC and platelet concentrates (PCs) are the main blood products transfused in the peri-transplant period. Many recommendations in this chapter are based on evidence from studies including a broad variety of diseases. Only a few studies addressed transfusion strategy specifically in patients undergoing HSCT (see review Christou et al. 2016). Many recommendations are derived from patients with cytopenia in non-transplant settings. There are both need and opportunity to address issues regarding transfusion of HSCT patients in clinical trials. So far, there is a paucity of studies on the impact of transfusion on HSCT-specific outcomes.

RBC, PC, and FFP for patients who are candidates for HSCT should be leukocyte-reduced, i.e., should contain $<1 \times 10^6$ leukocytes/unit. Leukocyte reduction reduces febrile non-hemolytic transfusion reactions and decreases the incidence of alloimmunization to leukocyte antigens and the risk of CMV transmission. Also all cellular blood components (RBC, PC, granulocyte transfusions) must be irradiated (see below).

23.2 Irradiation for Prevention of Transfusion-Associated GvHD (ta-GvHD)

Ta-GvHD is a rare complication of transfusion wherein viable donor T lymphocytes in cellular blood products mount an immune response against the recipient (Kopolovic et al. 2015). Some of the clinical presentations of ta-GvHD resemble that of GvHD (fever, cutaneous eruption, diarrhea, liver function abnormalities). Also many patients develop pancytopenia. Since mortality is high (>90%), prevention of ta-GvHD is critical (Kopolovic et al. 2015). HSCT recipients are at risk of ta-GvHD and should receive irradiated cellular blood products (Kopolovic et al. 2015). It is recommended that no part of the component receives a dose <25 Gy and >50 Gy (European Committee (Partial Agreement) on Blood Transfusion (CD-P-TS) 2017). Some pathogen-reduction technologies have been shown to inactivate lymphocytes, and additional gamma-irradiation is not required (Cid 2017).

There is no consensus on the duration of the use of irradiated blood products in HSCT recipients. Standard practice is (1) auto-HSCT, at

H. Schrezenmeier (✉) · S. Körper · B. Höchsmann
C. Weinstock
Institute of Clinical Transfusion Medicine
and Immunogenetics Ulm, German Red Cross Blood
Transfusion Service Baden-Württemberg-Hessen
and University Hospital Ulm, Ulm, Germany

Institute of Transfusion Medicine, University of Ulm,
Ulm, Germany
e-mail: h.schrezenmeier@blutspende.de

least 2 weeks prior to stem cell collection until at least 3 months after HSCT, and (2) allo-HSCT, at the latest starting with conditioning until at least 6 months after HSCT or until immune reconstitution. However, some centers recommend lifetime use of irradiated products since it is difficult to confirm complete and sustained immunological reconstitution.

23.3 Prevention of CMV Transmission

The highest risk of transfusion-transmitted CMV (TT-CMV) remains in CMV-seronegative recipients of matched CMV-negative HSCT (Ljungman 2014). Risk of TT-CMV can be reduced by transfusion of leukocyte-reduced blood products (i.e., <1 to 5 × 10^6 residual leukocytes per unit) or by transfusion of blood components from CMV-seronegative donors (Ziemann and Thiele 2017). However, it is unclear whether the "belt and suspender approach," i.e., the use of both leukocyte-reduced and seronegative products, further reduces the risk of TT-CMV. Donations from newly CMV-IgG-positive donors bear the highest risk for transmitting CMV infections (Ziemann and Thiele 2017). Currently no international consensus on risk mitigation for CMV transmission exists. A recent snapshot of current practice revealed that about half of the countries use either leukocyte-reduced or seronegative products and the other half use the combination of both (Lieberman et al. 2014). Also, there is no consensus how long CMV-seronegative products should be given to transplant recipients: the current practice ranges from 100 days after transplant till lifelong (or until CMV seroconversion) (Lieberman et al. 2014).

23.4 Red Blood Cell Concentrates (RBCs)

A restrictive RBC transfusion threshold of 7–8 g/dL hemoglobin is recommended for adult patients who are hemodynamically stable. A restrictive RBC transfusion threshold of 8 g/dL is recommended for patients with existing cardiovascular disease (Carson et al. 2016). These cutoffs are derived from studies on a broad range of indications. Only one randomized clinical trial is available specifically for patients undergoing HSCT (TRIST trial, NCT01237639). It compared a liberal strategy (Hb threshold <90 g/L) with a restrictive strategy (Hb threshold <70 g/L). Health-related quality of life was similar between groups, and no appreciable differences in HSCT-associated outcomes were reported (Tay et al. 2016). The median number of RBC units transfused was lower in the restrictive strategy compared to the liberal strategy group, but this did not reach statistical significance (Tay et al. 2016).

In adult recipients, one unit of RBC increases the hemoglobin concentration by about 1 g/dl. In children, the dose should be calculated by the formula:

Volume (mL RBC): Target Hb after transfusion (g/dL) − pretransfusion Hb (g/dL) × 4 × weight (kg)

In recent years, several randomized trials showed no evidence that transfusion of fresh RBC reduced morbidity or mortality compared to standard issue RBCs. Thus, the AABB recommends that patients should receive RBC selected at any point within their licensed dating period (Carson et al. 2016).

Chronic RBC transfusions result in iron overload. Hyperferritinemia and iron overload before HSCT are associated with reduced overall survival and incidence of non-relapse mortality after allo-HSCT. However, a meta-analysis (Armand et al. 2014) and a prospective cohort study suggest that iron overload, as assessed by liver iron content, is not a strong prognostic factor for overall survival in a general adult HSCT population. Thus, ferritin alone is an inadequate surrogate for iron overload in HSCT.

23.5 Platelet Concentrates (PCs)

PC should be transfused prophylactically to non-bleeding, nonfebrile patients when platelet counts are ≤10 × 10^9/L (Schiffer et al. 2018). Prophylactic platelet transfusions may be administered at higher counts based on clinical judgment (Schiffer et al. 2018). Patients with active bleeding, febrile conditions, or active infections should receive prophylactic PC transfusions at a threshold of 20×10^9/L. Also, in case of specific transplant-related toxicity which might increase the risk of bleeding (acute GvHD, mucositis, hemorrhagic cystitis, or diffuse alveolar hemorrhage), a threshold of 20×10^9/L or even higher, based on careful clinical observation, might be justified.

Two prospective randomized control trials comparing prophylactic versus therapeutic PC transfusion in adult patients (≥ 16 years) suggest that a therapeutic transfusion strategy might be feasible in patients after auto-PBSCT but cannot be easily transferred to other indications (AML, allo-HSCT) for whom special attention to the increased risk of bleeding, in particular, CNS bleeding, is needed (Stanworth et al. 2013; Wandt et al. 2012). The results may not be generalizable to children since a subset analysis of the PLADO trial demonstrated that bleeding rates were significantly increased among children, particularly among those undergoing autologous HSCT (Josephson et al. 2012).

The randomized PLADO trial compared different doses of PC transfusions ("low dose," "medium dose," and "high dose" defined as 1.1×10^{11}, 2.2×10^{11}, and 4.4×10^{11} platelets per m^2 BSA) (Slichter et al. 2010). While a strategy of "low-dose" transfusion significantly reduces the overall quantity of platelets transfused, patients required more frequent PC transfusion events (Slichter et al. 2010). At doses between 1.1×10^{11} and 4.4×10^{11} platelets/m^2, the number of platelets in the prophylactic transfusions had no effect on the incidence of bleeding.

Both apheresis PC and pooled PC from whole blood donations are safe and effective. Available data suggest equivalence of the products in non-allosensitized recipients (Schrezenmeier and Seifried 2010). A clear advantage of apheresis PCs can only be demonstrated in allosensitized patients with HLA- and/or HPA-antibodies who receive antigen-compatible apheresis PCs.

Some patients experience inadequate increment after PC transfusions, i.e., a corrected count increment (CCI) below 5000/μL at 1 h after transfusion of fresh, ABO-identical PCs on at least two subsequent transfusions. Refractoriness can be caused by non-immunological factors (>80%) or immunological factors (<20%) (Fig. 23.1). If platelet refractoriness is suspected and no apparent nonimmune causes can be identified, screening for the presence of HLA-Ab is recommended. If HLA-Ab are present, the patient should receive apheresis PCs from matched donors (Juskewitch et al. 2017; Stanworth et al. 2015): ideally all four antigens (HLA-A, HLA-B) of donor and

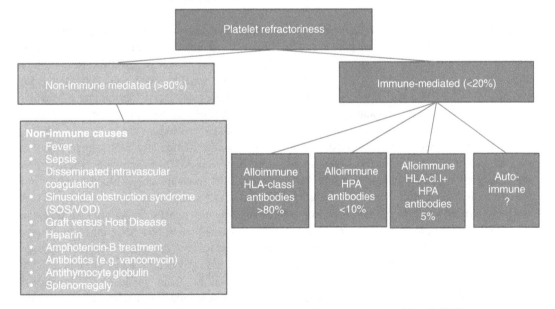

Fig. 23.1 Etiology of platelet transfusion refractoriness (modified according to Pavenski et al. 2012)

recipient are identical. Also PCs from donors expressing only antigens which are present in the recipient can be used. If PCs from such donors are not available, donors with "permissive" mismatches in HLA-A or HLA-B shall be selected (e.g., based on cross-reactive groups or computer algorithms that determine HLA compatibility at the epitope level). If no better-matched donor is available, antigen-negative platelets, i.e., not expressing the target antigen(s) of the recipients' HLA allo-Ab, can be transfused. Screening for antibodies against human platelet antigens (HPA) should be performed if refractoriness persists also after transfusion of HLA-matched PCs and nonimmune causes are unlikely. Approaches for patients without compatible platelet donors are autologous cryopreserved platelets (e.g., collected in remission prior to allogeneic HSCT), IS (e.g., rituximab), and high-dose IVIg and plasmapheresis.

23.6 Immunohematological Consequences of ABO-Mismatched Transplantation

About 40–50% of allo-HSCT are ABO mismatched. While transplantation across the ABO barrier is possible, immunohematological problems have to be taken into account. There is a risk that ABO incompatibility between donor and recipient causes hemolytic transfusion reactions. In case of major ABO mismatch and a recipient anti-donor isoagglutinin titer ≥1:32, the red cell contamination in PBSC graft should be kept <20 mL, and RBC depletion of BM grafts must be performed. If recipient anti-donor isoagglutinin titers are low (≤1:16), no manipulation of the PBSC graft is required, and RBC depletion of a BM graft might be considered in this situation but is not mandatory. In case of minor ABO incompatibility and a high donor anti-recipient isoagglutinin titer (≥1:256), plasma depletion of both PBSC and BM grafts should be performed. If the donor anti-recipient isoagglutinin titer is low (≤1:128), no manipulation of the PBSC graft is required, and plasma depletion of a BM graft might be considered but is not mandatory. In case of bidirectional ABO incompatibility and high

titers of anti-recipient isoagglutinins, both RBC and plasma depletion is required.

Delayed hemolysis can occur in minor ABO-mismatched HSCT, in particular after RIC, due to hemolysis of remaining recipient red cells by isoagglutinins produced by donor B lymphocytes.

Major or bidirectional ABO-incompatible HSCT can cause pure red cell aplasia (PRCA), delayed engraftment, and increased RBC transfusion requirement. The risk is higher if a group O recipient with high-titer anti-A isoagglutinins receives a group A graft. If no spontaneous remission of PRCA occurs and anti-donor isoagglutinins persist, various treatments to remove isoagglutinins, to reduce their production, or to stimulate erythropoiesis can be used (see review Worel 2016).

23.7 Transfusion in ABO- or RhD-Incompatible HSCT

The change of blood group and the persistence of recipient isoagglutinins require a special approach for transfusion support in ABO-incompatible HSCT considering several aspects: isoagglutinins might target engrafting progenitors and transfused platelets to which variable amounts of ABO antigens can be bound. ABO blood group antigens are expressed in many non-hematopoietic tissues which continue to express the recipients' ABO antigens also after engraftment. ABO antigens can be secreted into body fluids. If possible, exposure of HSC recipients to isoagglutinins should be avoided. RBCs which are ABO compatible with both HSC donor and recipient are mandatory. Plasma and PCs which are compatible with both the donor and the recipient should be preferred. Table 23.1 summarizes the recommendation for ABO preference of transfusions in ABO-incompatible HSCT.

For PCs, some choices of blood groups might not always be available. To reduce the risk of adverse events due to isoagglutinins, apheresis PC donors with high-titer ABO antibodies should be excluded. However, a preferred strategy is the use of plasma-reduced PC (both for apheresis PC and pooled PC from whole blood donations). These are suspended in platelet additive solution with only about 30% plasma volume remaining.

Table 23.1 RBC, platelet, and plasma transfusion support for patients undergoing ABO-incompatible HSCT

ABO incompatibility	Recipient	Donor	Phase I[c] All products	Phase II and phase III[c] RBC Choice[a]	Platelets First choice	Platelets Second choice[a]	Plasma First choice	Plasma Second choice
Major	O	A	Recipient	O	A	AB, B, O	A	AB
	O	B	Recipient	O	B	AB, A, O	B	AB
	O	AB	Recipient	O	AB	A, B, O	AB	–
	A	AB	Recipient	A, O	AB	A, B, O	AB	–
	B	AB	Recipient	B, O	AB	B, A, O	AB	–
Minor	A	O	Recipient	O	A[b]	AB, B, O	A	AB
	B	O	Recipient	O	B[b]	AB, A, O	B	AB
	AB	O	Recipient	O	AB[b]	A, B, O	AB	–
	AB	A	Recipient	A, O	AB[b]	A, B, O	AB	–
	AB	B	Recipient	B, O	AB[b]	B, A, O	AB	–
Bidirectional	A	B	Recipient	O	AB	B, A, O	AB	–
	B	A	Recipient	O	AB	A, B, O	AB	–

– not applicable

[a]Choices are listed in the order of preference

[b]For practical reasons, the use of donor type platelets might be defined as first choice, in phase III, i.e., after complete engraftment

[c]Phase I until preparative regimen, phase II until complete engraftment, phase III after complete engraftment.

HSC recipients should receive RhD-negative RBC and also RhD-negative PC except when both HSC donor and recipient are RhD-positive. If the HSC donor is RhD-positive and the recipient is RhD-negative, platelet transfusion can be switched to RhD-positive products after erythroid engraftment, i.e., appearance of RhD-positive red cells.

Whenever possible, RBC should be compatible both with HSCT donor and recipient for CcEe antigens. If Rh antigens of HSCT donor and recipient differ in a way that compatibility with both is not possible (e.g., recipient CCD.ee, donor ccD.EE), then RBC compatible with the recipient shall be chosen in the period until engraftment. After the appearance of donor-derived red cells, RBC supply should switch to compatibility with the graft. Patients should receive K-negative RBC except when both recipient and donor are K positive.

23.8 Granulocyte Concentrates

In life-threatening non-viral infections during neutropenia, the use of irradiated granulocyte transfusions should be considered. Response and survival after granulocyte transfusion correlate strongly with hematopoietic recovery. Thus, granulocyte transfusions may mainly bridge the gap between specific treatment and neutrophil recovery. Granulocyte transfusions can help to control active fungal infections in a very high-risk population of patients who otherwise are denied by transplant program. A retrospective study suggested that granulocyte transfusion might maintain the mucosal integrity and thus reduces bacterial translocation and triggers for GvHD. In the randomized RING trial, success rates for granulocyte and control arms did not differ within any infection type. The overall success rates for the control and granulocyte transfusion group were 41% and 49% (n.s.) (Price 2015). However, patients who received high dose ($\geq 0.6 \times 10^9$ granulocytes/kg per transfusion) fared better than patients who received lower doses. The collection center should ensure to provide a high-dose concentrate by appropriate donor selection, pre-collection stimulation, and apheresis techniques. The optimal number of granulocyte transfusions is unclear. Adverse events of granulocyte infusions are fever, chills, pulmonary reactions, and alloimmunization. Studies demonstrated that overall risk of alloimmunizations was low and there was no effect of alloimmunization on the primary outcome (survival, microbial response), the occurrence of transfusion reactions, or post transfusion neutrophil increments. Alloimmunization remains a problem because of its negative impact on increments after platelet transfusion and potential increase of graft failure after HSCT. Donor-specific HLA-Ab might be implicated in early graft failure (Spellman et al. 2010). If granulocyte transfusions are used prior to a planned unrelated HSCT, recipients should be monitored for the development of HLA-Ab, and the search algorithm for the UD should take into account donor-specific antibodies. All granulocyte concentrates must be gamma-irradiated and should be obtained from CMV-seronegative donors, ideally also confirmed by CMV-PCR to avoid donations in the serological window period.

Key Points

- Patients undergoing HSCT must be transfused with irradiated blood products (at least 2 weeks prior to stem cell collection in auto- and starting with the conditioning in allo-HSCT)
- A restrictive RBC transfusion threshold of 7–8 g/dL hemoglobin is recommended for adult patients who are hemodynamically stable
- RBC must be compatible with both the HSC donor and the recipients
- Platelet concentrates should be transfused to non-bleeding, nonfebrile patients when platelet counts are $\leq 10 \times 10^9$/L
- Prophylactic platelet transfusion remains the standard of care for thrombocytopenic patients undergoing allogeneic HSCT
- RBC must be compatible with both the HSC donor and the recipient

References

Armand P, Kim HT, Virtanen JM, et al. Iron overload in allogeneic hematopoietic cell transplantation outcome: a meta-analysis. Biol Blood Marrow Transplant. 2014;20:1248–51.

Carson JL, Guyatt G, Heddle NM, et al. Clinical practice guidelines from the AABB: red blood cell transfusion thresholds and storage. JAMA. 2016;316:2025–35.

Christou G, Iyengar A, Shorr R, et al. Optimal transfusion practices after allogeneic hematopoietic cell transplantation: a systematic scoping review of evidence from randomized controlled trials. Transfusion. 2016;56:2607–14.

Cid J. Prevention of transfusion-associated graft-versus-host disease with pathogen-reduced platelets with amotosalen and ultraviolet A light: a review. Vox Sang. 2017;112:607–13.

European Committee (Partial Agreement) on Blood Transfusion (CD-P-TS). Guide to the preparation, use and quality assurance of blood components. 19th. 2017. EDQM.

Josephson CD, Granger S, Assmann SF, et al. Bleeding risks are higher in children versus adults given prophylactic platelet transfusions for treatment-induced hypoproliferative thrombocytopenia. Blood. 2012;120:748–60.

Juskewitch JE, Norgan AP, De Goey SR, et al. How do I … manage the platelet transfusion-refractory patient? Transfusion. 2017;57:2828–35.

Kopolovic I, Ostro J, Tsubota H, et al. A systematic review of transfusion-associated graft-versus-host disease. Blood. 2015;126:406–14.

Lieberman L, Devine DV, Reesink HW, et al. Prevention of transfusion-transmitted cytomegalovirus (CMV) infection: standards of care. Vox Sang. 2014;107:276–311.

Ljungman P. The role of cytomegalovirus serostatus on outcome of hematopoietic stem cell transplantation. Curr Opin Hematol. 2014;21:466–9.

Pavenski K, Freedman J, Semple JW. HLA alloimmunization against platelet transfusions: pathophysiology, significance, prevention and management. Tissue Antigens. 2012;79:237–45.

Price TH, Boeckh M, Harrison RW, et al. Efficacy of transfusion with granulocytes from G-CSF/dexamethasone-treated donors in neutropenic patients with infection. Blood. 2015;126:2153–61.

Schiffer CA, Bohlke K, Delaney M, et al. Platelet transfusion for patients with cancer: American Society of Clinical Oncology clinical practice guideline update. J Clin Oncol. 2018;36:283–99.

Schrezenmeier H, Seifried E. Buffy-coat-derived pooled platelet concentrates and apheresis platelet concentrates: which product type should be preferred? Vox Sang. 2010;99:1–15.

Slichter SJ, Kaufman RM, Assmann SF, et al. Dose of prophylactic platelet transfusions and prevention of hemorrhage. N Engl J Med. 2010;362:600–13.

Spellman S, Bray R, Rosen-Bronson S, et al. The detection of donor-directed, HLA-specific alloantibodies in recipients of unrelated hematopoietic cell transplantation is predictive of graft failure. Blood. 2010;115:2704–8.

Stanworth SJ, Estcourt LJ, Powter G, et al. A no-prophylaxis platelet-transfusion strategy for hematologic cancers. N Engl J Med. 2013;368:1771–80.

Stanworth SJ, Navarrete C, Estcourt L, Marsh J. Platelet refractoriness–practical approaches and ongoing dilemmas in patient management. Br J Haematol. 2015;171:297–305.

Tay J, Allan DS, Chatelein E, et al. Transfusion of red cells in hematopoietic stem cell transplantation (TRIST study): a randomized controlled trial evaluating 2 red cell transfusion thresholds. Blood. 2016;128:1032.

Wandt H, Schaefer-Eckart K, Wendelin K, et al. Therapeutic platelet transfusion versus routine prophylactic transfusion in patients with haematological malignancies: an open-label, multicentre, randomised study. Lancet. 2012;380:1309–16.

Worel N. ABO-mismatched allogeneic hematopoietic stem cell transplantation. Transfus Med Hemother. 2016;43:3–12.

Ziemann M, Thiele T. Transfusion-transmitted CMV infection–current knowledge and future perspectives. Transfus Med. 2017;27:238–48.

Nutritional Support

Annic Baumgartner and Philipp Schuetz

24.1 Introduction

Patients undergoing HSCT, particularly allo-HSCT, are at risk for malnutrition (Fuji et al. 2012). Malnutrition is associated with poor clinical outcome, decreased OS, higher risk of infectious and immunologic complications, delayed neutrophil engraftment and prolonged hospital stay (Baumgartner et al. 2016, 2017). Importantly, most patients are well-nourished or even overweight upon admission to HSCT but experience rapid deterioration of nutritional status during treatment (Fuji et al. 2014). Weight loss results from a complex interplay of toxic, inflammatory and immunological mechanisms leading to caloric deficits by anorexia as well as a catabolism of the metabolism.

Nutritional support is meant to reduce caloric deficit and reduce the risks for negative metabolic effects. However, there is a lack of large-scale trials proving benefit of nutritional interventions in this setting (Baumgartner et al. 2017). The current nutritional approach is thus based on physiological considerations and results of observational and some smaller interventional trials and needs to be adapted to an individual patient's situation.

24.2 Screening for Malnutrition

Pre-existing malnutrition is an important additional risk factor in patients undergoing HSCT. International guidelines such as the European Society of Enteral and Parenteral Nutrition (ESPEN) recommend screening for malnutrition at admission for transplantation (Bozzetti et al. 2009). There is no international consensus on how to assess malnutrition in this patient population. For reasons of practicability, the use of the NRS 2002 is generally recommended (Bozzetti et al. 2009). In the acute setting, weight assessment may be inaccurate because of inflammatory fluid retention.

Based on "Supportive Care" in EBMT Handbook, 2009, by Tamás Masszi and Arno Mank.

A. Baumgartner (✉)
Internal Medicine and Endcrinology/Diabetology/
Clinical Nutrition and Metabolism, Medical
University Clinic of Kantonsspital Aarau, University
of Basel, Aarau, Switzerland
e-mail: annic.baumgartner@ksa.ch

P. Schuetz
Department of Endocrinology, Diabetes
and Metabolism and Internal Medicine, Kantonsspital
Aarau, University of Basel, Aarau, Switzerland

24.3 Nutritional Recommendations (See General Recommendations in Table 24.1 **and** Fig. 24.1; Monitoring in Table 24.2 and Nutritional Strategies in Fig. 24.1)

24.3.1 Nutrition in Allo-HSCT

24.3.1.1 Route of Administration

Due to its positive effects on GI integrity and microbiome, enteral nutritional (EN) support is generally preferred over parenteral nutrition (PN) in case of a functioning GI tract.

During allo-HSCT, patients often experience GI failure so PN is used instead. Yet, higher risk of central line infections as well as hyperglycaemia associated with PN demand restricted use (Seguy et al. 2012).

Small, prospective, non-randomized trials on EN found satisfying results on feasibility and safety with lower infection rates as well as beneficial effects such as earlier neutrophil engraftment and lower rates of severe GI GvHD (Seguy et al. 2012; Guièze et al. 2014). Some studies even report higher OS (Seguy et al. 2012). Results of a large prospective trial are expected (Lemal et al. 2015).

We encourage the use of EN as a first-line measure. Indication for PN should be limited to

Table 24.1 Summary of general recommendations for nutritional support

Screening for malnutrition	
Indication	All patients to estimate risk for pre-existing malnutrition
Tools	NRS 2002
Nutritional support	
General management	1. Early involvement of dietitians
	2. Consider placement of nasogastric tube on day +1
	3. Standardized monitoring of nutritional intake
	4. Nutritional reassessment every 3 days using the NRS 2002
Indication of intervention	1. Oral intake <60% for 3 days consecutively
	2. Consider nutritional support in all patients with preexisting malnutrition and/or BMI < 18
Discontinuation	Oral intake >50% for 3 days consecutively
Estimation of caloric needs	According to Harris Benedict formula (ideal body weight)
	OR BASA-ROT table/(25–30 kcal/kg ideal body weight)
Route of nutritional support	1. Intensification of oral nutrition
	2. Enteral nutrition
	3. Parenteral nutrition
Forms of nutritional support	
Intensified oral nutrition	*Indication*: Malnutrition or underweight (BMI < 18 kg/m^2) and preserved oral intake
	Options: Additional snacks rich in proteins and energy, protein or calorie enrichment of main courses, additional protein and energy drinks (ONS)
	Standardized supplementation: None
Enteral nutrition	*Indication*: If nutritional goals cannot be reached by oral support alone
	Standardized supplementation:
	Vitamin K once weekly
Parenteral nutrition	*Indication*: If nutritional goals cannot be reached in patients with gastrointestinal failure and/or intolerance for NGT
	Standardized supplementation:
	Lipid-soluble vitamins (ADEK)
	Water-soluble vitamins
	Trace elements
Vitamin and trace elements	Multivitamin generally recommended
	Vitamin D: Supplementation recommended (Bolus of 40000E at admission, maintenance therapy with 1500E orally per day
	Other vitamins or trace elements if overt deficiency
Immunonutrition	Generally not recommended

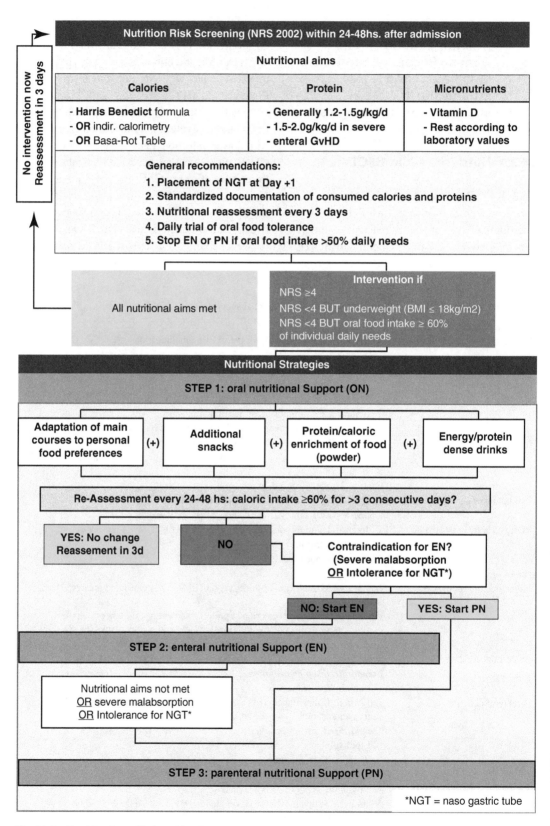

Fig. 24.1 Algorithm for guided nutritional support

intolerance for nasogastric tube and GI failure including severe malabsorption or limited gastroenteral passage.

24.3.1.2 Indications and Timing

There are few study data regarding optimal timing of nutrition. The ESPEN guidelines recommend implementation of nutritional support if oral caloric intake falls below 60–70% of basic requirements for 3 days consecutively (Bozzetti et al. 2009).

Discontinuation of EN or PN should be considered, if >50% of daily requirements are met by oral intake (Bozzetti et al. 2009). To enhance early return to oral food intake patients should be encouraged to maintain minimal oral intake throughout therapy.

24.3.1.3 Estimation of Caloric Needs

Most studies investigating energy expenditure by indirect calorimetry have been performed in small paediatric populations. Validity of the data for adults therefore is limited, and results are controversial (Sharma et al. 2012; Duro et al. 2008).

Determination of energy requirements based on calculations, e.g., by the BASA-ROT table or Harris-Benedict Formula, does not differ significantly from results by indirect calorimetry (Sharma et al. 2012; Valentini 2012; Harris 1918). Therefore, we recommend estimation of energy requirements according to an adjusted Harris-Benedict formula.

24.3.2 Nutrition in Auto-HSCT

In general, effects of auto-HSCT on nutritional status are less pronounced. Nutritional support is not generally recommended and has to be evaluated individually in patients experiencing severe complications or in patients with pre-existing malnutrition.

Table 24.2 Monitoring of nutritional parameters

Parameter	Frequency of assessment	Significance and implications
Anthropometry		
Weight	Daily	Correlation with fluid balance
		Evaluation of diuretics and
		Albumin supplementation
Bioimpedance assessment	Individually	Uncontrolled, unexplained weight loss
		Severe, prolonged inflammation
Nutritional assessment		
Oral food consumption	3× daily	Evaluation of nutritional support
Laboratory parameter		
Albumine	Weekly	Evaluation of supplementation in anasarca
Sodium, Potassium	Daily	Adaptation of potassium supplementation
Calcium, Magnesium, Phosphate	Twice weekly	Adaptation of supplementation
		CAVEAT refeeding, gastrointestinal loss
INR, Quick	Twice weekly	Evaluation of supplementation
		CAVEAT low content in certain products for EN/PN
Glucose	3–6× daily if PN or preexisting diabetes mellitus otherwise twice weekly	Adaptation of insulin dose
Creatinine	Daily	Correction of fluid balance
		CAVEAT toxic damage
Liver function tests	Twice weekly	Evaluation of toxic damage, infection, hepatic GvHD, VOD or relapse
Triglycerides	Twice weekly if PN	Adaptation of PN
Vitamin D	At admission	Begin routine supplementation
Vitamin B12	At admission	Supplementation pretransplantational individually

24.3.3 Nutrition in Acute Gastrointestinal GvHD

GvHD of the digestive tract leads to excessive diarrhoea, abdominal pain, nausea, vomiting, gastrointestinal bleeding, dysphagia and malabsorption. Patients experience malnutrition to a higher extent and show significantly more additional complications (van der Meij et al. 2013).

Caloric demands are mainly driven by energy loss through diarrhoea. Enteral solutions should be low in fibre and fat and not contain lactose. Maintaining a minimal amount of oral or enteral nutrition facilitates early dietary recovery (Imataki et al. 2006; Andermann et al. 2016). Complete bowel rest and total PN are indicated in severe GvHD grade IV and stool volume >1500 ml in 24 h (Bozzetti et al. 2009; Imataki et al. 2006).

Protein requirements are elevated. Recommendations range from 1.2 to 2.5 g/kg/day. We recommend aiming for 1.5–2 g/kg/day in the absence of severe renal impairment (Bozzetti et al. 2009; Muscaritoli et al. 2002).

Vitamin and trace elements are often deficient and need to be measured regularly to evaluate need of supplementation.

24.3.4 Low Bacterial Diet/Low Microbial Diet/Neutropenic Diet

A low microbial diet has been installed in the 1980s to prevent potential threat of food-borne infections from organisms colonizing the gastrointestinal tract.

There is no standardized protocol, and variations amongst centres, contradictions even, are high. Yet, there is no proof of efficacy in preventing infections or death.

In line with most current publications, we recommend safe food handling and strict hand hygiene as proposed by the FDA or the EC over a neutropenic diet.

24.4 Immunonutrition

A meta-analysis on glutamine found reduced severity and duration of mucositis and GvHD (Kota and Chamberlain 2017). To date, no randomized controlled trial showed a benefit on overall survival or reduction of infection rates (Crowther et al. 2009).

Pre- and probiotics may enhance diversity of the GI microbiome. So far, no study has evaluated their effects compared to placebo. Again, there might be a benefit on severity of GvHD (Ladas et al. 2016). Safety has been evaluated in a pilot study in children and adolescents and proved satisfying.

There are no randomized controlled trials assessing the benefits of omega-3 fatty acids or trace elements. Except for vitamin D, there is no proven benefit of a routine supplementation (Hall and Juckett 2013). Based on this data, we do not recommend routine use of immunonutrients.

24.5 Long-Term Follow-Up

Follow-up should include regular nutritional screening and documentation of weight, BMI, appetite and functional status based on patients' history. A balanced, Mediterranean diet can be recommended along with regular physical training to regain muscle mass. An increase in weight should be addressed early to avoid full development of a metabolic syndrome because of high baseline cardiovascular risk in transplanted patients.

Persisting malnutrition, especially in chronic GvHD, should be handled by an interdisciplinary team. Caloric needs seem to be elevated and often require in- and out-hospital nutritional support.

Key Points
- There is high risk for malnutrition upon HSCT treatment
- Malnutrition is an independent risk factor in these patients
- The potential benefit of all nutritional interventions remains largely unproven
- All dietary recommendations are based on physiological considerations and results of mainly observational trials
- Adherence to a systematic approach to nutritional support improves transparency, comparability and generally reduces use of unnecessary PN

- Oral and enteral nutritional support is recommended over parenteral support in case of functioning gastrointestinal tract
- A minimal oral or enteral food intake is beneficial for recovery of mucosa and microbiome
- Immunonutrients did not show significant beneficial effects and therefore are not recommended for routine use
- Neutropenic diets did not show a benefit over safe food handling approaches

References

Andermann TM, Rezvani A, Bhatt AS. Microbiota manipulation with prebiotics and probiotics in patients undergoing stem cell transplantation. Curr Hematol Malig Rep. 2016;11:19–28.

Baumgartner A, Bargetzi A, Zueger N, et al. Revisiting nutritional support for allogeneic hematologic stem cell transplantation—a systematic review. Bone Marrow Transplant. 2017;52:506–13.

Baumgartner A, Zueger N, Bargetzi A. Association of nutritional parameters with clinical outcomes in patients with acute myeloid leukemia undergoing hematopoietic stem cell transplantion. Ann Nutr Metab. 2016;69:89–98.

Bozzetti F, Arends J, Lundholm K, Micklewright A, Zurcher G, Muscaritoli M. ESPEN guidelines on parenteral nutrition: non-surgical oncology. Clin Nutr. 2009;28:445–54.

Crowther M, Avenell A, Culligan D. Systematic review and meta-analyses of studies of glutamine supplementation in haematopoietic stem cell transplantation. Bone Marrow Transplant. 2009;44:413–25.

Duro D, Bechard LJ, Feldman HA, et al. Weekly measurements accurately represent trends in resting energy expenditure in children undergoing hematopoietic stem cell transplantation. J Parenter Enter Nutr. 2008;32:427–32.

Fuji S, Mori T, Khattry N, et al. Severe weight loss in 3 months after allogeneic hematopoietic SCT was associated with an increased risk of subsequent non-relapse mortality. Bone Marrow Transplant. 2014;50:100–5.

Fuji S, Mori T, Lee V, et al. A multi-center international survey related to the nutritional support after hemato-poietic stem cell transplantation endorsed by the ASIA Pacific Blood and Marrow Transplantation (APBMT). Food Nutr Sci. 2012;3:417–21.

Guièze R, Lemal R, Cabrespine A, et al. Enteral versus parenteral nutritional support in allogeneic haematopoietic stem-cell transplantation. Clin Nutr. 2014;33:533–8.

Hall AC, Juckett MB. The role of vitamin D in hematologic disease and stem cell transplantation. Nutrients. 2013;5:2206–21.

Harris JA, Benedict FG. A biometric study of human basal metabolism. Proc Natl Acad Sci U S A. 1918;4:370–3.

Imataki O, Nakatani S, Hasegawa T, et al. Nutritional support for patients suffering from intestinal graft-versus-host disease after allogeneic hematopoietic stem cell transplantation. Am J Hematol. 2006;81:747–52.

Kota H, Chamberlain RS. Immunonutrition is associated with a decreased incidence of graft-versus-host disease in bone marrow transplant recipients: a meta-analysis. JPEN J Parenter Enteral Nutr. 2017;41:1286–92.

Ladas EJ, Bhatia M, Chen L, et al. The safety and feasibility of probiotics in children and adolescents undergoing hematopoietic cell transplantation. Bone Marrow Transplant. 2016;51:262–6.

Lemal R, Cabrespine A, Pereira B, et al. Could enteral nutrition improve the outcome of patients with haematological malignancies undergoing allogeneic haematopoietic stem cell transplantation? A study protocol for a randomized controlled trial (the NEPHA study). Trials. 2015;16:136.

Muscaritoli M, Grieco G, Capria S, Iori AP, Rossi Fanelli F. Nutritional and metabolic support in patients undergoing bone marrow transplantation. Am J Clin Nutr. 2002;75:183–90.

Seguy D, Duhamel A, Rejeb MB, et al. Better outcome of patients undergoing enteral tube feeding after myeloablative conditioning for allogeneic stem cell transplantation. Transplantation. 2012;94:287–94.

Sharma TS, Bechard LJ, Feldman HA, et al. Effect of titrated parenteral nutrition on body composition after allogeneic hematopoietic stem cell transplantation in children: a double-blind, randomized, multicenter trial. Am J Clin Nutr. 2012;95:342–51.

Valentini L. The BASA-ROT table: an arithmetic-hypothetical concept for easy BMI-, age-, and sex-adjusted bedside estimation of energy expenditure. Nutrition. 2012;28:773–8.

van der Meij BS, de Graaf P, Wierdsma NJ, et al. Nutritional support in patients with GVHD of the digestive tract: state of the art. Bone Marrow Transplant. 2013;48:474–82.

GVHD Prophylaxis (Immunosuppression)

David Michonneau and Gérard Socié

25.1 Introduction

The most life-threatening complication of allo-HSCT is the graft-versus-host disease (GVHD) which occurs when T cells from the recipient recognize the host as foreign. Despite 50 years of history and nearly half a million of procedures performed worldwide, GVHD remains the most challenging issue physicians are facing on a daily basis.

Overall, 30–50% of the patients will develop acute GVHD, and around 15% will have severe GVHD (grades III–IV). The main risk factor for developing chronic GVHD is the previous development of the acute form of the disease.

The pathophysiology, diagnosis, and management of both acute and chronic GVHD will be covered by other chapters in this Handbook (Chaps. 43 and 44). This chapter will summarize the use of IS to prevent the development of acute GVHD since attempt to prevent chronic GVHD basically rely on the ability to prevent the acute disease. Readers with interest on a more detailed overview of the acute GVHD biological process, prevention, and therapy can

D. Michonneau · G. Socié (✉)
Hematology/Transplantation, AP/HP Hospital St Louis, Paris, France

University Paris VII, Denis Diderot, Paris, France

INSERM UMR 1160, Paris, France
e-mail: gerard.socie@aphp.fr

refer to an excellent recent review (Zeiser and Blazar 2017).

25.2 GVHD Prophylaxis After MAC; The "Gold" Standard; CNI in Combination with MTX

Back in the mid-1980s, Storb and colleagues reported that the combination of CSA/MTX (Table 25.1) was superior to CSA in a series of prospective randomized phase 3 trials (Storb et al. 1986). This gold standard regimen remains the most widely used in Europe today as prophylaxis regimen especially after MAC.

In the late 1990s, another CNI-based prophylactic regimen using tacrolimus (TAC) in conjunction with MTX was developed, and two randomized phase 3 trials were published after MAC in HLA-identical and URD, respectively (Ratanatharathorn et al. 1998; Nash et al. 2000). Although both reported a significant decreased in the incidence of grade II–IV acute GVHD, none of the two could demonstrate an improved survival rate with TAC/MTX as compared to CSA/MTX. The reasons for this lack of improvement are twofold: (1) in the trial performed from HLA-identical sibling D, there was an imbalanced of disease risk among the two groups with higher risk patients with leukemia among patients receiving TAC/MTX, and (2) for the trial in URD, the HLA-typing methodology at

Table 25.1 CSA/MTX for GVHD prophylaxis

	Cyclosporine	Methotrexate
Drug posology	3 mg/kg/day IV till engraftment then orally	15 mg/m² day +1 10 mg/m² day +3, +6, +11
Adjusting dose	Target dose to 150–200 ng/mL; adjust to renal function	Day 11 may be omitted if grade III/IV mucositis
Interaction	Numerous; ++ with azoles	
Secondary effects	Numerous Renal insufficiency, CNS, and endothelial toxicities	Mucositis

that time was serologically based and thus included a very high proportion of patients with almost certainly high degree of mismatching. Nevertheless it should be stressed that the TAC/MTX regimen is currently considered as the American gold standard, while it never reached popularity in Europe.

CSA and TAC inhibit GVHD by preventing the activation of the nuclear factor of activated T-cell (NFAT) family of transcription factors, thereby reducing the transcription of interleukin-2 and the activation of effector T cells, albeit with a concurrent reduction in levels of interleukin-2-dependent anti-inflammatory Tregs.

25.3 GVHD Prophylaxis After RIC; Is CNI Plus MMF Standard?

From the early development of the RIC, two regimens have been used in the setting of RIC, CSA (or TAC) alone or in combination with MMF (reviewed in; Zeiser and Blazar 2017). Somewhat surprisingly the association of CSA/MMF while largely used worldwide has never been tested stringently in the setting of a large randomized prospective randomized trial. CNI in this setting are usually used at the same dose (and share the same toxicity profile) as after MAC. MMF's toxicity mainly relies on sometimes unpredictable hematological toxicity. Attention must be paid to the use of ganciclovir (for CMV reactivation) in addition to MMF because of the risk of severe pancytopenia. MMF is usually delivered at the

dose of 30 mg/kg/day split into two to three doses. Anecdotal evidence suggests depending on the transplant situation (i.e., HLA-identical vs. URD) that MMF should be delivered (till day + 80?) in recipients from URD.

25.4 Can PT-CY Be Considered as Standard GVHD Prophylaxis in Transplantation from Haploidentical Donors and Beyond?

There is a recent bloom in the use of haploidentical donor during the past few years worldwide. While initial attempt was to use megadose of CD34+ selected HSC, the advent of PT-CY has really revolutionized this procedure. The PT-CY designed by Baltimore's group includes CY 50 mg/kg on day +3 and +4 followed by TAC/MMF. Toxicities include those associated with CNI and MMF. Specific toxicity associated with CY includes hemorrhagic cystitis and the rare but potentially serious early cardiologic dysfunction. Although the incidence of acute GVHD remains significant (in around 1/3 of the patients), there is now some evidence that PT-CY might be associated with low rate of chronic GVHD (reviewed in; Fuchs 2017).

Furthermore, beyond the setting of haploidentical transplant, PT-CY has gained popularity in other setting including transplantation from URD and HLA-identical sibling. Although it seems unlikely today that any formal randomized trial (vs. ATG) will be launched after haplo-HSCT, it would be of major scientific interest to prospectively compare within a phase 3 trial ATG vs. PT-CY.

Finally, whether PT-CY is equally effective after RIC and MAC regimen is currently unknown as it is unknown if other combination like sirolimus (SIR) + MMF can be as effective as (or less effective as) CNI/MMF in addition to PT-CY in the haploidentical situation or even if PT-CY can safely be used as a single agent after HLA-identical sibling transplants, as recently reported (Mielcarek et al. 2016).

CY administered in two doses scheduled soon after transplantation depletes highly proliferating alloreactive conventional T cells while helping to preserve Tregs.

25.5 ATG or Alemtuzumab for GVHD Prophylaxis in HSCT

Since almost two decades, both ATG and alemtuzumab (ALEM) have been used to prevent GVHD especially after transplantation from URD. ALEM although efficacious in preventing acute GVHD has never been tested prospectively in a randomized phase 3 trial and has almost exclusively been developed in the UK. ATG however has been tested in four prospective randomized phase 3 trials. Three out of these four used anti-T-lymphocyte globulin (ATLG) and one rabbit ATG (rATG). However, the design, the time period, patients' selection, donor type, and primary end point of these four randomized trials differ (see Table 25.2 for references). From the perspective of GVHD prophylaxis efficacy, all four trials demonstrated a significant decrease in chronic GVHD rate and in three out of the four a statistical significant decrease in the rate of acute GVHD. Other end points varied among the four trials. In particular the American trial by Soiffer et al. was the only one in which patients who received ATLG experienced an increased rate of relapse mainly in patients with AML who received TBI as part of a MAC pre-transplant.

25.6 New Immunosuppressive Regimens for GVHD Prophylaxis

With current treatment strategies summarized above, the rate of moderate to severe acute GVHD remains of concern in the range of 20–50%. As reviewed elsewhere in the Handbook, the treatment of acute and of chronic GVHD with high-dose steroids remains unsatisfactory with 30–50% of the patients being steroid resistant or dependent. There is thus an unmet clinical need in GVHD prophylaxis. After years of lack of new agent in this setting, the better knowledge of basic T-cell immunology, of the pathophysiology of the disease, and new drug development by the industry, new agents have been tested mostly in phase 2 trials which appeared to be promising. This section summarized the drugs with most advanced development that reported an acute GVHD incidence in the 20% range (i.e., a range that may warrant development of subsequent phase 3 trials). Readers with interest on a more detailed portfolio of current drug development and new targets could refer to a recent review (Zeiser and Blazar 2017).

In contrast to CNI, SIR, an mTOR inhibitor, is a more potent suppressor of the expansion of conventional T cells than Tregs, owing to the greater dependence of conventional T cells on the mTOR-protein kinase B pathway. This was the basis of the development by the Dana-Farber Cancer Institute (DFCI) group of a regimen that leads to an estimated cumulative incidence of acute GVHD grades II–IV of 20.5% and of less than 5%

Table 25.2 Four randomized trials using ATG as a GVHD prophylaxis

	Finke et al. (2009)	Kroger et al. (2016)	Soiffer et al. (2017)	Walker et al. (2016)
N	202	168	254	203
Product	ATLG	ATLG	ATLG	rATG
Primary end point	GVHD	cGVHD	cGVHD-free survival	Freedom from all IST
Conditioning	MAC	MAC	MAC	MAC+RIC
Donor	URD	Id. Sibling	URD	URD
GvHD prophylaxis	CSA +MTX	CSA +MTX	TAC +MTX	CSA or TAC+MTX or MMF
Acute GVHD	33 vs. 51% (grade II–IV)	11 vs. 18% (grade II–IV)	23 vs. 40% (grade II–IV)	50 vs. 65% (any grade)
Chronic GVHD	Decreased	Decreased	Decreased	Decreased

grades III–IV. This prompted a large trial of the BMTCTN comparing TAC/SIR to TAC/MTX. The primary end point of the trial was to compare grade II–IV acute GVHD-free survival using an intention-to-treat analysis of 304 randomized subjects. There was no difference in the probability of day 114 grade II–IV acute GVHD-free survival (67% vs. 62%, $P = 0.38$). Grade II–IV GVHD was similar in the TAC/SIR and TAC/MTX arms (26% vs. 34%, $P = 0.48$) (Cutler et al. 2014). A smaller randomized single-center phase 2 study found however less cumulative incidence with 43% grade II–IV after TAC/SIR (as compared to an unexpected high rate of 89% after TAC/MTX) (Pidala et al. 2012).

Encouraging rates have also been reported by two other compounds: Bortezomib (BOR) (Koreth et al. 2012) and Maraviroc in 2012 (Reshef et al. 2012) delivered in addition to TAC/MTX. These two drugs as well as CY have been then tested in randomized phase 2 trials in the setting of HSCT (BMTCTN 1203 trial) after RIC in a pick-the-winner-designed trial (i.e., aimed to test in a multicenter setting the three drugs) and compared to prospective contemporary cohort of patients who received TAC/MTX. The final results of this trial closed for recruitment will be available in 2018. Finally, in an open-label three-arm phase 2 randomized controlled trial, investigator at the DFCI compared grade II–IV acute GVHD between conventional TAC/MTX (A) vs. BOR/TAC/MTX (B) and vs. BOR/SIR/TAC (C), in RIC-HSCT recipients from URD in 138 patients. Day +180 grade II–IV acute GVHD rates were similar (A 32.6%, B 31.1%, C 21%) as was the 2-year NRM. Overall, the BOR-based regimens evaluated did not seem to improve outcomes compared with TAC/MTX therapy (Koreth et al. 2018).

Finally, based on preclinical works in mice models, two drugs Vorinostat and Tocilizumab provided exciting results and were supported by ancillary biological data in humans.

- Vorinostat, a histone deacetylase inhibitor, at low concentration has anti-inflammatory and immunoregulatory effects. Pavan Reddy's group in Michigan provided compelling evidences that in preclinical models Vorinostat reduced GVHD rate, suppressed pro-inflammatory cytokines, regulated APCs, and enhanced Treg functions. In two separate trials (Choi et al. 2014, 2017), authors translated their findings in the clinical setting. In one trial where Vorinostat was added to standard prophylaxis after RIC in HLA-identical siblings, acute GVHD grade II–IV rate was 22% and that of grades III–IV of 6%. In another trial after MAC in URD, the acute GVHD rates were similar.

- The addition of Tocilizumab to CNI+ MTX standard prophylaxis has been tested by two different groups (Kenedy et al. 2014; Dorobyski et al. 2018). Tocilizumab is a humanized anti-IL-6 receptor monoclonal antibody. IL-6 levels are increased early during GVHD and are present in all target tissues. Blockade of the IL-6 signaling pathway has been shown to reduce the severity of GVHD and to prolong survival in experimental models. Investigators in Milwaukee and in Brisbane conducted two separate phase 2 trials using Tocilizumab, and both found very low rate of grade II–IV acute GVHD (less than 15%).

Other new agents are currently either tested in preclinical models or are in the early stage of development in clinical trials (reviewed in Zeiser and Blazar 2017). New strategies that have shown efficacy in preclinical models of GVHD include the inhibition of Janus kinase (JAK) and rho-associated protein kinase 1 (ROCK-1). The blockade of phosphatidylinositol 3-kinase (PI3K), mitogen-activated protein kinase (MEK) proteins 1 and 2, aurora A kinase, and cyclin-dependent kinase 2 (CDK2) have been shown to reduce acute GVHD in murine models.

25.7 Conclusion and Perspective

Despite decades of experience with transplantation, GVHD still occurs in over 40% of the patients. When acute GVHD develops, the main treatment is high-dose steroids. However around one third of the patients will be steroid resistant.

Steroid resistance remains associated with a dismal prognosis (30–40% 1-year survival). These data urge for developing new strategies to prevent GVHD. Fortunately enough, based on preclinical findings and improved knowledge on the immune biology of HSCT, recent drug combination opens the gate for future development.

Key Points

- Current GVHD prophylaxis relies on CNI + short-term MTX after MAC and of CSA ± MMF after RIC
- ATG has been demonstrated to decrease acute GVHD after URD transplant and of chronic GVHD
- Despite the above two points, new prophylactic regimens are clearly warranted since severe GVHD rates still lie on the 25% range

References

Choi SW, Braun T, Chang L, et al. Vorinostat plus tacrolimus and mycophenolate to prevent graft-versus-host disease after related-donor reduced intensity conditioning allogeneic haematopoietic stem-cell transplantation. Lancet Oncol. 2014;15:87–95.

Choi SW, Braun T, Henig I, et al. Vorinostat plus tacrolimus/methotrexate to prevent GVHD after myeloablative conditioning, unrelated donor HSCT. Blood. 2017;130:1760–7.

Cutler C, Logan B, Nakamura R, et al. Tacrolimus/sirolimus vs tacrolimus/methotrexate as GVHD prophylaxis after matched, related donor allogeneic HCT. Blood. 2014;124:1372–7.

Dorobyski WR, Szabo A, Zhu F, et al. Tocilizumab, tacrolimus and methotrexate for prevention of acute graft-versus-host disease: low incidence of lower gastrointestinal tract disease. Haematologica. 2018;103:717–27.

Finke J, Bethge WA, Schmoor C, et al. Standard graft-versus-host disease prophylaxis with or without anti-T-cell globulin in haematopoietic cell transplantation from matched unrelated donors: a randomised, open-label, multicentre phase 3 trial. Lancet Oncol. 2009;10:855–64.

Fuchs EJ. Related haploidentical donors are better choice than matched unrelated donors: point. Blood Adv. 2017;1:397–400.

Kenedy GA, Varelias A, Vuckovic S, et al. Addition of interleukin-6 inhibition with tocilizumab to standard graft-versus-host disease prophylaxis after allogeneic stem-cell transplantation: a phase 1/2 trial. Lancet Oncol. 2014;15:1451–9.

Koreth J, Kim HT, Lange PB, et al. Bortezomib-based immunosuppression after reduced-intensity conditioning hematopoietic stem cell transplantation: randomized phase II results. Haematologica. 2018;103:522–30.

Koreth J, Stevenson KE, Kim HT, et al. Bortezomib-based graft-versus-host disease prophylaxis in HLA-mismatched unrelated donor transplantation. J Clin Oncol. 2012;30:3202–8.

Kroger N, Solano C, Wolschke C, et al. Antilymphocyte globulin for prevention of chronic graft-versus-host disease. N Engl J Med. 2016;374:43–53.

Mielcarek M, Furlong T, O'Donnell PV, et al. Post-transplant cyclophosphamide for prevention of graft-versus-host disease after HLA-matched mobilized blood cell transplantation. Blood. 2016;127:1502–8.

Nash RA, Antin JH, Karanes C, Fay JW, et al. Phase 3 study comparing methotrexate and tacrolimus with methotrexate and cyclosporine for prophylaxis of acute graft-versus-host disease after marrow transplantation from unrelated donors. Blood. 2000;96:2062–8.

Pidala J, Kim J, Jim H, et al. A randomized phase II study to evaluate tacrolimus in combination with sirolimus or methotrexate after allogeneic hematopoietic cell transplantation. Haematologica. 2012;97:1882–9.

Ratanatharathorn V, Nash RA, Przepiorka D, et al. Phase III study comparing methotrexate and tacrolimus (prograf, FK506) with methotrexate and cyclosporine for graft-versus-host disease prophylaxis after HLA-identical sibling bone marrow transplantation. Blood. 1998;92:2303–14.

Reshef R, Luger SM, Hexner EO, et al. Blockade of lymphocyte chemotaxis in visceral graft-versus-host disease. N Engl J Med. 2012;367:135–45.

Soiffer RJ, Kim HT, McGuirk J, et al. Prospective, randomized, double-blind, phase III clinical trial of anti-T-lymphocyte globulin to assess impact on chronic graft-versus-host disease–free survival in patients undergoing HLA-matched unrelated myeloablative hematopoietic cell transplantation. J Clin Oncol. 2017;35:4003–11.

Storb R, Deeg HJ, Whitehead J, et al. Methotrexate and cyclosporine compared with cyclosporine alone for prophylaxis of acute graft versus host disease after marrow transplantation for leukemia. N Engl J Med. 1986;314:729–35.

Walker I, Panzarella T, Couban S, et al. Pre-treatment with anti-thymocyte globulin versus no anti-thymocyte globulin in patients with haematological malignancies undergoing haemopoietic cell transplantation from unrelated donors: a randomised, controlled, open-label, phase 3, multicentre trial. Lancet Oncol. 2016;17:164–73.

Zeiser R, Blazar BR. Acute graft-versus-host disease; biologic process, prevention and therapy. N Engl J Med. 2017;377:2167–79.

Management ATG (SIRS)

Francesca Bonifazi

26.1 Introduction

Currently horse and rabbit anti-lymphoglobulins (ATLG) or antithymocyte globulin (ATG) is available; the main, although not exclusive, use is for the treatment of aplastic anemia (horse) and for GVHD prophylaxis (rabbit). They differ in the manufacturing process (i.e., used animal, pulsed antigens, antibody specificities, and cellular targets): for this reason, dose, timing, and setting cannot be interchangeable, and also clinical results are different. As they are polyclonal serum-derived products from nonhuman organisms, they can cause serum sickness and infusion reactions.

26.2 ATLG/ATG Infusion Protocol (See Table 26.1)

ATLG/ATG infusion should be performed in trained centers. Standard hygienic handling of the injection site, careful evaluation of the infusion speed, and appropriate choice of the venous access are crucial. Medical personnel should carefully watch over patients for adverse events not only during but also after infusion.

F. Bonifazi (✉)
Institute of Hematology "Seràgnoli", University Hospital S. Orsola-Malpighi, Bologna University, Bologna, Italy
e-mail: francesca.bonifazi@unibo.it

During administration, the patient needs to be monitored for symptoms related to infusion reactions or anaphylaxis. The first dose should be administered at a reduced speed for the first 30 min. If no symptoms of intolerance occur, infusion rate may be increased. In case of anaphylactic or anaphylactoid reactions, physicians must be prepared to promptly manage this event, and appropriate medical treatment has to be implemented.

A central venous catheter is preferred, although a peripheral large high-flow access may be acceptable, if a central line is not available. Thrombophlebitis is the major risk when a peripheral vein is used. The availability of a high-flow access is important in case of treatment of infusion reactions.

Premedication is mandatory in order to improve systemic and local tolerance (see later). Stability, compatibility, and dilution are different for each product, and specific manufacturer recommendations should be followed carefully.

Preinfusion intraepidermal tests are not yet validated for rabbit ATG but, according to manufacturer indications, are recommended for horse ATLG.

— Although standard infusion time is between 4 and 12 h, a longer administration time correlates with milder side effects, thus making infusions of 12 h highly advised.

Table 26.1 Infusion of ATLG/ATG

Factors	Comments
Infusion site	– Central line is highly preferred – Risk of thrombophlebitis and drug precipitation are higher in peripheral veins
Dilution	Avoid to inject undiluted preparation; follow the manufacturer instructions for each ATLG/ATG type
Compatibility	– rATLG-Grafalon: avoid to mix concentrate solution with glucose, blood, blood derivatives, sodium heparin, and lipid-containing solutions – rATG-Thymoglobulin: avoid dilutions with other than saline and dextrose – Horse ATGAM: avoid dextrose injection or acidic solution because of precipitation or instability
Stability	Diluted solutions up to 24 h (infusion time included) stored in refrigerator
Duration of infusion	4–12 h – Slower infusion results in a lower incidence and severity of infusion reactions; therefore ≥12 h infusion is recommended Start first administration at low infusion rate (at least for the first 30–60 min)
Drug interactions	Not reported
Premedication	Mandatory; steroids, acetaminophen, antihistamines
Preinfusion test	– Not advised for rabbit sera – Recommended for ATGAM – Skin and conjunctival tests not extensively validated
Criteria for permanent discontinuation	Anaphylaxis: severe anaphylaxis, always. De-sensitization protocols: not validated
What does D/C stand for?	SIRS: depending on grading and clinical evaluation of pros and cons. In case of rechallenge, more stringent monitoring is required

26.3 ATLG/ATG Dose

Dose and timing of ATLG/ATG administration vary substantially among transplant centers (Bacigalupo et al. 2001; Finke et al. 2009; Walker et al. 2016; Kröger et al. 2016; Soiffer et al. 2017).

The currently used doses of ATLG/ATG are calculated and validated in clinical trials, according to body weight. A strong rationale and some preliminary data (Admiraal et al. 2017) suggest that calculating the ATG/ATLG dose according to the cellular target, i.e., the number of total lymphocyte before infusion of the first dose, can provide the optimal drug exposure and therefore maximize the benefit (GVHD decrease) over the potential risks (increase of relapses and infections). Since ATLG and ATG are different preparations arising from different manufacturing processes and different pulsed antigens, no dose equivalence can be established.

26.4 Infusion Reactions

ATLG/ATG administration can be complicated by several infusion reactions including fever, chills, erythema, dyspnea, oxygen desaturation, nausea/vomiting, diarrhea, abdominal pain, hyperkalemia, tachycardia, hypo- or hypertension, malaise, rash, urticaria, headache, arthralgia, myalgia (serum sickness, after 5–15 days from infusion), hepatic cytolysis, and even systemic anaphylaxis.

Even if the NCI Terminology Criteria for Adverse Events (CTCAE) use different scales for grading reactions to infusion of chemotherapy and allergic/anaphylaxis reactions, there are no specific symptoms enabling to distinguish "standard" infusion reaction from an allergic one that can evolve to anaphylaxis.

Anaphylaxis and acute allergic reactions are based on IgE effect and histamine release by mastocytes, but the vast majority of symptoms can be attributed to the cytokine release syndrome (CRS) and are generally reversible. CRS is a form of systemic inflammatory response syndrome (SIRS) (Matsuda and Hattori 2006; Balk 2014). CRS can follow not only ATG/ATLG infusion but also chemotherapy, MoAb (Remberger et al. 1999; Feng et al. 2014), bispecific antibodies, or CAR-T cell therapies (Lee et al. 2014). All these (both allergic and nonallergic, such as CRS) are infusion reactions. Serum sickness is a hypersensitivity phenomenon that can develop after 5–15 days after the infusion, and it is well responsive to steroid treatment.

26.5   SIRS

SIRS is a clinical syndrome due to dysregulated inflammation. SIRS may occur in several conditions, such as infection, autoimmune disorders, vasculitis, thromboembolism, chemotherapy infusion, surgery, and burns. The denomination originates from changes of some parameters (temperature, heart and respiratory rates, and white blood cell count) occurring after infection/sepsis according to Bone (Bone et al. 1992). A pediatric version tailored on patient age is also available (Goldstein 2005). More recently, some authors (Lee et al. 2014) revised the classification of the cytokine release syndrome according to the treatment required (oxygen, vasopressors, organ toxicity).

26.5.1 Risk Factors for SIRS

SIRS after ATLG/ATG infusion cannot be predicted and the risk factors are not well known.

The binding of ATLG/ATG to the surface of target cells (lymphocytes, monocytes, dendritic cells) elicits cytokine production and systemic inflammation (Bone et al. 1992).

Thus, that the higher the number of lymphocytes at the moment of the (first) infusion, the more likely is the risk of systemic activation of inflammation and then SIRS.

Accordingly, RIC regimens are reported to be associated with greater cytokine release syndrome (Remberger and Sundberg 2004) because of the likely higher number of residual lymphocytes in RIC in comparison with MAC regimens.

26.5.2 Management of SIRS

26.5.2.1   Prophylaxis
ATLG/ATG infusion reactions can be reduced in frequency and severity by two factors: premedication and speed of infusion. Premedication is performed with steroids, antihistamine, and acetaminophen. The optimal schedule of premedication is not yet well established. Doses of prednisolone of 250 mg (higher than 1 mg/kg), given before the first infusion and followed by an additional dose in the same day, reduce the incidence of infusion reactions and cytokine release as reported (Pihusch et al. 2002).

The rate of infusion is one of the most important factors to reduce the incidence and severity of infusion reactions since lower infusion rates are associated with a lower incidence and the severity of reactions. Administration time ≥ 12 h is the preferred schedule to yield high compliance to ATLG/ATG infusion.

26.5.2.2   Treatment
If symptoms of SIRS appear, the drug should be discontinued, at least temporarily.

Treatment is symptomatic and depends upon the clinical manifestations. Intensive care for respiratory and hemodynamic support should be given according to international guidelines for critical patients, and the intervention of an intensive specialist may be requested. SIRS after ATLG/ATG is different from sepsis-induced SIRS where steroids failed to achieve a significant benefit (Cronin et al. 1995). Symptoms due to ATLG/ATG-related SIRS are more pronounced on day +1 and then tend to decrease. Steroids, widely used preemptively, provide high response rates also as a treatment measure.

Permanent Discontinuation/Rechallenge

Rechallenge after anaphylaxis and after standard infusion reactions >3 is strongly discouraged.

Non-controlled life-threatening infections are contraindications to transplant and should not modify ATLG/ATG administration per se.

Desensitization protocols are not yet clearly validated.

Key Points

- SIRS is a systemic reaction related to cytokine release after ATLG/ATG infusion.
- The infusion reactions can be reduced by premedication (steroids, antihistamines, and acetaminophen) and by a low infusion rate (12 h or longer).

References

Admiraal R, Nierkens S, de Witte MA, et al. Association between anti-thymocyte globulin exposure and survival outcomes in adult unrelated haemopoietic cell transplantation: a multicentre, retrospective, pharmacodynamic cohort analysis. Lancet Haematol. 2017;4:e183–91.

Bacigalupo A, Lamparelli T, Bruzzi P, et al. Antithymocyte globulin for graft-versus-host disease prophylaxis in transplants from unrelated donors: 2 randomized studies from Gruppo Italiano Trapianti Midollo Osseo (GITMO). Blood. 2001;98:2942–7.

Balk RA. Systemic inflammatory response syndrome (SIRS): where did it come from and is it still relevant today? Virulence. 2014;5:20–6.

Bone RC, Balk RA, Cerra FB, et al. American College of Chest Physicians/Society of Critical Care Medicine Consensus Conference: definitions for sepsis and organ failure and guidelines for the use of innovative therapies in sepsis. Crit Care Med. 1992;20:864–74.

Cronin L, Cook DJ, Carlet J, et al. Corticosteroid treatment for sepsis: a critical appraisal and meta-analysis of the literature. Crit Care Med. 1995;23:1430–9.

Feng X, Scheinberg P, Biancotto A, et al. In vivo effects of horse and rabbit antithymocyte globulin in patients with severe aplastic anemia. Haematologica. 2014;99:1433–40.

Finke J, Bethge WA, Schmoor C, et al. Standard graft-versus-host disease prophylaxis with or without anti-T-cell globulin in haematopoietic cell transplantation from matched unrelated donors: a randomised, open-label, multicentre phase 3 trial. Lancet Oncol. 2009;10:855–64.

Goldstein B, Giroir B, Randolph A, International Consensus Conference on Pediatric Sepsis. International pediatric sepsis consensus conference: definitions for sepsis and organ dysfunction in pediatrics. Pediatr Crit Care Med. 2005;6:2–8.

Kröger N, Solano C, Wolschke C, et al. Antilymphocyte globulin for prevention of chronic graft-versus-host disease. N Engl J Med. 2016;374:43–53.

Lee DW, Gardner R, Porter DL, et al. Current concepts in the diagnosis and management of cytokine release syndrome. Blood. 2014;124:188–95.

Matsuda N, Hattori Y. Systemic inflammatory response syndrome (SIRS): molecular pathophysiology and gene therapy. J Pharmacol Sci. 2006;101:189–98.

Pihusch R, Holler E, Mühlbayer D, et al. The impact of antithymocyte globulin on short-term toxicity after allogeneic stem cell transplantation. Bone Marrow Transplant. 2002;30:347–54.

Remberger M, Sundberg B. Cytokine production during myeloablative and reduced intensity therapy before allogeneic stem cell transplantation. Haematologica. 2004;89:710–6.

Remberger M, Svahn BM, Hentschke P, et al. Effect on cytokine release and graft-versus-host disease of different anti-T cell antibodies during conditioning for unrelated haematopoietic stem cell transplantation. Bone Marrow Transplant. 1999;24:823–30.

Soiffer RJ, Kim HT, McGuirk J, et al. Prospective, randomized, double-blind, phase III clinical trial of anti-t-lymphocyte globulin to assess impact on chronic graft-versus-host disease-free survival in patients undergoing HLA-matched unrelated myeloablative hematopoietic cell transplantation. J Clin Oncol. 2017;35:4003–11.

Walker I, Panzarella T, Couban S, et al. Pretreatment with anti-thymocyte globulin versus no anti-thymocyte globulin in patients with haematological malignancies undergoing haemopoietic cell transplantation from unrelated donors: a randomised, controlled, open-label, phase 3, multicentre trial. Lancet Oncol. 2016;17:164–73.

Infection Control and Isolation Procedures

Malgorzata Mikulska

27.1 Introduction

Infection control is defined as a set of measures aimed at preventing or stopping the spread of infections in healthcare settings. All HSCT recipients should follow general guidelines (e.g. CDC) for preventing healthcare-associated infections through hand hygiene, disinfection and sterilization, environmental infection control, isolation precautions and prevention of intravascular catheter-related infection (Sehulster et al. 2004; Guidelines for Hand Hygiene in Healthcare Settings (2002), Guideline for Isolation Precautions: Preventing Transmission of Infectious Agents in Healthcare Settings (2007), Guidelines for Environmental Infection Control in Health-Care Facilities (2003), all available at https://www.cdc.gov/infectioncontrol/guidelines/index.html; Freifeld et al. 2011).

Dedicated and detailed international recommendations for HSCT recipients on preventing infectious complications have been published in 2009 (Tomblyn et al. 2009; Yokoe et al. 2009). As there were no well-executed randomized or con-

trolled trials and little evidence to hand from cohort case-controlled or multiple time-series studies or uncontrolled experiments, reliance had to be placed on descriptive studies, reports of expert committees or on the opinions of respected authorities. Hence, most of these recommendations on infection control could only be graded as level III.

Isolation procedures in HSCT recipient comprise precautions universal for all healthcare settings (Standard Precautions and Transmission-Based Precautions) and those specific for HSCT and employed to prevent transmission of spores of filamentous fungi, mainly *Aspergillus*, with unfiltered air.

There is no consensus on specific *protective environment*, called also reverse isolation, for neutropenic patients. HSCT recipients should be placed in single-patient room, with adequate ventilation system (see below), if possible. However, no clear benefit of routine footwear exchange, or use of disposable gloves and gowns on the rate of infections have been demonstrated, and procedures vary significantly between institutions, with routine use of masks and disposable gloves and gowns in some but not others. On the contrary, the negative effect of strict protective isolation on patient's quality of life and well-being should be acknowledged and weighted against the evidence of benefits of single protective measures (Abad et al. 2010).

M. Mikulska (✉)
Division of Infectious Diseases, Department
of Health Sciences (DISSAL), IRCCS Ospedale
Policlinico San Martino, University of Genova,
Genova, Italy
e-mail: m.mikulska@unige.it

27.2 Standard Precautions

Should be used universally for all patients and they include:

1. Proper hand hygiene
2. Use of standard personal protective equipment (PPE)
3. Appropriate cleaning and disinfection protocols (including those for shared equipment or toys and play areas in paediatric units)
4. Safe injection practices
5. Infection control practices for special procedures (e.g. surgical masks for lumbar puncture)

27.2.1 Hand Hygiene

It is by far the most effective means of prevention of pathogen transmission (Freifeld et al. 2011; Tomblyn et al. 2009). The preferred method of hand decontamination is with an alcohol-based hand rub, due to its superior convenience and reduced drying of the skin. Handwashing with soap and water is recommended if hands are visibly soiled, for example, with blood or body fluids, or after potential contact with spores of *Clostridium difficile* or with *Norovirus*. Of note, 15–30 s is the minimum necessary handwashing time.

PPE used routinely by healthcare workers during patient care and procedures are gloves, gowns (used if direct contact with patient's fluids is expected) and mouth, nose and eye protection (used during procedures which are likely to generate splashes or sprays of blood, body fluids, secretions and excretions). Routine donning of gowns upon entrance into a high-risk unit, including HSCT unit, is not indicated.

27.3 Transmission-Based Precautions

These are the measures used in addition to standard precautions for patients with documented or suspected infection or colonization with highly transmissible or epidemiologically important pathogens for which additional precautions are

necessary to prevent transmission. The main types of transmission-based precautions are *contact* precautions, *airborne* precautions and *droplet* precautions. The specific PPE and the examples of pathogens which require each type of transmission-based precautions are outlined in Table 27.1.

Contact precaution should be also applied in a *pre-emptive* way, e.g. in case of patients transferred from high-risk facilities, pending the results of surveillance cultures. Clear criteria should be provided for appropriate discontinuation of contact precautions (usually when three different swabs from a known multidrug-resistant (MDR) positive site, taken 1–7 days apart, are negative). In case of contact precautions, and particularly if a patient is still colonized with a resistant pathogen, this information should be clearly stated on the discharge information form for the centres which will care for this patient subsequently. In case of MDR Gram-negative pathogens, full antibiotic susceptibility results should be provided to allow appropriate empirical therapy in case of severe subsequent infection.

Cough etiquette should be promoted. Additionally, transplant recipients, particularly those with respiratory symptoms, should use surgical masks and maintain special separation from others in common waiting areas, ideally a distance of at least 1 m.

Upon entering HSCT unit, *visitors* should be screened for the presence of symptoms of easily transmissible diseases such as *viral respiratory tract infections*, gastroenteritis, etc. and, if present, advised to postpone their visit until no longer symptomatic. Also, healthcare workers with respiratory symptoms should refrain from direct patient care until the symptoms resolve. Seronegative persons who were exposed to communicable diseases such as measles or chickenpox should refrain from contact with HSCT recipients or transplant candidates until the incubation period passes without developing the disease. Instructional materials for patients and visitors on recommended hand hygiene, respiratory hygiene/cough etiquette practices and the application of transmission-based precautions should be provided. Vaccination of healthcare workers

Table 27.1 Transmission-based precautions, to be applied in addition to standard precautions

Type of precaution	Patients placement and PPE to be used by patients	PPE for healthcare personnel	Example of pathogens and comments
Contact	– Single room; if not available, cohorting of those colonized/infected by the same pathogen – During transport, cover patient's colonized/infected areas	– Disposable gloves and gowns – Use patient-dedicated or disposable equipment; if not feasible, clean and disinfect thoroughly	– Infection with *Clostridium difficile* – Colonization or infection with MDR pathogens – Infectious diarrhoea due to pathogens such as *Salmonella*, *Norovirus*, *Rotavirus*, etc All the units or other hospitals involved in patient's care should be notified about all the isolated pathogens requiring contact precautions
Droplet	– Single room; if not available, cohorting of those infected by the same pathogen – Surgical mask – Follow CDC's respiratory hygiene/cough etiquette in healthcare setting	– Mask (surgical) – Disposable gloves and gowns	– Pathogens transmitted by respiratory droplets (i.e. large-particle droplets >5 μ in size) that are generated by a patient who is coughing, sneezing or talking, e.g. influenza or other respiratory viruses In case of transplant recipients, the duration of precautions should be extended due to the possibility of prolonged shedding caused by immunodeficiency
Airborne	– Rooms with at least 6 (existing facility) or 12 (new construction/renovation) air changes per hour and direct exhaust of air to the outside (if not possible, the air may be returned to the air-handling system or adjacent spaces if all air is directed through HEPA filters) – Surgical mask – Follow CDC's respiratory hygiene/cough etiquette in healthcare setting	– N95 or higher-level respirator for respiratory protection	– *Mycobacterium tuberculosis* (patients with respiratory tuberculosis and sputum with direct evidence of mycobacteria) – Measles, chickenpox and disseminated herpes zoster

HEPA high-efficiency particulate air, *MDR* multidrug resistant, *PPE* personal protective equipment

and household contacts is paramount and discussed in the dedicated chapter.

27.4 Management of the Threat of MDR Bacteria

In the era of increasing bacterial resistance, an important part of infection control deals with *prevention of colonization and infection with MDR bacteria* (Siegel et al. 2007). Active surveillance, for example, with rectal swabs for detecting colonization with vancomycin-resistant enterococci (VRE) or carbapenem-resistant *Enterobacteriaceae* or nasal swabs for methicillin-resistant *Staphylococcus aureus*, should be performed in institutions where

these pathogens are regularly encountered or in patients coming from such institutions.

The need for screening for different pathogens may vary according to local epidemiology. For instance, Italian statement on the management of carbapenem-resistant *Klebsiella pneumoniae* (CR-*Kp*) infections in HSCT was published (Girmenia et al. 2015). Briefly, they recommended active detection of CR-*Kp* carriers before and after HSCT, since the carriers have approximately 30% risk of developing CR-*Kp* bloodstream infection; staff education and monitoring of adherence to contact precautions; a cautious approach to declare a patient no longer colonized and a need for coordinated effort to intra- or inter-hospital transmission. HSCT is not contraindicated in MDR carriers, but establishing upfront the appropriate empirical therapy to be administered in case of fever during neutropenia is mandatory, and careful evaluation of the possibility of decolonization in selected cases through oral administration of non-absorbable molecules or faecal microbiota transplantation is warranted (Girmenia et al. 2015; Bilinski et al. 2017).

In order to counteract the threat of MDR pathogens and the shortage of agents active against Gram-negative MDR bacteria, *antimicrobial stewardship program* should be implemented in every centre (Gyssens et al. 2013). Additionally, national systems for surveillance, with obligation for notification and recommendations for containment and infection control measures, should be put in place (Tacconelli et al. 2014).

The aim of *antimicrobial stewardship* is to limit the negative impact of MDR pathogens on patients' outcome, and its *main elements* are detailed in Table 27.2.

Successful implementation of antimicrobial stewardship is based on a multidisciplinary approach and close collaboration between the treating haematologists, microbiology laboratory and infectious diseases consultation service, including infection control unit, hospital pharmacy and hospital authorities who should recognize that this is an important step in high-quality management of infectious complications after HSCT.

Surveillance of effectiveness of infection control practices should be put in place, with regular monitoring of adherence. In case of contact-transmission pathogens, such as *Clostridium difficile* or MDR bacteria, laboratory data should be regularly analysed to detect any trends indicating possible increase in transmission.

27.5   HSCT Environment

Flowers, fountains, water leaks and water-retaining bath toys carry the risk of *water-associated infections* with Gram-negative bacilli such as *Pseudomonas aeruginosa* or *Legionella* and thus should be avoided in the areas where

Table 27.2 Main elements of antimicrobial stewardship program

1. Regularly updated (e.g. every 6–12 months) surveillance of local epidemiology of infections in HSCT recipients, through reports on:
   (a) Resistance rates to main antibiotics in top 10 most frequent pathogens
   (b) Data on antibiotic consumption
   (c) Data on patient outcomes in case of most frequent/difficult infections
2. Implementation of updated diagnostic methods and prompt reporting of microbiologic results by the laboratory in order to provide clinicians with
   (a) Correct and timely diagnosis (e.g. of viral or fungal infections or *Clostridium difficile*, which may allow to avoid unnecessary antibiotic therapy)
   (b) Rapid results of antimicrobial susceptibility testing to allow choosing the best targeted antibiotic therapy
3. Promoting appropriate antibiotic use, for example
   (a) Implementing timely de-escalation or discontinuation of antibiotic treatment, particularly during neutropenia
   (b) Appropriate dosing for different indications
   (c) Optimized infusion strategies for time- and dose-dependent molecules, e.g. use of extended or continuous infusion of time-dependent molecules such as beta-lactams
4. Establishing and regularly updating protocols for prevention and treatment of infections, e.g. identifying antibiotic and antifungal regimens for empirical therapy in accordance with local epidemiology (e.g. prevalence of extended spectrum beta-lactamase (ESBL) producing Enterobacteriaceae, methicillin-resistant staphylococci, azole-resistant aspergilli, etc.)

severely immunocompromised patients are being cared for (Yokoe et al. 2009). In addition, there are issues specific for HSCT recipients, such as room ventilation, intensified protective measures applied during hospital construction and renovations, avoidance of contact with soil (including potted plants) and avoidance of dust both permanently (e.g. non-carpeting and no porous surfaces) and while cleaning, all aimed at decreasing the risk of invasive aspergillosis (Yokoe et al. 2009).

CIBMTR/ASBMT/EBMT global recommendations on protective environment concerning hospital *room design and ventilation* are available (Yokoe et al. 2009). Briefly, allo-HSCT recipients should ideally be placed in protective environment rooms that incorporate several features including central or point-of-use HEPA (high-efficiency particulate air) filters with 99.97% efficiency for removing particles ≤0.3 μm in diameter and ≥12 air exchanges/hours, with directed airflow and consistent positive air pressure differential between the patient's room and the hallway ≥2.5 Pa. All these measures remove airborne fungal spores and are aimed at preventing airborne infections with filamentous fungi such as aspergilli. The efficacy of protective isolation measures in case of auto-HSCT recipients is less well established.

Currently *HEPA-filtered rooms* are probably available in almost all centres, while few centres-fulfilled all the CIBMTR/ASBMT/EBMT requirements. However, the knowledge on the details and maintenance of protective environments in the HSCT setting was recently found inadequate, requiring education efforts and cooperation with hospital infection control and the hospital maintenance services (Styczynski et al. 2018).

During *construction and renovations*, due to high density of fungal spores, protective environmental measures are particularly important, and mould-control measures should be intensified and filtration efficiency should be monitored frequently to best determine appropriate time for replacement. Specific recommendations are available and should be followed (Sehulster et al. 2004). For example, construction and renovation areas should have negative air pressure relative to HSCT patient care areas to ensure that air flows from patient care areas toward construction areas, and a portable, industrial-grade HEPA filter should be used between a construction zone and the HSCT unit if a large area is under construction and negative pressure differential cannot be guaranteed. In addition, HSCT recipients may benefit from wearing N95 respirators outside HEPA-filtered areas, particularly during ongoing constructions, since unlike surgical masks, higher efficiency ones offer protection against *Aspergillus* spores. Active monitoring of cases of invasive mould infections should be performed in order to detect any possible outbreak.

27.6 Food Safety in Transplant Recipients

Drinking *water* should be safe; thus boiled or bottled water is to be preferred. Tap water in highly populated areas is usually regarded as safe from bacterial contamination because regularly tested for it. However, it may still contain *Cryptosporidiums*. Water from private wells should be avoided.

The use of *low-microbial diet*, which prohibits fresh fruits and vegetables and unprocessed food, did not result in a decreased incidence of infections in neutropenic patients (Sonbol et al. 2015; van Dalen et al. 2016). Standard food safety practices that emphasize safe handling and washing or thoroughly cooking food were found to be just as safe and produced no increase in infection rates or incidence of neutropenic fever. Similarly, to other immunocompromised patients, HSCT recipients should avoid foods possibly contaminated by *Listeria monocytogenes*, *Campylobacter jejuni*, *Salmonella enteritidis*, *Toxoplasma gondii*, etc. *Main high-risk foods* to avoid include:

- Raw or undercooked meat, poultry, fish or shellfish
- Refrigerated smoked fish
- Unpasteurized milk
- Foods with raw or undercooked eggs
- Unwashed fruits and vegetables
- Raw sprouts
- Soft cheeses made from unpasteurized milk like brie, camembert and blue-veined and fresh cheese (can be eaten if cooked)
- Hot dogs, deli meats and luncheon meats that have not been reheated to steaming hot or to 75 °C
- Unsafe water and ice made of it

Food safety practices for food handling should be followed, and specific information for cancer patients is available online (https://www.fda.gov/downloads/Food/FoodborneIllnessContaminants/

UCM312793.pdf). Too restrictive diet recommendations, in the absence of the clear benefit of avoiding foods other than abovementioned, may have negative impact on patient's nutritional status and/or quality of life.

Key Points

- General guidelines for preventing healthcare-associated infections should be followed, and hand hygiene is the single most effective measure.
- Mandatory isolation procedures comprise Standard Precautions and Transmission-Based Precautions if appropriate: airborne, contact or droplets.
- Specific recommendations on ventilation, room design and protective environment during construction/renovation are provided to protect HSCT from transmission of spores of filamentous fungi, mainly *Aspergillus*.
- Protocols for prevention of colonization and infection with multidrug-resistant bacteria should be put in place, particularly in centres where these bacteria are already present.
- Antimicrobial stewardship program should be implemented in every centre to promote optimal use of antibiotics.
- Standard food safety practices should be applied, and only selected foods should be avoided (e.g. raw/undercook/underheated meat, fish or eggs, unpasteurized milk, unwashed fruits and vegetables, unsafe water).

References

Abad C, Fearday A, Safdar N. Adverse effects of isolation in hospitalised patients: a systematic review. J Hosp Infect. 2010;76:97–102.

Bilinski J, Grzesiowski P, Sorensen N, et al. Fecal microbiota transplantation in patients with blood disorders inhibits gut colonization with antibiotic-resistant bacteria: results of a prospective, single-center study. Clin Infect Dis. 2017;65:364–70.

Centers for Disease Control and Prevention. Guideline for hand hygiene in health-care settings: recommendations of the Healthcare Infection Control Practices Advisory Committee and the HICPAC/SHEA/APIC/IDSA Hand Hygiene Task Force. MMWR Recomm Rep. 2002;51(RR16):1.

Freifeld AG, Bow EJ, Sepkowitz KA, et al. Clinical practice guideline for the use of antimicrobial agents in neutropenic patients with cancer: 2010 update by the Infectious Diseases Society of America. Clin Infect Dis. 2011;52:427–31.

Girmenia C, Viscoli C, Piciocchi A, et al. Management of carbapenem resistant Klebsiella pneumoniae infections in stem cell transplant recipients: an Italian multidisciplinary consensus statement. Haematologica. 2015;100:e375.

Gyssens IC, Kern WV, Livermore DM, ECIL-4, a joint venture of EBMT, EORTC, ICHS and ESGICH of ESCMID. The role of antibiotic stewardship in limiting antibacterial resistance among hematology patients. Haematologica. 2013;98:1821–5.

Sehulster LM, Chinn RYW, Arduino MJ, et al. Guidelines for environmental infection control in health-care facilities. Recommendations from CDC and the Healthcare Infection Control Practices Advisory Committee (HICPAC). Chicago: American Society for Healthcare Engineering/American Hospital Association; 2004.

Siegel JD, Rhinehart E, Jackson M, Chiarello L, Healthcare Infection Control Practices Advisory Committee. Guideline for isolation precautions: preventing transmission of infectious agents in healthcare settings. 2007. http://www.cdc.gov/ncidod/dhqp/pdf/isolation2007.pdf.

Sonbol MG, Firwana B, Diab M, et al. The effect of a neutropenic diet on infection and mortality rates in cancer patients: a meta-analysis. Nutr Cancer. 2015;67:1230–8.

Styczynski J, Tridello G, Donnelly P, et al. Protective environment for hematopoietic cell transplant (HSCT) recipients: the Infectious Diseases Working Party EBMT analysis of global recommendations on healthcare facilities. Bone Marrow Transplant. 2018;53:1131. https://doi.org/10.1038/s41409-018-0141-5.

Tacconelli E, Cataldo MA, Dancer SJ, et al. ESCMID guidelines for the management of the infection control measures to reduce transmission of multidrug-resistant Gram-negative bacteria in hospitalized patients. Clin Microbiol Infect. 2014;20(Suppl 1):1–55.

Tomblyn M, Chiller T, Einsele H, et al. Guidelines for preventing infectious complications among hematopoietic cell transplantation recipients: a global perspective. Biol Blood Marrow Transplant. 2009;15:1143–38.

van Dalen EC, Mank A, Leclercq E, et al. Low bacterial diet versus control diet to prevent infection in cancer patients treated with chemotherapy causing episodes of neutropenia. Cochrane Database Syst Rev. 2016;4:CD006247.

Yokoe D, Casper C, Dubberke E, et al. Infection prevention and control in health-care facilities in which hematopoietic cell transplant recipients are treated. Bone Marrow Transplant. 2009;44:495–7.

General Management of the Patient: Specific Aspects of Children

Francesca Riccardi and Elio Castagnola

28.1 Introduction

Many of the conditions requiring allo-HSCT and related complications are similar in adults and children and are covered in other chapters of this handbook.

However, since pediatric age is a continuum between newborns and adults, there are at least two aspects, psychological and infectious disease issues, that may require a dedicated approach for the following reason:

1. *Psychological aspects.* Childhood encompasses different ages and consequently different cognitive, decisional, and emotional capacities that make psychological intervention far more faceted than in adults. In addition, psychological intervention should also take in charge at higher extent the needs and the expectations of the patient's family.
2. *Infectious diseases.* Data on epidemiology and management of infections in children are far less numerous and consistent than in adults. In addition most of the available data are derived from studies in adults, and they

cannot always simply be transposed to children for an effective application.

In the following paragraphs, we will analyze the specific approaches related to these aspects in children undergoing HSCT.

28.2 Psychological Aspects (Table 28.1)

Children who undergo HSCT experience several *numerous psychological reactions*: anxiety, depression, behavioral and social problems, and post-traumatic stress symptoms. In the stages before HSCT, anxiety increases, and the emotional distress continues to rise until 1 week after transplant, whereas depression is heightened by hospitalization and physical isolation. Age (<7 years) and severity of the illness influence the level of emotional reactions. Especially, children <5 years are more likely to withdraw and to be deprived of their self-help skills and even of their mobility and speech skills. The level of pre-HSCT emotional disturbance is strongly predictive of post-HSCT emotional functioning; therefore early intervention appears of critical importance (Packman et al. 2010).

The most studied psychological treatments for children with cancer are *cognitive behavioral therapies* (CBT) that are considered to improve emotional adjustment, compliance with medical

F. Riccardi
Consultant Hematology Unit, Hemato-Oncology and SCT Pole, Istituto Giannina Gaslini, Genoa, Italy

E. Castagnola (✉)
Infectious Diseases Unit, Department of Pediatrics, Istituto Giannina Gaslini, Genoa, Italy
e-mail: eliocastagnola@gaslini.org

Table 28.1 Main psychological problems in HSCT in pediatric age

	Problems	Suggested intervention
Patients	*Emotional disturbance*: anxiety, depression, behavioral and social problems, post traumatic stess symptoms *HRQOL*: compromission is evident before and soon after HSCT. Start to improve between 4 and 6 months after HSCT *Neurocognitive area*: impairment is associated with younger age at diagnosis and treatment. Adaptive skills and social competence are affected in the first year after HSCT	– Individual therapies to improve emotional adjustment, compliance with medical treatment and behavioral problems associated with HSCT – Guided imagery, distraction, rhythmic breathing, relaxation to decrease the distress due to medical procedures – Clinical assessment is recommended: before the recovery period 1 year after HSCT annually thereafter
Siblings	Post-traumatic stress reactions, anxiety, low self-esteem, feelings of guilt and school problems	Open communication Facilitate the access of sibling to the hospital
Parents	Parental distress, anxiety, depression, post traumatic stress symptoms. Take care of additional burden due to medical complications	Familial intervention Crisis intervention approach Stress and coping models

treatment, and behavioral problems associated with HSCT. Effective interventions are clearly largely dependent on social skills and emotional well-being. Techniques such as guided imagery, distraction, rhythmic breathing, and relaxation are commonly used to decrease the acute psychological distress due to medical procedures including HSCT (Packman et al. 2010). Psychiatric assessment and pharmacological approach should be advisable when other approaches are not sufficient for children with preexisting psychiatric diagnoses who are vulnerable to worsening of the psychiatric disorders (Steele et al. 2015).

Health-related quality of life (HRQOL) compromission is usually evident prior to and soon after transplant and starts to improve between 4 and 6 months after HSCT. Child psychosocial problems, caregiver stress, and social support emerged as significant predictors of physical and emotional outcome after discharging. Indeed, high level of stress of caregivers and/or low perceived social support was associated with higher risk of psychologically complicated outcome. On the contrary emotional and behavioral problems of the child at discharge were not associated to substantially slower improvements in overall HRQOL that usually occurred between 3 and 9 months after discharge. This is because reestablishment of usual activities that were precluded during HSCT outbalances emotional

problems due to the return to "normal" life (Loiselle et al. 2016).

As for neurocognitive functions, long-term studies are not fully concordant, but some findings (Kelly et al. 2018) seem to suggest that *children's intelligence quotient* (IQ) scores post HSCT are inferior to those before HSCT. In particular adaptive skills and social competence domains are affected in the first year after HSCT and so do self-esteem and emotional well-being. Impairment in neurocognitive area is associated with younger age at diagnosis and treatment and may occur even if school performance remains in normal ranges. Children may also experience decrements in executive functioning skills, like deficits in fine motor abilities usually seen in patients who received cranial irradiation at younger age. Clinical assessment is recommended before the recovery period, at 1 year after HSCT and annually thereafter, or, at least, at the beginning of each stage of education. In the post-HSCT assessment, clinicians should also consider the impact of factors such as isolation, missed schooling, and impaired socialization with peers. Encouraging results in cognitive rehabilitation come from intensive therapist-delivered training since the systematic use of computer-based training appeared to improve working memory and processing speed (Kelly et al. 2018).

Siblings, either donors or non-donors, are at risk of developing emotional disturbances such as post-traumatic stress reactions, anxiety, low self-esteem, feelings of guilt, and school problems. Indeed, researches are needed to identify the most useful intervention to cope with negative effects of HSCT on siblings (Packman et al. 2010; Gerhardt et al. 2015). Currently adopted strategies include open communication about the patient's medical situation and transplant process, favoring the idea of accepting help from friends and family members, and facilitating the access of sibling to the hospital arranging visits in a way that they look like a special event or assigning a sibling a special role (Gerhardt et al. 2015; White et al. 2017).

Parental distress, anxiety, and depression levels are often increased as a result of their child undergoing HSCT. The distress and anxiety may be even greater for parents whose healthy child also becomes part of the HSCT process through donating his/her marrow (Packman et al. 2010). Significant determinants of parental distress include prior parent and patient experience of distress associated with the child's illness, the child's tendency of internalizing or externalizing behavior problems, the family's attitude to provide support, and a parental proneness toward avoidant coping behaviors (Phipps et al. 2005). Parents mostly experience post-traumatic stress symptoms that manifest in cognitive and behavioral efforts to avoid reminders of the HSCT and intrusive thoughts about it (Virtue et al. 2014).

Early and late HSCT medical complications significantly increase the psychological involvement of the caregiver. HSCT healthcare professionals should also take care of the additional burden that complications generate on the parents and should proactively link parents to resources aimed to help them coping with this extra load (Heinze et al. 2015). Despite the recognized needs, very few caregivers seek out psychological service. The most frequent barriers are that clinicians prioritize medical patient's needs and cover tasks usually deemed to social support, lack of adequate locations, and embarrassment about seeking psychological counseling (Devine et al. 2016).

Familial interventions aimed to enhance protective factors, improve communication, and decrease parental anxiety and depression are crucial. In this respect, cancer-specific psychological interventions may serve as a template to delivering HSCT-tailored interventions (Packman et al. 2010). Traditional individual therapy is very useful even if in adapted forms. Usually it includes crisis intervention approach and stress and coping models to reduce HSCT-related stress. CBT can encompass different strategies such as the expression of emotional feelings, identification of distorted automatic thoughts, the use of problem-focused coping skills, discussion of psychosocial impact on the family, and training in assertiveness and communication skills (Steele et al. 2015).

28.3 Infectious Diseases

Infections represent one of the most frequently occurring and feared complications of HSCT.

Antibacterial prophylaxis for febrile neutropenia is frequently administered in pediatric HSCT but never specifically analyzed in a randomized clinical trial. Its use can be associated with selection of resistant strains.

In the pre-engraftment phases, *empirical antibiotic therapy* for febrile neutropenia could be represented by monotherapy with an anti-*Pseudomonas* beta-lactam, but it is mandatory its adaptation to local epidemiological data (Lehrnbecher et al. 2017). Moreover, empirical antibiotic therapy should be considered also after engraftment because of the important risk of morbidity and mortality. Antibiotic-resistant pathogens represent a new challenge because of the high mortality rates (>50%) observed in pediatric HSCT (Girmenia et al. 2015; Caselli et al. 2016).

Clostridium difficile may represent a cause of severe, and sometimes recurrent, disease, but it must be kept in mind that children aged below 2 years may harbor this pathogen in their intestinal tract (Lees et al. 2016;

Enoch et al. 2011) and that other pathogens (e.g., viruses or *Cryptosporidium*) could be the cause of gastroenteritis (Castagnola et al. 2016). Table 28.2 summarizes antibacterial drugs for prophylaxis and treatment of invasive diseases.

Invasive fungal disease (IFD) is associated with high mortality in pediatric HSCT (Cesaro et al. 2017; Castagnola et al. 2018b). Increasing age has been identified as a risk factor for the development of IFD (Fisher et al. 2017), but recent multivariable analyses showed that age is no longer significant in the presence of severe acute or chronic extensive GvHD or in cases of primary graft failure or rejection (Castagnola et al. 2014, 2018a).

Primary prophylaxis should be implemented in the highest-risk groups like patients with primary graft failure or rejection, or with severe acute or chronic extensive GvHD, or in centers with high incidence of IFD (Groll et al. 2014).

Table 28.2 Prophylaxis and therapy of invasive bacterial infections in children undergoing allogeneic HSCT

Prophylaxis for febrile neutropenia	
Ciprofloxacin	Oral or IV until neutrophil recovery or start of empirical therapy for febrile neutropenia
	Notes: Never analyzed in a randomized clinical trial in HSCT. Risk of selection of resistant strains
Amoxicillin-clavulanate	Oral or IV until neutrophil recovery or start of empirical therapy for febrile neutropenia
	Notes: Never analyzed in a randomized clinical trial in HSCT. Risk of selection of resistant strains
Empirical therapy for febrile neutropenia, or fever after engraftment, especially in presence of GvHD	
Pipera-tazo	100 mg/kg (max 4000 mg) of piperacillin q6h
Cefepime	33 mg/kg (max 2000 mg) q8h
Ceftazidime	33 mg/kg (max 2000 mg)
Meropenem	20 mg/kg (max 1000 mg) q8h
	Notes: Risk of selection of resistant Gram-negatives or *C. difficile* associated disease. Higher doses could be necessary for treatment of carbapenem resistant pathogen when MIC is ≤16 mg/L. For higher MIC values carbapenems are not indicated
Combination therapy	Aminoglycoside [e.g. amikacin 20 mg/kg (max 1500 mg) q24h] + beta-lactam
	Notes: According to local susceptibility, and proportions of resistance to beta-lactams indicated for monotherapy
Documented infections: according with localizations and antibiotic susceptibility tests	
Antibiotics for resistant pathogens, combinations could be needed	*Gram-positives*: vancomycin, teicoplanin daptomycin, linezolid, tigecycline, fosfomycin
	Gram-negatives: ciprofloxacin, colistin, tigecycline (not active against P. aeruginosas), fosfomycin, ceftazidime-avibactam (not active against metallo beta-lactamases), ceftolozane-tazobactam (not active against carbapenemases)
	Notes:
	– According to ATB susceptibility tests in documented infections
	– Beta-lactams should be preferred to glycopeptides in case of infections due to oxacillin-susceptible staphylococci
	– Do not use empirical glycopeptides for persistent fever without signs of localizations attributable to Gram-positives or high suspicion or risk by patient's history or local epidemiology of oxacillin-resistant staphylococci or ampicillin-resistant enterococci
	– For vancomycin resistant staphylococci or enterococci daptomycin, linezolid or tigecycline could represent therapeutic options
	– No PK data for ceftazidime-avibactam or ceftolozane-tazobactam available in children
Clostridium difficile associated disease	
Vancomycin, metronidazole, fidaxomicin	Oral therapy, vancomycin 10 mg/kg (max 125 mg) q6h as 1st choice
	Fidaxomicin is not registered for <18 years
	Notes: No data are available for fecal transplantation in immunocompromised children. Different dosages proposed for recurrent disease

MIC minimally inhibitory concentration, *GvHD* graft vs. host disease, *Pipera-tazo* Piperacillin-Tazobactam

Diagnosis of IFD is based on isolation of fungal pathogens from cultures of sterile sites or tissue invasion demonstrated by histology or by the presence of fungal antigens in blood or cerebrospinal fluid or bronchoalveolar lavage, associated with suggestive imaging (Castagnola et al. 2016; Tomà et al. 2016) in children with a compatible clinical picture. Detection of galactomannan and 1-3-beta-D-glucan is widely used for the diagnosis of (probable) IFD also in children. However, a recent meta-analysis (Lehrnbecher et al. 2016) and new clinical data (Calitri et al. 2017) showed highly variable and generally poor sensitivity, specificity, and predictive values of these tests, especially when used for screening. PCR should still be considered as an investigative test (Lehrnbecher et al. 2016). Also, for the use of antifungal drugs, there are caveats.

Treatment: Voriconazole frequently needs to be administered at higher dosages in the youngest patients (<5 years) to achieve and maintain effective plasma concentrations (Xu et al. 2016; Soler-Palacın et al. 2012; Neely et al. 2015; Castagnola and Mesini 2018). Inflammation, steroid administration, or obesity can further modify its concentrations (Castagnola and Mesini 2018; Natale et al. 2017) and so do genetic factors (Teusink et al. 2016). Finally, severe cutaneous adverse events can be observed also in children when voriconazole is administered for prolonged periods, especially in concomitance with sun exposure (Goyal et al. 2014; Bernhard et al. 2012). Posaconazole oral suspension has variable absorption implying the risk of sub-therapeutic concentrations (Jancel et al. 2017), especially in the presence of intestinal acute GvHD (Heinz et al. 2016). This can be at least partially avoided by fatty meal and/or other "bundle" measures or using doses based on body surface area (Castagnola and Mesini 2018). Posaconazole tablets have no absorption problems, and pediatric pharmacological data show that their use determines effective

concentrations also in children (Castagnola and Mesini 2018). However, tablets are slightly less than 2 cm long and should be swallowed whole with water and should not be crushed, chewed, or broken (EMA 2018) thus limiting their use in youngest patients, but alternate day administration could represent an effective strategy (Mesini et al. 2018). Triazoles have also many drug interactions that must be kept in mind during their use. For all these reasons, therapeutic drug monitoring is mandatory both for prophylactic and therapeutic uses (Groll et al. 2014).

Pneumocystis jirovecii pneumonia is a severe, life-threatening fungal infection in allo-HSCT recipients. Primary prophylaxis is highly recommended in children undergoing allo-HSCT at least in the post-engraftment. Prophylaxis is highly effective, and in case of documented failure, especially in adolescents, compliance must be checked (Castagnola and Mesini 2018). Table 28.3 summarizes dosages of drugs for prevention or treatment of IFD in children.

Viral Infections No major differences between children and adults are expected. However, primary viral infections are more frequent in pediatrics, and in this setting, it must be stressed that healthy household contacts and healthcare workers may represent important sources, with possible hospital spreading.

Screening and Isolation Application of bundle procedures for patients as well as correct hand hygiene, correct vascular access manipulation, correct isolation procedures according to the via of pathogen spreading, and the use of HEPA filters can be all of great utility in the prevention of difficult to treat infections in HSCT.

Vaccines represent also an important tool for prevention of viral and bacterial (*S. pneumoniae*) infections in the post transplant setting.

Table 28.3 Prophylaxis and therapy of IFI in children undergoing allogeneic HSCT

Voriconazole

Spectrum of activity: molds, yeasts

Prophylaxis: No evidence to support this indication in children. Dosage in children aged 2 to <12 years or 12–14 years with weight <50 kg: 9 mg/kg q12h; In children aged ≥15 years or 12–14 years and with weight ≥50 kg: 4 mg/kg q12h (1st day, 6 mg/kg). Target concentration >1 and <6 mg/L at steady state

Therapy: Dosage in children aged 2 to <12 years or 12–14 years with weight <50 kg: 9 mg/kg q12h; In children aged ≥15 years or 12–14 years with weight ≥50 kg: 4 mg/kg q12h (1st day, 6 mg/kg). Target concentration >1 and <6 mg/L at steady state.

Notes: Measure serum concentrations (mandatory) before the 5th dose (2 days of treatment); before the 5th dose following any dose adjustment; routinely every 1–2 weeks after achievement of steady-state; when interacting drugs start or stop in case of potential clinical or laboratory manifestations of toxicity

Posaconazole

Spectrum of activity: molds, yeasts

Prophylaxis: Oral suspension: 120 mg/m² q8h for children who can not swallow tablets. Tablets: loading dose of 300 mg q12h (1st day) then maintenance 300 q24h, independently from meal. According with BW:

Body weight	Load (1st day)	Maintenance
15–21 kg	150 mg q12h	100 mg q24h
22–30 kg	150 mg q12h	150 mg q24h
31–35 kg	200 mg q12h	200 mg q24h
35–40 kg	250 mg q12h	250 mg q24h
>40 kg or 13 years	300 mg q12h	300 mg q24h

Target concentration for prophylaxis 0.7 mg/L at steady state. Not registered for use <18 years

Therapy: Oral suspension: 120 mg/m² q8h for children who cannot swallow tablets. Tablets: loading dose of 300 mg q12h (1st day) then maintenance 300 q24h, independently from meal. According with BW:

Body weight	Load (1st day)	Maintenance
15–21 kg	150 mg q12h	100 mg q24h
22–30 kg	150 mg q12h	150 mg q24h
31–35 kg	200 mg q12h	200 mg q24h
35–40 kg	250 mg q12h	250 mg q24h
>40 kg or 13 years	300 mg q12h	300 mg q24h

Target concentration for therapy ≥1 mg/L at steady state. Not registered for use <18 years

Notes: When using oral suspension remove acid suppression if possible and use "posaconazole bundle":
– ascorbic acid 500 mg per os with each dose of posaconazole
– 120–180 mL of carbonated soda beverage (i.e.: cola or ginger ale) or acidic fruit juice (e.g.: cranberry or orange juice) with each dose of posaconazole
– heavy snack or food with each dose, preferably high-fat, including
– use a more fractionated schedule (q 6-8h)

With any formulation measure serum concentrations (mandatory): 7 days after initiation of therapy or following dose adjustment or when interacting drugs start or stop or in case of concerns about GI absorption, especially for prolonged periods of time or in case of potential clinical or laboratory manifestations of toxicity

Itraconazole

Spectrum of activity: molds, yeasts

Prophylaxis: Moderate evidence to support a recommendation in children. Oral solution 2.5 mg/kg per day orally (in children aged ≥2 years) q12h, with empty stomach. Target concentration for prophylaxis 0.5 mg/L at steady state

Notes: Measure serum concentrations. For oral administration use oral solution. Administer with empty stomach

Fluconazole

Spectrum of activity: yeast

Prophylaxis: Not highly recommendable because of the narrow spectrum (yeasts only). 6 mg/kg/ day (maximum 400 mg/ day) intravenously or orally q24h

Therapy: 10–20 mg/kg/day, maximum 800 mg/day) intravenously or orally q24h

Liposomal amphotericin B

Spectrum of activity: molds, yeasts

Prophylaxis: Moderate evidence to support intravenous, no evidence for nebulized administration Intravenous: 1 mg/ kg q24h every other day or 2.5 mg/kg q24h twice weekly; Nebulized: 25 mg q12h on 2 consecutive days per week associated with fluconazole

Therapy: Intravenous: 3–5 mg/kg according to etiology. Doses up to 10 mg/kg have been proposed for mucormycosis

Table 28.3 (continued)

Micafungin
Spectrum of activity: yeast (not *Cryptococcus*) (molds?)
Prophylaxis: Not highly recommendable because of the narrow spectrum (yeasts only)
1 mg/kg (in children weighing ≥50 kg, 50 mg) q24h
Therapy: 2–4 mg/kg (max 100 mg/kg) q24h
Isavuconazole
Spectrum of action: molds, yeasts
Prophylaxis: No evidence for this indication. No data for pediatric use and dosage. Not registered <18 years
Therapy: No data for pediatric use and dosage. Not registered <18 years
Corimoxazole, dapsone, atovaquone, pentamidine
Spectrum of action: P. Jirovecii
Prophylaxis: Cotrimoxazole 1st choice: 2.5 mg/kg of trimethoprim (max 180 mg) q12h, 1–3 days/week
Therapy: Cotrimoxazole 1st choice: 5 mg/kg of trimethoprim q8h
Notes: In case op pneumonia add prednisone at 2 mg/kg/day. Nebulized pentamidine requires special tools for administration

IFI invasive fungal infection

Key Points

Many of the conditions requiring allo-HSCT and related complications are similar in adults and children and are covered in other chapters of this handbook.

However, since pediatric age is a continuum between newborns and adults, there are at least two aspects:

- Psychological aspects. Childhood encompasses different ages and consequently different cognitive, decisional, and emotional capacities that make psychological intervention far more faceted than in adults.
- Infectious diseases. Data on epidemiology and management of infections in children are far less numerous and consistent than in adults. Despite that there are many differential aspects in its management.

References

Bernhard S, Kernland Lang K, et al. Voriconazole-induced phototoxicity in children. Pediatr Infect Dis J. 2012;31:769–71.

Calitri C, Caviglia I, Cangemi G, et al. Performance of 1,3-β-D-glucan for diagnosing invasive fungal diseases in children. Mycoses. 2017;60:789–95.

Caselli D, Cesaro S, Fagioli F, et al. Incidence of colonization and bloodstream infection with carbapenem-resistant Enterobacteriaceae in children receiving antineoplastic chemotherapy in Italy. Infect Dis (Lond). 2016;48:152–3.

Castagnola E, Bagnasco F, Amoroso L, et al. Role of management strategies in reducing mortality from invasive fungal disease in children with cancer or receiving hemopoietic stem cell transplant: a single center 30-year experience. Pediatr Infect Dis J. 2014;33:233–7.

Castagnola E, Bagnasco F, Menoni S, et al. Risk factors associated with development and mortality by invasive fungal diseases in pediatric allogeneic stem cell transplantation. A pediatric subgroup analysis of data from a prospective study of the Gruppo Italiano Trapianto di Midollo Osseo (GITMO). Bone Marrow Transplat. 2018;53:1193. https://doi.org/10.1038/s41409-018-0160-2.

Castagnola E, Mesini A. Antifungal prophylaxis in children receiving antineoplastic chemotherapy. Curr Fungal Infect Rep. 2018;12:78. https://doi.org/10.1007/s12281-018-0311-3.

Castagnola E, Ruberto E, Guarino A. Gastrointestinal and liver infections in children undergoing antineoplastic chemotherapy in the years 2000. World J Gastroenterol. 2016;22:5853–66.

Cesaro S, Tridello G, Castagnola E, et al. Retrospective study on the incidence and outcome of proven and probable invasive fungal infections in high-risk pediatric onco-hematological patients. Eur J Haematol. 2017;99:240–8.

Devine KA, Manne SL, Mee L, et al. Barriers to psychological care among primary caregivers of children undergoing hematopoietic stem cell transplantation. Support Care Cancer. 2016;24:2235–42.

Enoch DA, Butler MJ, Pai S, et al. Clostridium difficile in children: colonisation and disease. J Infect. 2011;63:105–13.

European Medicine Agency. Posaconazole summary of product characteristics. www.ema.europa.eu. Last check 15 Mar 2018.

Fisher BT, Robinson PD, Lehrnbecher T, et al. Risk factors for invasive fungal disease in pediatric cancer and hematopoietic stem cell transplantation: a systematic review. J Pediatr Infect Dis Soc. 2017. https://doi.org/10.1093/jpids/pix030. [Epub ahead of print].

Gerhardt CA, Lehmann V, Long KA, Alderfer MA. Supporting siblings as a standard of care in pediatric oncology. Pediatr Blood Cancer. 2015;62(Suppl 5):S750–804.

Girmenia C, Rossolini GM, Piciocchi A, et al. Infections by carbapenem-resistant Klebsiella pneumoniae in SCT recipients: a nationwide retrospective survey from Italy. Bone Marrow Transplant. 2015;50:282–8.

Goyal RK, Gehris RP, Howrie D. Phototoxic dermatoses in pediatric BMT patients receiving voriconazole. Pediatr Blood Cancer. 2014;61:1325–8.

Groll AH, Castagnola E, Cesaro S, et al. Fourth European Conference on Infections in Leukaemia (ECIL-4): guidelines for diagnosis, prevention, and treatment of invasive fungal diseases in paediatric patients with cancer or allogeneic haemopoietic stem-cell transplantation. Lancet Oncol. 2014;15(8):e327–40.

Heinz WJ, Cabanillas Stanchi KM, Klinker H, et al. Posaconazole plasma concentration in pediatric patients receiving antifungal prophylaxis after allogeneic hematopoietic stem cell transplantation. Med Mycol. 2016;54:128–37.

Heinze KE, Rodday AM, Nolan MT, et al. The impact of pediatric blood and marrow transplant on parents: introduction of the parent impact scale. Health Qual Life Outcomes. 2015;13:46.

Jancel T, Shaw PA, Hallahan CW, et al. Therapeutic drug monitoring of posaconazole oral suspension in paediatric patients younger than 13 years of age: a retrospective analysis and literature review. J Clin Pharm Ther. 2017;42:75–9.

Kelly DL, Buchbinder D, Duarte RF, et al. Neurocognitive dysfunction in hematopoietic cell transplant recipients: expert review from the late effects and Quality of Life Working Committee of the Center for International Blood and Marrow Transplant Research and complications and Quality of Life Working Party of the European Society for Blood and Marrow Transplantation. Biol Blood Marrow Transplant. 2018;24:228–41.

Lees EA, Miyajima F, Pirmohamed M, Carroll ED. The role of Clostridium difficile in the paediatric and neonatal gut—a narrative review. Eur J Clin Microbiol Infect Dis. 2016;35:1047–57.

Lehrnbecher T, Robinson PD, Fisher BT, et al. Galactomannan, β-D-glucan, and polymerase chain reaction–based assays for the diagnosis of invasive fungal disease in pediatric cancer and hematopoietic stem cell transplantation: a systematic review and meta-analysis. Clin Infect Dis. 2016;63:1340–8.

Lehrnbecher T, Robinson P, Fisher B, et al. Guideline for the management of fever and neutropenia in children with cancer and hematopoietic stem-cell transplantation recipients: 2017 update. J Clin Oncol. 2017;35:2082–94.

Loiselle KA, Rausch JR, Bidwell S, et al. Predictors of health-related quality of life over time among pediatric hematopoietic stem cell transplant recipients. Pediatr Blood Cancer. 2016;63:1834–9.

Mesini A, Faraci M, Giardino S, et al.. Alternate day dosing of posaconazole tablets in children leads to efficient plasma levels. Eur J Haematol. 2018 Mar 15. https://doi.org/10.1111/ejh.13063. [Epub ahead of print].

Natale S, Bradley J, Huy Nguyen W, et al. Pediatric obesity: pharmacokinetic alterations and effects on antimicrobial dosing. Pharmacotherapy. 2017;37:361–78.

Neely M, Margol A, Fu X, et al. Achieving target voriconazole concentrations more accurately in children and adolescents. Antimicrob Agents Chemother. 2015;59:3090–7.

Packman W, Weber S, Wallace J, Bugescu N. Psychological effects of hematopoietic SCT on pediatric patients, siblings and parents: a review. Bone Marrow Transplant. 2010;45:1134–46.

Phipps S, Dunavant M, Lensing S, Rai SN. Psychosocial predictors of distress in parents of children undergoing stem cell or bone marrow transplantation. J Pediatr Psychol. 2005;30:139–53.

Soler-Palacın P, Frick MA, Martın-Nalda A, et al. Voriconazole drug monitoring in the management of invasive fungal infection in immunocompromised children: a prospective study. J Antimicrob Chemother. 2012;67:700–6.

Steele AC, Mullins LL, Mullins AJ, Muriel AC. Psychosocial interventions and therapeutic support as a standard of care in pediatric oncology. Pediatr Blood Cancer. 2015;62(Suppl 5):S585–618.

Teusink A, Vinks A, Zhang K, et al. Genotype-directed dosing leads to optimized voriconazole levels in pediatric patients receiving hematopoietic stem cell transplantation. Biol Blood Marrow Transplant. 2016;22(3):482–6. e-pub ahead of print 2015/12/01. https://doi.org/10.1016/j.bbmt.2015.11.011.

Tomà P, Bertaina A, Castagnola E, et al. Fungal infections of the lung in children. Pediatr Radiol. 2016;46:1856–65.

Virtue SM, Manne SL, Mee L, et al. Psychological distress and psychiatric diagnoses among primary caregivers of children undergoing hematopoietic stem cell transplant: an examination of prevalence, correlates, and racial/ethnic differences. Gen Hosp Psychiatry. 2014;36:620–6.

White TE, Hendershot KA, Dixon MD, et al. Family strategies to support siblings of pediatric hematopoietic stem cell transplant patients. Pediatrics. 2017;139(2):e20161057. e-pub ahead of print 2017/01/26. https://doi.org/10.1542/peds.2016-1057.

Xu G, Zhu L, Ge T, Liao S, Qi F. Pharmacokinetic/pharmacodynamic analysis of voriconazole against Candida spp. and Aspergillus spp. in children, adolescents and adults by Monte Carlo simulation. Int J Antimicrob Agents. 2016;47:439–45.

Vaccinations

Rafael de la Cámara

29.1 General Concepts

Vaccination should be considered a *routine practice for all HSCT receptors*, either autologous or allogeneic, adults or children. It should be implemented in all HSCT programs. Adult cover is particularly important as they represent 90% of HSCTs. To obtain this objective, the following are necessary:

To have in place a standardized program specific for HSCT patients.

- The collaboration of the Preventive Department of the hospital and primary care physicians.
- The program must be simple, with a clear chronology, and convenient for the patient and physician (no increase in the number of visits).
- FACT-JACIE Standards (version 7.0, March 2018) require that policies/SOP are in place for post transplant vaccination schedules and indications.

The vaccination program should include not only the patient but also those who live with the patient and the healthcare workers (HCWs).

R. de la Cámara (✉)
Department of Hematology, Hospital de la Princesa, Madrid, Spain
e-mail: jrcamara@telefonica.net

There is no a unique vaccine schedule for all HSCT patients. Each center should discuss and adapt a specific vaccine program.

- The practical application of the immunization programs shows important variations across centers (Miller et al. 2017).
- Auto-HSCT is generally vaccinated with the schedule used for allogeneic patients with small differences (see Tables 29.1 and 29.2).

Reasons for universal vaccination of HSCT patients:

- *General interest*: as a general healthcare principle, all the population should be cor rectly vaccinated, including adults and of course HSCT patients. If an increasing col lective of patients, like HSCT, is not well vaccinated, that can generate holes of immu nity that can be a risk for the health of the general population.
- *Individual interest for each HSCT patient* vaccination protects the patient against infec tions that can cause important morbi-mortal ity. There are frequent infections in HSCT that have safe vaccines (pneumococcus, influenza, HBV) and other rare infections associated with high mortality that have an unsatisfactory prevention/treatment but can be prevented by immunization (tetanus, diphtheria, measles, polio).

Table 29.1 International consensus recommendations (Ljungman et al. 2009)

Vaccine	No. of doses	Time post-HSCT to initiate vaccine	Grading
Influenza (inactivated)	1 2 for children <9 years, or if <6 m from HSCT (C III)	4–6 months, yearly, lifelong seasonal vaccination	AII
Measles[a]	1 (2 in children)	24 months	AII children BII seronegative adults
Mumps[a]			CIII
Rubella[a] (in adults for sero(-) females with pregnancy potential)			BIII
Hepatitis B virus (HBV) (follow country recommendations for general population)[b]	3	6–12 months	BII
Human papillomavirus	Follow recommendations for general population in each country		CIII
Inactivated polio	3	6–12 months	BII
Pneumococcal conjugate (PCV)	3	3–6 months	BI
– polysaccharide pneumococcal vaccine (PPS)	1	6 months after last PCV	BII
– in case of GVHD, use PCV instead of PPS for this 4th dose	1		CIII
Meningococcal conjugate (follow country recommend for general population)	1	6–12 months	BII
Haemophilus influenzae conjugate	3	6–12 months	BII
Diphtheria-tetanus (DT preferred over Td)	3	6–12 months	BII
Pertussis (acellular) (DTaP preferred over Tdap)	3	6–12 months	CIII

[a]MMR. These vaccines are contraindicated (EIII) before 24 months post-HSCT or in case of active GVHD or IS. These vaccines are usually given together as a combination vaccine

[b]VHB. Vaccination is recommended for HBV surface Ag-negative or HBV core Ab-positive patients, as vaccination can reduce the risk of reverse seroconversion (BII). For HBV surface Ag-negative or HBV core Ab-negative HSCT patients, recommendations for the general population in their country of residence should be followed

29.2 General Principles of Vaccination in HSCT Patients

29.2.1 The Pretransplant Vaccination

The pretransplant vaccination is not effective to maintain a prolonged post transplant immunity. In other to protect the HSCT patient, a complete series of post transplant vaccinations is required. This is different from what is recommended for solid organ transplant (SOT) recipients for whom pretransplant vaccination is an essential part of the vaccination program. Post-HSCT patients should be viewed as "never vaccinated" regardless of the pre-HSCT vaccination history of the patient or the donor (Rubin et al. 2014).

29.2.2 The Pre-HSCT Immunity

The pre-HSCT immunity for a specific pathogen is not a reason to withhold vaccination after transplant. The majority of patients will lose their immunity after HSCT.

As general rule, *live vaccines should be considered contraindicated* (there are exceptions, see later). The inactivated, subunit, or protein/polysaccharide vaccines can be safely administered.

There are few randomized trials in HSCT patients, and many of the studies have been done in patients transplanted with BM/PB, using

Table 29.2 ECIL recommendations for allo-HSCT recipients (Cordonnier et al. 2017)

Vaccine	No. of doses[a]	Time post-HSCT to initiate vaccine	Grading
Influenza (inactivated)	1 (or 2, special cases)[b]	>6 months	AIIr
		As long as patient is judged to be IS	BIIr
		Yearly, lifelong from 3 months in case of a community outbreak	BIIr
Measles–mumps–rubella			
• Measles	1 (2 in children) MMR	≥24 months	BIIu
In sero(-) patients, with no GVHD, no IS, no REL of underlying disease, and no IGIV at least 8 months		≥12 months in case of measles outbreak in patients with low grade IS	CIII
• Rubella	1 MMR	≥24 months	CIIu
In sero(-) women and of childbearing potential, with same precautions as for measles vaccine			
Virus hepatitis B[c]			
• Sero(-) patients before HSCT and patients vaccinated pre-HSCT but lost their immunity at 6 months)	3[d]	6–12 months	BIIt
• Previously infected and anti-HBs <10 IU/L		6–12 months	BIII
• Sero(-) patients with a donor with positive anti-HBc		Vaccine before transplant	BIII
Human papilloma virus (HPV) Follow recommendations for general population in each country	According to official label	From 6–12 months	BIIu
Inactivated polio	3[e]	6–12 months	BIIu
Live-attenuated varicella vaccine	1	Can be considered in sero(-) patients, with ALL the following: >24 m from HSCT, no GVHD, no IS, no REL of the underlying disease, and no IGIV in the last 8 months	BIIr
	2	The addition of a second dose in adults may be considered in patients who were sero(-) before HSCT or had no history of VZ infect	
Live-attenuated zoster vaccine	Not recommended		DIII
Pneumococcal conjugate (PCV)	3	3 months	AI
Polysaccharidic vaccine In case of GVHD, use PCV instead of PPS for this 4th dose (BIIr)	1	12 months (no earlier than 8 weeks after last PCV)	BI
Meningococcal conjugate (in accordance with country recommendations and local prevalence)	2	From 6 months	
		For men-C or tetravalent vaccine	BIIu
		For men-B vaccine	BIII
Haemophilus influenzae conjugate	3	3 months or 6 months	BIIr
Diphtheria-tetanus (DT is preferred to Td)	3[e]	From 6 months	BIu
Pertussis (acellular) (DTaP is preferred over Tdap)	3	From 6–12 months	CIII

[a]If not specified otherwise, the interval between dose is 1 month
[b]Influenza: A second dose of influenza vaccine, after 3–4 weeks from the first, may have a marginal benefit and should preferably be considered in patients with severe GVHD or low lymphocyte count (B II r) and also for the patients vaccinated early (from 3 months after transplant) (B II r). Children ≥6 months through 8 years, receiving influenza for the first time after transplant, should receive a second dose at least 4 weeks after the first dose
[c]HBV. After post transplant vaccination, if anti-HBs is <10 mIU/ml, an additional three doses should be considered, but the benefit of this second series of vaccination is uncertain. IDSA guidelines (Rubin et al. 2014) give the same recommendations (strong, low). For adolescents and adults, a high dose of vaccine (40 μg) is recommended for these booster doses (strong, low)
[d]Three doses: interval 0, 1, and 6 months
[e]At 1–2 months interval
Note for auto-HSCT: same recommendations but grading changes for some vaccines: influenza BIIr (instead AII); PCV BIII (instead AI)

MAC. The experience with other sources (CBU), conditioning regimens (RIC), and donors (haplo) is scarce.

Many vaccines are administered by *intramuscular route*, which can be a problem for severe thrombocytopenic patients (less than 50×10^9 platelets/L). For severe thrombocytopenic patients, some vaccines can be safely administered SC (inactivated poliomyelitis, conjugate pneumococcal vaccine) or even intradermic route (for influenza vaccine). Clinical experience suggests that intramuscular injections are safe if the platelet count is ≥ 30 to 50×10^9/L, a ≤ 23-gauge needle is used, and constant pressure is maintained at the injection site for 2 min (Rubin et al. 2014).

29.2.3 The Dose of Vaccine

The dose of vaccine used is the same for general population, with some exceptions (see Table 29.2). A uniform specific interval between doses cannot be recommended, as various intervals have been used in studies. As a general guideline, a minimum of 1 month between doses may be reasonable.

29.2.4 Several Patient and Vaccine Characteristics Impact on the Vaccine Response

Time from Transplantation As a general rule, the later time a vaccine is administered, the better response is obtained (there are exceptions; see pneumococcal vaccine section). Usually >12 months from transplant is associated with better responses.

Type of Vaccine T-cell-dependent vaccine obtains better response than T-cell-independent vaccines, because it triggers memory response that leads to a longer protection compared with T-cell-independent vaccine.

The presence of GVHD or ongoing IS treatment has been associated with a decrease in

vaccine response, particularly for polysaccharide-based vaccines.

- Some vaccine responses seem to be not impaired by the presence of GVHD/IS treatment. This is the case of conjugated *Haemophilus* vaccine, conjugated pneumococcal vaccine, conjugated meningococcal vaccine, inactivated polio vaccine, and diphtheria-tetanus vaccine.
- International guidelines recommend different attitudes in patients with GVHD for the moment of vaccine administration.
- The international consensus guidelines (Ljungman et al. 2009) recommend to not postpone vaccinations with non-live vaccines in patients with ongoing active or resolved cGVHD of any severity grade.
- However, the International Consensus Conference on Clinical Practice in chronic GVHD (Hilgendorf et al. 2011) recommends postponing vaccination in patients with GVHD: if patients receive prednisone >0.5 mg/kg bodyweight as part of a combination therapy or a three-agent IS treatment is given, vaccination may be postponed until IS is reduced to a double combination or prednisone <0.5 mg/kg bodyweight in order to achieve better vaccine response. In any case, IS therapy should not lead to postponing vaccination for more than 3 months, and this applies for patients with ongoing active or resolved cGVHD of any severity grade.
- In practices, the majority of centers seems to delay vaccinations if GVHD is present (Miller et al. 2017).

The use of rituximab decreases serological vaccine response at least to tetanus and influenza.

- ECIL 2017 guidelines (Cordonnier et al. 2017): patients who have received rituximab from transplant should have their vaccine program delayed at least more than 6 months after the last dose.

- As the antibody response is uncertain, specific antibody assessment after vaccination can be helpful.

29.2.5 Types of Vaccines in HSCT Patients

Generally recommended for all HSCT (auto and allogeneic)

- Influenza (inactivated/subunit), poliomyelitis (inactivated), human papillomavirus, pneumococcus, *Haemophilus influenzae*, hepatitis B, meningococcus, tetanus, diphtheria, pertussis, and measles–mumps–rubella (special conditions, see Sects. 29.4 and 29.5).

Optional/special situations, to cover situations such as after disease exposure or before travel to areas endemic for infections:

- Hepatitis A, tick-borne encephalitis, Japanese B encephalitis, rabies, yellow fever (live), varicella (Varivax®, live).

Contraindicated: As general rule, *all live vaccines*:

- Oral polio vaccine, bacillus Calmette-Guérin, oral typhoid, zoster vaccine (Zostavax®), intranasal influenza vaccine, oral rotavirus vaccine.
- The exceptions for this rule are live vaccines for measles–mumps–rubella that are recommended following strict safety rules (see Sect. 29.4), yellow fever (live) (see specific section), and varicella (Varivax®, live); all these vaccines are contraindicated (EIII) before 24 m post-HSCT or in case of active GVHD or IS.

Use of IVIG and Vaccines For inactivated vaccines, Ig do not inhibit immune responses. For live virus vaccines, vaccination should be delayed 8 months after the last dose of Ig administration.

29.3 Benefits and Risks of Vaccination in HSCT Patients

29.3.1 Benefits

Direct Benefits The prevention of the specific infectious disease, as shown by influenza and varicella vaccination. Nonetheless, the majority of the efficacy studies in HSCT patients are based on surrogate markers (serology response) and not on the demonstration of a reduced risk of the infectious disease.

Indirect Benefits The benefits of vaccination can go beyond the prevention of a particular infection, as shown by influenza vaccine. Influenza immunization with inactivated vaccine is recommended by cardiologists as part of comprehensive secondary prevention with the same enthusiasm as the control of cholesterol, blood pressure, and other modifiable risk factors (Davis et al. 2006). It reduces cardiovascular mortality (risk ratio (RR) 0.45) (Clar et al. 2015), all-cause mortality (odds ratio (OR) 0.61), myocardial infarction (OR 0.73), and major adverse cardiovascular events (OR 0.47) (Loomba et al. 2012). Although all these studies were performed in general population, it is logical to assume a similar trend in HSCT patients.

29.3.2 Risks

Limited evidence indicates that *inactivated vaccines* have the same safety profile in immunocompromised patients as in immunocompetent individuals (Beck et al. 2012; Rubin et al. 2014; Cordonnier et al. 2017), and there is no evidence that they induce or aggravate GVHD (Cordonnier et al. 2017).

Live vaccines represent a real risk for HSCT and should not be used except in special situations with strict requirements (see section of varicella vaccine and ECIL vaccination guidelines table). Fatal disseminated VZV infections due to vaccine strain have been reported in HSCT patients after varicella vaccine and zoster vaccine, even when vaccine was administered several years after transplant (Cordonnier et al. 2017).

29.4 Vaccination Recommendations

There are several international recommendations focused on HSCT patients. The best known are those by the Infectious Disease Working Party (IDWP) of the EBMT, ECIL, CDC, and Infectious Diseases Society of America (IDSA).

The IDWP of the EBMT was one of the first cooperative groups that published recommendations specific for HSCT patients. The first ones were published in 1995, with updates in 1999 and 2005. In 2017 guidelines were reviewed and updated under the umbrella of the ECIL group, available online (Cordonnier et al. 2017) (Table 29.2).

In 2009 an international consensus guideline was published cosponsored by the main groups involved in HSCT and immunocompromised hosts (Ljungman et al. 2009) and probably is the most widely used in practice (Table 29.1).

The IDSA published their last recommendations in 2014 (Rubin et al. 2014).

There are other more specific guidelines focused on one pathogen (Engelhard et al. 2013) or on patients with GVHD (Hilgendorf et al. 2011).

29.5 Specific Vaccines

29.5.1 Influenza

29.5.1.1 Clinical Manifestations
(Ljungman et al. 2011; Engelhard et al. 2013)

Twenty percent of HSCT with confirmed influenza are afebrile.

It is a serious disease in HSCT: One third develop pneumonia, 10% require mechanical ventilation, and 6% died (Ljungman et al. 2011) (i.e., 100–300 times higher the mortality of influenza in general population). Other complications include encephalitis that can be lethal and myocarditis.

29.5.1.2 Influenza and Cardiovascular Disease (CVD)

The majority of influenza deaths are related to lung complications. Nonetheless, in general population up to a third of deaths related to influenza are CV deaths (Loomba et al. 2012).

The risk of acute myocardial infarction is significantly increased after laboratory-confirmed influenza infection (Kwong et al. 2018).

HSCT patients are at high risk of developing CVD. At 10 years, 8% will develop CVD (Armenian et al. 2012).

29.5.1.3 Vaccine

Evidence of Vaccine Efficacy
- A retrospective study showed a protection rate of 80% in the rates of virologically confirmed influenza (Machado et al. 2005).
- A systematic review and meta-analysis showed significantly lower odds of influenza-like illness after vaccination in transplant recipients (HSCT and SOT) compared with patients receiving placebo or no vaccination (Beck et al. 2012). Seroconversion and seroprotection were lower in transplant recipients compared with immunocompetent controls.
- Given the suboptimal immunogenicity in HSCT patients, family members and healthcare professionals involved in the care of these populations should be vaccinated.

Vaccine Response (Engelhard et al. 2013; Cordonnier et al. 2017)
- Longer interval from transplant is associated with better serology response. Vaccination within the first 6 months after transplant produces poor serology responses. Nonetheless, seasonal vaccination against

influenza can boost the cellular immune response in HSCT patients as early as 3 months after HSCT, but the protective effect is lower compared with healthy controls (Engelhard et al. 2013).

- Conflicting data exist on the benefit of a second dose of vaccine, and marginal benefit was seen with the use of GM-CSF.
- In HSCT the superiority of high-dose influenza vaccine has not been demonstrated (Halasa et al. 2016).
- Rituximab administration during the year before vaccination was associated with a lack of seroprotective titer.
- Active GVHD and low lymphocyte counts at vaccination are associated with poor immune response.

Live, attenuated influenza vaccine is contraindicated in HSCT patients (Rubin et al. 2014).

There is a difference in *the duration of influenza vaccine recommendation* in the European (Cordonnier et al. 2017) and US guidelines (Rubin et al. 2014):

- ECIL recommends vaccination as long as patient is judged to be immunosuppressed (A II r) although considered, with a lower strength, the use of yearly, lifelong (B II r) (Cordonnier et al. 2017).
- IDSA recommends lifelong immunization (Rubin et al. 2014).
- There are no trials to support one or other recommendations, but a lifelong immunization seems logical as fatal influenza illness can occur several years after HSCT, without clear risk factors in some patients, particularly in auto-HSCT (Ljungman et al. 2011), and the proved safety of influenza vaccine in this population. Moreover, for general population, the CDC recommends routine annual influenza vaccination for all persons aged ≥6 months (Grohskopf et al. 2017).

For severe thrombocytopenic patients, the intradermic influenza vaccine can be safely administered although it has not yet been evaluated in transplant recipients.

29.5.2 Measles, Mumps, and Rubella

The clinical impact and the reasons for immunization in HSCT patients differ among these viruses:

- *Measles*: Severe and also fatal measles infections (pneumonia, encephalitis) have been reported in SCT recipients. The aim of vaccination is to protect the patient of severe consequences of infection.
- *Rubella*: There are no reports of severe rubella disease occurring in HSCT recipients. The main indication for rubella vaccination is prevention of congenital rubella in fertile women.
- *Mumps*: There are no reports of severe mumps occurring in HSCT recipients. The indication for mumps vaccination is therefore weak. There is no indication for routine mumps vaccination after HSCT. However, mumps is included in combination vaccines with measles and rubella.

Vaccines Only live-attenuated vaccines are available. Presentations: measles alone, combined measles–mumps–rubella, combined measles–mumps–rubella–varicella (live).

29.5.3 Hepatitis B Virus (HBV)

Prevention of infection and reverse seroconversion:

- Approximately 40–70% of HSCT patients obtain a titer of anti-HBs of >10 mIU/mL after post-HSCT vaccination, a rather low response compared with healthy controls. Even those who fail to obtain a response may benefit from vaccination as it can prevent reverse seroconversion.
- Patients that have evidence of a previously resolved hepatitis B infection prior to the transplant (i.e., HBsAg negative but anti-HBs and/or anti-HBc) are at risk or reverse seroconversion.

- Immunization for HBV can prevent HBV reverse seroconversion even in non-responders to hepatitis B vaccine after allo-HSCT (Takahata et al. 2014). Probably, antigen-specific memory T cells and cytotoxic T cells induced by hepatitis B vaccine are largely responsible for prevention of reverse seroconversion in non-responders to the vaccine. This reinforces the need of HBV vaccination.

29.5.4 Human Papilloma Virus (HPV)

In HSCT women nearly 40% will have genital HPV infection in long-term follow-up (Shanis et al. 2018). HPV is associated with cervical, vulvar, and vaginal cancer in females, penile cancer in males, and anal cancer and oropharyngeal cancer in both females and males.

In long-term survivors, second neoplasias are a significant complication after allo-HSCT. Cervix cancer is one of the most frequent. Squamous cell cancers, the commonest post transplant solid tumors, are associated with HPV infection. Genital HPV disease is a significant late complication of allo-HSCT, occurring in one third of women. Prolonged systemic IS treatment for cGVHD is associated with a higher risk of developing HPV-related squamous intraepithelial lesions.

Regular gynecologic examination, cervical cytology, and HPV testing after HSCT is recommended for all women (Majhail et al. 2012) as preventing measure for HPV-related cancer and as a tool for early diagnose and treatment of genital GVHD.

29.5.4.1 Vaccine
- HPV vaccine is a noninfectious, virus-like particle (VLP) vaccine. There are three formulations of HPV vaccines that differ in the number of HPV covered: a 9-valent HPV vaccine (6, 11, 16, 18, 31, 33, 45, 52, and 58 VLPs) (Gardasil 9®), quadrivalent HPV vaccine (6, 11, 16, and 18 VLPs) (Gardasil®), and bivalent vaccine (16, 18 VLPs) (Cervarix®).
- The experience with HPV vaccine in HSCT is limited, 20 children (MacIntyre et al. 2016)

and 64 adults (Stratton et al. 2018), but shows a good immune response, similar to health women, with no specific safety issue.
- HPV vaccine is recommended in all guidelines (Ljungman et al. 2009; Hilgendorf et al. 2011; Rubin et al. 2014; Cordonnier et al. 2017) but with a low grade of recommendation (B II u to C III) due to the limited experience in HSCT patients. The recommended number of doses is three (Hilgendorf et al. 2011; Rubin et al. 2014).

29.5.5 Poliovirus

The WHO European Region was declared polio-free in 2002. Imported wild-type and vaccine-type polioviruses still remain a threat to unvaccinated people in the EU/EEA. Maintaining high vaccination coverage in all population groups remain an essential tool for keeping Europe polio-free.

Only inactivated poliovirus vaccines are used in all EU/EEA countries.

Oral polio vaccine (OPV) is contraindicated for HSCT patients due to the risk of paralytic poliomyelitis. This complication has occurred after vaccination of patients with severe combined immune deficiency but has not been described in HSCT patients.

29.5.6 Varicella Zoster Virus (VZV)

Prevention of VZV After HSCT Antiviral prophylaxis (acyclovir/valacyclovir) is the primary mode of prevention. It should be given for at least 1 year after allo-HSCT and for 3–6 months after auto-HSCT (Cordonnier et al. 2017).

Types of Vaccines There are three types of available vaccines and one not commercially available. None is licensed for use in IS patients.

- Live-attenuated varicella vaccine, a low-titer VZV vaccine (Varivax®, Varilix®). It is also available in combination in the same vaccine with measles, mumps, and rubella.

- Varicella vaccine can be used in HSCT following strict requirements (see ECIL and IDSA vaccination guidelines) (Cordonnier et al. 2017; Rubin et al. 2014). Although vaccination with varicella-attenuated vaccine is indicated/considered in guidelines, in practice it is rarely used due to concerns of safety, particularly in adults (Miller et al. 2017). The commercial availability of the VZ subunit vaccine and maybe in the future the inactivated vaccine will make the use of the attenuated vaccines even lower.
- Live-attenuated zoster vaccine, a high-titer vaccine (Zostavax®). It contains more than 14 times more virus than varicella vaccine. In all guidelines, this vaccine is contraindicated in HSCT patients.
- New phase III studies with new VZL vaccines in auto-HSCT.
  - *Adjuvanted VZV subunit vaccine* (Shingrix®) (de la Serna et al. 2018; Sullivan et al. 2018) consists of recombinant VZV gE antigen mixed with AS01B adjuvant. It was recently approved by the FDA (October 2017) and EMA (March 2018) for prevention of herpes zoster (HZ) and post-herpetic neuralgia, in adults 50 years of age or older. It is administered IM in two doses separated by 60 days.
  - *Inactivated VZV-vaccine (V212), in auto-HSCT* (Winston et al. 2018), is not yet commercially available. It is administered in four doses by SC injection, beginning ~5 days prior to chemotherapy or ~30 days prior to auto-HSCT and the remaining doses being administered at 30, 60, and 90 days later.
  - Both vaccines showed a high vaccine efficacy for preventing zoster which was 68–64%, post-herpetic neuralgia 89–84%, VZV-related hospitalizations 85%, and for other VZV complications 78–75%. The positive results of these studies probably are going to change the prevention of VZV complications after auto-HSCT.

29.5.7 Pneumococcus

Pneumococcus is a frequent and *serious complication in HSCT*. The incidence of invasive pneumococcal disease (IPD) in HSCT is 50 times higher compared to the general population (Shigayeva et al. 2016). In spite of this high incidence of IPD, less than one in five HSCT patients with IPD had received pneumococcal vaccine.

29.5.7.1 Types of Vaccine
- Polysaccharidic (PS) vaccine
  - 23-valent polysaccharidic (PS) vaccine (Pneumo 23®, Pneumovax23®): poor immunogenic, T-cell-independent response, no boost benefit
  - Poor responses, particularly in patients with GVHD
  - PS after PCV vaccine increases and expands the response obtained with PCV. Some non-responders to PCV will achieve a response with PS vaccine.
- Conjugate vaccine (PCV): highly immunogenic, T-cell-dependent response, with boost benefit
  - 13-valent in the majority of countries (Prevenar 13r®) (that replace the previous 7-valent vaccine) or 10-valent available in some countries (Synflorix®).
  - Five trials have shown a good response to PCV after three doses (range 54–98%). Four trials used 7-valent conjugated vaccine and one the 13-valent vaccine (Cordonnier et al. 2017). These responses are much better compared with what is obtained with PS vaccine.
  - Early vaccination at 3 months is not inferior to late vaccination (9 months) after allo-HSCT.
  - PCV should always be administered before PS vaccine.

29.5.8 Diphtheria-Tetanus-Pertussis

The exposure to *tetanus* in the environment is a real risk for HSCT patients, so the aim of vaccination after transplant is to protect the patient.

Diphtheria has essentially been eradicated but ongoing vaccination is critical for immunity. Diphtheria cases are still happening in Europe with an increase of 280% from 2009 to 2014. The reappearance of diphtheria cases in countries like Spain diphtheria-free for more than 30 years (Jane et al. 2018) is alarming and another reason to vaccine all our HSCT patients.

There are very limited published data of *pertussis* in HSCT and no reported case of severe or fatal pertussis infection after SCT in adults. Therefore, the objective of vaccination in these patients is avoiding pertussis transmission by HSCT patients.

29.6 Vaccinations Before Travel to Areas Endemic for Infections
(See Table 29.3)
(Ljungman et al. 2009)

29.7 Serological Testing

For the majority of vaccines, no pre- or postvaccination serology is recommended. Nonetheless, there are exceptions for this rule (Ljungman et al. 2009).

29.7.1 Pre-Vaccination

Testing for Abs to measles is recommended in adults, with vaccination performed only if the patient is seronegative (CIII).

If vaccination against varicella is contemplated, testing of immunity should be carried out and vaccination should be administered to seronegative patients only (CIII).

29.7.2 Postvaccination

Pneumococcal vaccine: Testing to assess the response to vaccination is recommended at

Table 29.3 Vaccinations before travel to areas endemic for infections (Ljungman et al. 2009)

If contraindications for the vaccine exist, the patient should be advised not to travel to endemic areas (CIII)
Vaccination is one of the precautions that the HSCT patients should observe. There are other equal important measures that should be followed: chemoprophylaxis against malaria; mosquito-oriented precautions; food safety to prevent traveler's diarrhea; avoiding sun exposure, particularly for those under treatments associated with photosensitivity (like voriconazole)

Tick-borne and Japanese B encephalitis	• According to local policy in endemic areas (CIII)No data exist regarding the time after HCT when vaccination can be expected to induce an immune response
Rabies	• Rabies vaccine is made from killed virus and cannot cause rabies. Nonetheless, there are no data regarding safety, immunogenicity, or efficacy among HCT recipients • Preexposure rabies vaccination should probably be delayed until 12–24 months after HCT • Postexposure administration of rabies vaccine with human rabies Ig can be administered any time after HCT, as indicated
Yellow fever (live)	• Limited data regarding safety and efficacy (C III). Yellow fever vaccine has been safely administered to a limited number of post-HSCT patients (Rubin et al. 2014) • The risk–benefit balance may favor the use of the vaccine in patients residing in or traveling to endemic areas
Hepatitis A	• Follow recommendations for general population in each country (CIII) • Ig should be administered to hepatitis A-susceptible HCT recipients who anticipate hepatitis A exposure (for example, during travel to endemic areas) and for postexposure prophylaxis
Typhoid (IM), inactivated vaccine	• No data were found regarding safety, immunogenicity, or efficacy among HCT recipients. DIII. Remember that typhoid oral vaccine is live attenuated and is contraindicated in HSCT patients (EIII)
Cholera	• No data were found regarding safety and immunogenicity among HCT recipients. Vaccine is not recommended (DIII)

1 month or later after the third or fourth dose of pneumococcal vaccine (BIII). As a widely accepted definition of adequate response to pneumococcal vaccine is lacking, guidelines for revaccination of non-responders are not given. Testing for immunity to pneumococcus might reasonably be repeated every 2 years for the first 4 years (BIII).

Hepatitis B: Testing should be carried out 1 month or later after the third vaccine dose (BIII). A second three-dose vaccination schedule is recommended in non-responders (CIII)

Testing should be conducted approximately every 4–5 years to assess for immunity to HBV, measles, tetanus, diphtheria, and polio (BIII).

29.8 Vaccinations for Donors, Close Contacts/Family, and HCWs of HSCT Recipients (See Table 29.4) (Ljungman et al. 2009; Cordonnier et al. 2017; Rubin et al. 2014)

Table 29.4 Vaccinations for donors, close contacts/family, and HCWs of HCT recipients

General comments	
Inactivated vaccines can be safely given for donors, close contacts, and HCWs of HSCT patients	
For live vaccines a careful evaluation should be done (see below). Some have no safety issues for HSCT recipients but other can cause severe damage	
Donors	
Guidelines do not recommend donor vaccination for the benefit of the recipient[a,b]	

- Only vaccines that are indicated and recommended based on the donor's age, vaccination history, and exposure history should be administered
- Nonetheless, vaccination of the donor has been shown to improve the post transplant immunity of the patient in the case of tetanus, diphtheria, 7-valent pneumococcal conjugate vaccine (PCV), and *Haemophilus influenzae* type b-conjugate vaccines. Donation is an opportunity to update the donor vaccination calendar. If the donor has to receive any of these vaccines in his/her own interest, the administration of at least one dose pre-collection of stem cells could benefit also the receptor

Administration of MMR, MMRV, varicella, and zoster vaccines should be avoided within 4 weeks of stem cell harvest[b]. By extension, all live vaccines should be avoided before stem cell collection due to the risk of transmission of the pathogen with the graft[c]

Vaccines recommended for close contacts and HCWs of HSCT recipients

Who?	Vaccine	Dose/notes
All	Influenza, inactivated	•Annually, as long as there is contact with an IS recipient[a]: Close contacts: AII[a]-AIII[c]; HCWs: AI[a]-AIIt[c]
All sero(-) VZ	Varicella: AIII[a]	• 2 doses, separated by at least 28 days
HCWs Sero(-)	Measles	• AIII[a]; recommended, not graded[b,c]

Live vaccines given for *close contacts or HCWs* of HCST patients: precautions

Intranasal influenza vaccine	• If live influenza vaccine is administered to a close contact/HCWs, contact between the IS patient and household member should be avoided for 7 days (weak, very low)[b]
Measles-mumps-rubella	• No risk for the HSCT patient
Varicella	• The vaccination dose or doses should be completed >4 weeks before the conditioning regimen begins or >6 weeks (42 days) before contact with the HCT recipient is planned (BIII)[a]
	• If a varicella vaccinee develops a postvaccination rash within 42 days of vaccination, the vaccinee should avoid contact with HCT recipients until all rash lesions are crusted or the rash has resolved[a]

(continued)

Table 29.4 (continued)

Oral polio vaccine (OPV)	• Oral polio vaccine (OPV) should not be administered to individuals who live in a household with IS patients (strong, moderate)[b]. These vaccinated contacts shed the live-attenuated poliovirus strains of the vaccine in the stools that can induce paralytic poliomyelitis in immunocompromised patients like HSCT • If live-attenuated oral polio vaccine, that is still available in some non-US/non-European countries, is given to a household contact, a 4- to 6-week furlough is advised
Rotavirus	• Rotavirus vaccine is included in the children vaccine calendar of many countries, so it will be frequent that a HSCT patient has a child candidate for the vaccine • Virus is shed in stools for 2–4 weeks after vaccination. Transmission from vaccinated to IS person has been confirmed, but there are no reported cases of symptomatic infection in contacts • Highly IS patients should avoid handling diapers of infants who have been vaccinated with rotavirus vaccine for 4 weeks after vaccination (strong, very low) • HSCT recipients should have no contact with the stools or diapers of vaccinated children for 4 weeks following vaccination[c]
Vaccines for travel: yellow fever vaccine; oral typhoid vaccine	• Can safely be administered[b]

HCWs healthcare workers
[a]Ljungman et al. (2009)
[b]Rubin et al. (2014)
[c]Cordonnier et al. (2017)

Key Points

- Vaccination should be considered a routine practice for all HSCT receptors, either autologous or allogeneic, adults or children. It should be implemented in all HSCT programs.
- There is no a unique vaccine schedule for all HSCT patients. Each center should discuss and adapt a specific vaccine program.
- To obtain this objective, it is necessary to have in place a standardized program specific for HSCT patients with a simple and clear chronology and the collaboration of the Preventive Department of the hospital and primary care physicians.
- The vaccination program should include not only the patient but also those who live with the patient and the healthcare workers (HCWs).
- There are two main reasons for universal vaccination of HSCT patients: (a) the general interest as all the population should be correctly vaccinated to avoid holes of immunity that can be a risk for the health of the general population and (b) individual interest for each HSCT patient.

References

Armenian SH, Sun CL, Vase T, et al. Cardiovascular risk factors in hematopoietic cell transplantation (HCT) survivors: role in development of subsequent cardiovascular disease. Blood. 2012;120:4505–12.

Beck CR, McKenzie BC, Hashim AB, et al. Influenza vaccination for immunocompromised patients: systematic review and meta-analysis by aetiology. J Infect Dis. 2012;206:1250–9.

Clar C, Oseni Z, Flowers N, et al. Influenza vaccines for preventing cardiovascular disease. Cochrane Database Syst Rev. 2015;5:CD005050.

Cordonnier C, Cesaro S, De Lavallade H, et al. Guidelines for vaccination of patients with hematological malignancies and HSCT recipient. ECIL 2017. 2017; Published online 4-10-2017. www.ecil-leukaemia.com.

Davis MM, Taubert K, Benin AL, et al. Influenza vaccination as secondary prevention for cardiovascular disease: a science advisory from the American Heart Association/American College of Cardiology. J Am Coll Cardiol. 2006;48:1498–502.

Engelhard D, Mohty B, de la Camara R, et al. European guidelines for prevention and management of influenza in hematopoietic stem cell transplantation and leukemia patients: summary of ECIL-4 (2011), on behalf of ECIL, a joint venture of EBMT, EORTC, ICHS, and ELN. Transpl Infect Dis. 2013;15:219–32.

Grohskopf LA, Sokolow LZ, Broder KR, Walter EB, Bresee JS, Fry AM, et al. Prevention and control of seasonal influenza with vaccines: recommendations of the Advisory Committee on Immunization Practices - United States, 2017-18 influenza season. MMWR Recomm Rep. 2017;66:1–20.

Halasa NB, Savani BN, Asokan I, et al. Randomized double-blind study of the safety and immunogenicity of standard-dose trivalent inactivated influenza vaccine versus high-dose trivalent inactivated influenza vaccine in adult hematopoietic stem cell transplantation patients. Biol Blood Marrow Transplant. 2016;22:528–35.

Hilgendorf I, Freund M, Jilg W, et al. Vaccination of allogeneic haematopoietic stem cell transplant recipients: report from the international consensus conference on clinical practice in chronic GVHD. Vaccine. 2011;29:2825–33.

Jane M, Vidal MJ, Camps N, et al. A case of respiratory toxigenic diphtheria: contact tracing results and considerations following a 30-year disease-free interval, Catalonia, Spain, 2015. Euro Surveill. 2018;23. https://doi.org/10.2807/1560-7917.

Kwong JC, Schwartz KL, Campitelli MA, et al. Acute myocardial infarction after laboratory-confirmed influenza infection. N Engl J Med. 2018;378:345–53.

de la Serna J, Campora L, Chandrasekar P, et al. Efficacy and safety of an adjuvanted herpes zoster subunit vaccine in autologous hematopoietic stem cell transplant recipients 18 years of age or older: first results of the phase 3 randomized, placebo-controlled ZOEHSCT clinical trial. 2018. Late break abstract. BMT TANDEM meeting 2018, Salt Lake City.

Ljungman P, Cordonnier C, Einsele H, et al. Vaccination of hematopoietic cell transplant recipients. Bone Marrow Transplant. 2009;44:521–6.

Ljungman P, de la Camara R, Perez-Bercoff L, et al. Outcome of pandemic H1N1 infections in hematopoietic stem cell transplant recipients. Haematologica. 2011;96:1231–5.

Loomba RS, Aggarwal S, Shah PH, Arora RR. Influenza vaccination and cardiovascular morbidity and mortality. J Cardiovasc Pharmacol Ther. 2012;17:277–83.

Machado CM, Cardoso MR, da Rocha IF, et al. The benefit of influenza vaccination after bone marrow transplantation. Bone Marrow Transplant. 2005;36:897–900.

MacIntyre CR, Shaw P, Mackie FE, et al. Immunogenicity and persistence of immunity of a quadrivalent Human Papillomavirus (HPV) vaccine in immunocompromised children. Vaccine. 2016;34:4343–50.

Majhail NS, Rizzo JD, Lee SJ, et al. Recommended screening and preventive practices for long-term survivors after hematopoietic cell transplantation. Bone Marrow Transplant. 2012;47:337–41.

Miller PDE, de Silva TI, Skinner R, et al. Routine vaccination practice after adult and paediatric allogeneic haematopoietic stem cell transplant: a survey of UK NHS programmes. Bone Marrow Transplant. 2017;52:775–7.

Rubin LG, Levin MJ, Ljungman P, et al. 2013 IDSA clinical practice guideline for vaccination of the immunocompromised host. Clin Infect Dis. 2014;58: e44–100.

Shanis D, Anandi P, Grant C, et al. Risks factors and timing of genital human papillomavirus (HPV) infection in female stem cell transplant survivors: a longitudinal study. Bone Marrow Transplant. 2018;53:78–83.

Shigayeva A, Rudnick W, Green K, et al. Invasive pneumococcal disease among immunocompromised persons: implications for vaccination programs. Clin Infect Dis. 2016;62:139–47.

Stratton P, Battiwalla M, Abdelazim S, et al. Immunogenicity of HPV quadrivalent vaccine in women after allogeneic HCT is comparable to healthy volunteers. BMT TANDEM meeting 2018, Salt Lake City. Biol Blood Marrow Transplant. 2018;24: S85–6.

Sullivan K, Abhyankar A, Campora L, et al. Immunogenicity and safety of an adjuvanted herpes zoster subunit vaccine in adult autologous hematopoietic stem cell transplant recipients: phase 3, randomized, placebo-controlled, ZOE-HSCT clinical trial. 44th annual meeting of the European Society for Blood and Marrow Transplantation 18-21 March, Lisbon, Portugal; 2018.

Takahata M, Hashino S, Onozawa M, et al. Hepatitis B virus (HBV) reverse seroconversion (RS) can be prevented even in non-responders to hepatitis B vaccine after allogeneic stem cell transplantation: long-term analysis of intervention in RS with vaccine for patients with previous HBV infection. Transpl Infect Dis. 2014;16:797–801.

Winston DJ, Mullane KM, Cornely OA, Boeckh MJ, Brown JW, Pergam SA, et al. Inactivated varicella zoster vaccine in autologous haemopoietic stem-cell transplant recipients: an international, multicentre, randomised, double-blind, placebo-controlled trial. Lancet. 2018;391:2116–27.

Psychological Morbidity and Support

Alice Polomeni, Enrique Moreno,
and Frank Schulz-Kindermann

30.1 Introduction

Allo-HSCT is associated with significant physical
and psychological morbidity that may have a negative impact on patients' and on their relatives'
health-related quality of life (HRQoL) (Majhail
and Rizzo 2013). Patients suffer a broad range of
acute and chronic impairments of health-related
quality of life (HRQoL), concerning physical,
emotional, cognitive and social constraints.
Psychosocial difficulties have been identified
throughout the HSCT process, from pre-transplant to recovery phase and even for long-term
survivors. Insofar, psychological support of
HSCT recipients and caregivers is based on a—
where ever possible—preventive, concrete and
sustainable approach, comprising a broad range
of aspects of HRQoL. Psychooncological interventions are planned and conducted regularly in

A. Polomeni (✉)
Service d'Hématologie clinique et thérapie cellulaire,
Hôpital Saint Antoine - Assistance Publique-
Hôpitaux de Paris, Paris, France
e-mail: alice.polomeni@aphp.fr

E. Moreno
Department of Psychology, Asleuval (Valencian
Association of Leukemia), Valencia, Spain

F. Schulz-Kindermann
Pychooncological Outpatient Department,
Institute of Medical Psychology, University Cancer
Center Hamburg, University of Hamburg,
Hamburg, Germany

an interdisciplinary approach, taking into consid
eration medical, social and nursing issues.

30.2 The Period Preceding HSCT

Since HSCT often appears to be the only therapeu
tic cure, this can cause high expectations in patients
and their families, who may overestimate HSCT's
benefits and underestimate the procedure's mor
bidity and mortality risks. Several authors are ada
mant about the importance of pragmatic
information, specifically regarding prognosis, post
transplant effects and the impact of HSCT on
QOL. This information not only could guide
patients in their decision to undergo the treatment
(or not) but could also help them and their close
relatives to face the persistent side effects post-
HSCT (Jim et al. 2014). Studies show that specific
pre-transplant distress predicts psychosocial prob
lems during and after HSCT (Schulz-Kindermann
et al. 2002). This suggests a thorough medical as
well as psychosocial preparation about risks and
challenges with concomitant illustration of possi
ble coping resources. Understanding of the infor
mation about the prognosis can be associated with
depression and a worsening QOL over time
(Applebaum et al. 2016).

Frequently described are anxious-depressive
symptoms and sleep disruption pre-HSCT, linked
to the burden of uncertainty about treatment out
comes. Baseline anxiety and depression predict

worsening HRQoL during hospitalisation and post-treatment adjustment, even identifying these symptoms as risk factors for survival (Artherholt et al. 2014). This suggests a thorough survey of the psychosocial anamnesis and a brief screening in the course of treatment and survivorship. To avoid evitable strain, short instruments to measure distress, anxiety, depression and HRQoL—like the Distress Thermometer, Patient Health Questionnaire, Cancer Treatment-Related Distress Scale and EORTC QLQ-C30—should be implemented. Attention should always involve caregivers as well as minor children of patients. Finally, HSCT teams should screen patients' and families' met and unmet needs, including psychosocial support. Regarding preparation for HSCT, patients who are in a fairly stable physical state should take advantage of psychological support before admission to inpatient treatment. Psychological interventions cover different approaches like psychodynamic interviews, introduction in relaxation techniques, communication skills (regarding problem-focused communication with staff and with caregivers) and coping with side effects (pain, nausea, fatigue, restlessness, sleep disorder; see Syrjala et al. 2012).

30.3 Hospitalisation for HSCT

During hospitalisation, patients grapple with considerable changes, including a loss of physical abilities and autonomy. HSCT hospitalisation constraints, combined with poor physical condition, may increase patients' feelings of isolation and dependence, negatively affecting psychological well-being (Tecchio et al. 2013). Symptoms of depression, anxiety, sleep disruption and adjustment disorders are frequently reported (El Jawahri 2015). Unlike anxiety, which does not change over time, depression levels increase more than twofold after 2 weeks of isolation (Tecchio et al. 2013).

These symptoms can go unrecognised and have been known to interfere with HSCT medical treatment. Depression during hospitalisation is associated with longer hospital stay, increased

risk of mortality (Prieto et al. 2005), post transplant anxio-depressive symptoms and post traumatic stress syndrome (PTSS) (El-Jawahri et al. 2016).

Depressive symptoms are risk factors for a poorer outcome after HSCT. It is noteworthy to follow a precise diagnostic process, differentiating depression and demoralisation. The latter focuses on an attitude of senselessness and hopelessness, while depression has a pronounced somatic level, overlapping with fatigue. Recent research has explored psychoneuroendocrinology and psychoneuroimmunology to identify pathways that may mediate between psychosocial factors and disease outcomes (Costanzo et al. 2013). These authors have recommended the treatment of sleep and circadian disturbances, as well as the option of psychotropic medications and cognitive-behavioural interventions in the HSCT setting.

A significantly positive correlation between the presence of a family caregiver (FC) during hospitalisation and HSCT survival has been established (Foster et al. 2013). The support provided by the HSCT team can also help patients to better cope with hospitalisation and facilitate psychological adjustment after discharge, reducing difficulties in the transition towards outpatient care.

Psychooncological interventions concerning depressive and anxious symptomatology rely on psychoeducational, psychodynamic and biobehavioural approaches, incorporating adequate coping potential. Specific techniques to ameliorate anxiety but also side effects like pain, sleeplessness, nausea or restlessness comprise relaxation, imagery and hypnotherapeutic approaches. Particularly in cases of fear and panic, pharmacological approaches with benzodiazepines and certain antidepressants should be taken into account.

Precise and repeated pain diagnostics are paramount, deriving multidisciplinary pain management, including medication, ongoing information about pain management and psychological interventions. There is some evidence for effectiveness of relaxation, imagery, hypnosis and cognitive-behavioral therapy (Syrjala 2014).

30.4   Post-HSCT

Data show that patients in remission for 2–5 years post-HSCT have a high probability of long-term survival. Nevertheless, HSCT-related morbidity is substantial, negatively affecting psychological functioning and social integration. HSCT's late effects on physical and psychic well-being have been well described, notably for chronic graft versus host disease, the severity of which is significantly related to impaired psychosocial functioning and diminished QOL (Majhail and Rizzo 2013).

Regarding psychopathology post-HSCT, several studies reported high rates of anxiety and depression, even several years after transplantation. Notwithstanding, research on psychological issues after HSCT has shown inconsistent results due to varying outcome measures, participation biases and cohort size and composition (Sun et al. 2011).

Although some studies have shown that depression and anxiety rates do not differ significantly from those of siblings or population norms, others reveal rates of psychological distress of 14% to 90% in survivors of HSCT (Sun et al. 2011). Even though some results demonstrate that physical morbidity tends to decrease by 1-year post-HSCT and psychosocial condition improves gradually over 1–5 years (Sun et al. 2013), other research reports depressive symptoms as long as 5 or even 10 years after HSCT (Jim et al. 2016). An unsettling fact is that depression post-HSCT has been associated with higher mortality and increased risk of suicide (Tichelli et al. 2013).

Depressive symptoms and sleep disorders are related to cognitive dysfunctions. Sleep disruption remains an issue for 43% of HSCT patients after transplant (Jim et al. 2016). These rates of disruption are substantially higher than those of the general population. Incidence of cognitive dysfunction in the first 5 years after HSCT is up to 60% (Scherwath et al. 2013). Poor neurocognitive functioning and psychosocial outcomes lead to lax medication management and adherence to recommended monitoring guidelines, which in turn may increase post-treatment morbi-mortality risks (Mayo et al. 2016).

Psychological interventions for depressive symptoms focus on dysfunctional, exaggerated cognitions and on an increase of activities. Psychopharmacological treatment is often recommended additionally, offering a broad range of substances, which can and should be adapted to respective indications and to the broad range of further medication. In the case of severe demoralisation, existential and meaning-centred approaches are advisable and show some evidence.

Concerning lasting traumatic experiences, in cross-sectional studies between 5 and 19% fulfilled a diagnosis of post-traumatic stress disorder (PTSD). In one of the rare prospective studies, PTSD symptomatology was observable at all time points (Esser et al. 2017a). Therefore, psychological support should not only be offered in the acute phase but already before HSCT and in the long term. Impairment by pain and pain intensity were risk factors for elevated levels of PTSD symptomatology. This highlights the importance of informing patients early enough that pain might occur and to introduce techniques for dealing with it. Since medical complications predicted severity of PTSD symptomatology 1 year after HSCT, medical professionals should be aware of psychological strain among patients suffering from long-term medical complications.

Psychosocial issues have also been explored in QOL research. Some studies in this domain stated that even if medical problems remain, the patients' emotional well-being seems to improve throughout the rehabilitation period. Nonetheless, fatigue, sleep disorders, neurocognitive impairment, neurobehavioural problems and sexual dysfunction persist. Esser et al. (2017b) identified in a prospective study three stable symptom complexes: exhausted (incl. fatigue), affective (incl. irritability and depressive symptoms) and gastrointestinal (incl. nausea). Fatigue was most persistent and also most severe and predictive for HRQoL. Fear of relapse, feelings of disability and barriers to social rehabilitation are frequent concerns, even several years after the procedure, with only a minority of disease-free transplant survivors consider themselves having 'returned to normal' (Syrjala et al. 2012).

These psychosocial difficulties are not systematically approached in current HSCT follow-up: despite their incidence, anxious-depressive symptoms are not often reported which should be treated by HSCT physicians. Barriers to approaching psychosocial issues are, on one hand, patients' fear of being stigmatised and, on the other hand, doctors who tend to prioritise strictly medical aspects. Health professionals often poorly evaluate psychological symptoms: anxiety is overrated, depression is underestimated, and consistency between the patients and the medical team's evaluations seems insufficient. Most patients receive prescriptions for these lingering symptoms, even over long periods, yet half of them benefit of follow-up by specialised professionals due to organisational and emotional obstacles (Mosher et al. 2010).

Anxieties after HSCT may be treated in a cognitive-behavioural approach, relying on working directly with fear-related contents and applying this to the broad range of oversimplified anxieties. For progression anxiety, manualised psychooncological therapies are well-tried, combining psychoeducational elements with group-format psychological therapy. Cognitive-behavioural therapy has demonstrated effectiveness in the treatment of PTSD with cancer patients in a significant number of studies, including patients with HSCT (DuHamel et al. 2010). Concerning fatigue, there are several promising approaches combining psychosocial counselling with physical training.

30.5 Close Relatives

Family caregivers (FC) can contribute to patients' recovery and to better survival following HSCT (Ehrlich et al. 2016). That said, the HSCT impact on FC has not been sufficiently explored, with most studies suffering from limitations due to small and heterogeneous samples.

Current research shows that FC experience a significant burden across the treatment trajectory. At the time of transplant, FC report high levels of fatigue, sleep disorders, depression and anxiety (El Jawahri 2015). FC may have more emotional difficulties than patients, and their well-being can be impaired well past post transplant. FC face negative effects in their own family and professional and social lives and express marital dissatisfaction after HSCT (Langer et al. 2017).

Qualitative data indicate that the main FC difficulties are related to long-term HSCT consequences and the unpredictable, uncertain character of their evolution. Assuming not only daily tasks but also the patients' psychological support, FC may feel overwhelmed by the complex demands of the caregiving role and the social impact of a lengthy rehabilitation (Applebaum et al. 2016).

In spite of the obstacles met during this post transplant period, FC rarely benefit from regular psychosocial support. Attention should also involve patients' minor children. The current trend has been to outsource part of the patient care. Research should better explore FC's real-life experience in order to propose targeted interventions during HSCT's various stages.

30.6 Related Donors

Related donors (RDs) deserve particular attention. Although positive effects of related donation have been demonstrated—such as deep personal satisfaction and a higher degree of self-esteem—there is also a negative impact. The incidence of pain and depressive symptoms is higher in RDs than in unrelated donors. Unexplained chronic pain could be associated with psychological distress related to the recipient's medical condition and HSCT outcomes. Data suggest that psychological support and follow-up should also be offered to RD (Garcia et al. 2013).

Like for patients, sufficient information, preparation and guidance should be available for FC and RD. That is, not only the tremendous task should be emphasised but also probable problems and risks, as well as available resources of care. Several interventions were developed to support FC, like problem-solving skills, cognitive-behavioural interventions and expressive talking (Applebaum et al. 2016).

30.7 Adolescents and Young Adults (AYA)

The adolescent and young adult group (AYA) represents a particular group that significantly varies from non-AYA patients, especially in psychosocial aspects (Pulewka et al. 2017). Research reveals that a quarter of AYA patients who experienced HSCT reported depression and anxiety symptoms, with nearly half meeting the criteria for post-traumatic stress (Syrjala et al. 2012).

HSCT appears to be a risk factor for poor health-related quality of life (HRQoL) and social functioning in AYA cancer survivors (Tremolada et al. 2016). Qualitative studies show that this population encounters difficulties in physical (sexuality and fatigue), psychological (depression, adherence and dependency issues, fear of the future, uncertainty) and social domains (changes in roles and relationships, educations and financial issues, family problems). Evidence-based psychosocial interventions in this population are sparse and should include specific problems, such as family relationships and social integration (school and work). Recent approaches use group formats enhancing self-help resources of peers, activity coaching and motivational interviewing.

30.8 Paediatric Patients

In their review of the literature, Packman et al. (2010) shows that HSCT paediatric patients experience acute psychological symptoms such as anxiety and depression before and during hospitalisation, as well as significant peer isolation, behavioural problems and post-traumatic stress symptoms after HSCT. Declines in cognitive abilities, social functioning and self-esteem have also been observed.

It is noteworthy that the accord between parent and child is better regarding physical conditions than it is with psychological issues. This discrepancy between the child's and the parents' evaluations also holds true regarding HRQoL post-HSCT (Chang et al. 2012).

HSCT may lead to disruptions in family life: parents and siblings (notably, donors) also report high levels of anxiety, depression and post-traumatic stress symptoms (Packman et al. 2010).

Paediatric HSCT survivors report psychosocial difficulties and decreased QOL with a high risk for anxiety, depression and behavioural problems. Childhood survivors' specific issues are related to sexual dysfunction, impoverished self-image and social adjustment. As follow-up of childhood HSCT patients is fundamental, special attention should be paid to the risk of withdrawal as they journey towards adulthood (Cupit et al. 2016).

Key Points
- The previously discussed rates of psychological morbidity in HSCT patients emphasise the need for clinical assessment throughout the procedure and at regular intervals.
- Given their vital role in the patients' recovery process, HSCT teams should also assess FC for psychological adjustment and family functioning.
- Particular attention should be given to RDs, who do not benefit systematically from a medical and psychological follow-up.
- Regardless of the overwhelming evidence of psychological morbidity in HSCT patients and in FC, barriers still exist in discussing psychosocial issues in routine care.
- Systematic screening may contribute to stimulate discussion of psychological symptoms, but quality psychosocial

care requires team training and an effective multidisciplinary approach.

- Psychological support should be installed low threshold and as far as possible attached to the transplant centre.
- Effectiveness of psychooncological interventions is proven widely and should be adapted to patients and FCs all along the course of HSCT.

References

Applebaum AJ, Bevans M, Son T, et al. A scoping review of caregiver burden during allogeneic HSCT: lessons learned and future directions. Bone Marrow Transplant. 2016;51:1416–22.

Artherholt SB, Hong F, Berry DL, Fann JR. Risk factors for depression in patients undergoing hematopoietic cell transplantation. Biol Blood Marrow Transplant. 2014;20:946–50.

Chang G, Ratichek SJ, Recklitis C, et al. Children's psychological distress during pediatric HSCT: parent and child perspectives. Pediatr Blood Cancer. 2012;58:289–96.

Costanzo ES, Juckett MB, Coe CL, et al. Biobehavioral influences on recovery following hematopoietic stem cell transplantation. Brain Behav Immun. 2013;30(Suppl):S68–74.

Cupit MC, Duncan C, Savani BN, et al. Childhood to adult transition and long-term follow-up after blood and marrow transplantation. Bone Marrow Transplant. 2016;51:176–81.

DuHamel KN, Mosher CE, Winkel G, et al. Randomized clinical trial of telephone-administered cognitive-behavioral therapy to reduce posttraumatic stress disorder and distress symptoms after hematopoietic stem-cell transplantation. J Clin Oncol. 2010;28:3754–61.

Ehrlich KB, Miller GE, Scheide T, et al. Pre-transplant emotional support is associated with longer survival after allogeneic hematopoietic stem cell transplantation. Bone Marrow Transplant. 2016;51:1594–8.

El-Jawahri AR, Traeger LN, Kuzmuk K, et al. Quality of life and mood of patients and family caregivers during hospitalization for hematopoietic stem cell transplantation. Cancer, 2015. 121(6): p. 951–9.

El-Jawahri AR, Vandusen HB, Traeger LN, et al. Quality of life and mood predict posttraumatic stress disorder after hematopoietic stem cell transplantation. Cancer. 2016;122:806–12.

Esser P, Kuba K, Scherwath A, et al. Posttraumatic stress disorder symptomatology in the course of allogeneic HSCT: a prospective study. J Cancer Surviv. 2017a;11:203–10.

Esser P, Kuba K, Scherwath A, et al. Stability and priority of symptoms and symptom clusters among allogeneic HSCT patients within a 5-year longitudinal study. J Pain Symptom Manag. 2017b;54:493–500.

Foster LW, McLellan L, Rybicki L, et al. Validating the positive impact of in-hospital lay care-partner support on patient survival in allogeneic BMT: a prospective study. Bone Marrow Transplant. 2013;48:671–7.

Garcia MC, Chapman JR, Shaw PJ, et al. Motivations, experiences, and perspectives of bone marrow and peripheral blood stem cell donors: thematic synthesis of qualitative studies. Biol Blood Marrow Transplant. 2013;19:1046–58.

Jim HS, Quinn GP, Gwede CK, et al. Patient education in allogeneic hematopoietic cell transplant: what patients wish they had known about quality of life. Bone Marrow Transplant. 2014;49:299–303.

Jim HSL, Sutton SK, Jacobsen PB, et al. Risk factors for depression and fatigue among survivors of hematopoietic cell transplantation. Cancer. 2016;122:1290–7.

Langer S, Lehane C, Yi J. Patient and caregiver adjustment to hematopoietic stem cell transplantation: a systematic review of dyad-based studies. Curr Hematol Malig Rep. 2017;12:324–34.

Majhail NS, Rizzo D. Surviving the cure: long term follow up of hematopoietic cell transplant recipients. Bone Marrow Transplant. 2013;48:1145–51.

Mayo S, Messner HA, Rourke SB, et al. Relationship between neurocognitive functioning and medication management ability over the first 6 months following allogeneic stem cell transplantation. Bone Marrow Transplant. 2016;51:841–7.

Mosher CE, KN DuHamel KN, Rini CM, et al. Barriers to mental health service use among hematopoietic SCT survivors. Bone Marrow Transplant. 2010;45:570–9.

Packman W, Weber S, Wallace J, et al. Psychological effects of hematopoietic SCT on pediatric patients, siblings and parents: a review. Bone Marrow Transplant. 2010;45:1134–46.

Prieto JM, Atala J, Blanch J, et al. Role of depression as a predictor of mortality among cancer patients after stem-cell transplantation. J Clin Oncol. 2005;23:6063–71.

Pulewka K, Wolff D, Herzberg PY, et al. Physical and psychosocial aspects of adolescent and young adults after allogeneic hematopoietic stem-cell transplantation: results from a prospective multicenter trial. J Cancer Res Clin Oncol. 2017;143:1613–9.

Scherwath A, Schirmer L, Kruse M, et al. Cognitive functioning in allogeneic hematopoietic stem cell transplantation recipients and its medical correlates: a prospective multicenter study. Psychooncology. 2013;22:1509–16.

Schulz-Kindermann F, Hennings U, Ramm G, et al. The role of biomedical and psychosocial factors for the prediction of pain and distress in patients undergoing high-dose therapy and BMT/PBSCT. Bone Marrow Transplant. 2002;29:341–51.

Sun CL, Francisco L, Baker KS, et al. Adverse psychological outcomes in long-term survivors of hematopoietic cell transplantation: a report from the Bone

Marrow Transplant Survivor Study (BMTSS). Blood. 2011;118:4723–31.

Sun CL, Kersey JH, Francisco L, et al. Burden of morbidity in 10+ year survivors of hematopoietic cell transplantation: report from the bone marrow transplantation survivor study. Biol Blood Marrow Transplant. 2013;19:1073–80.

Syrjala K, Martin PJ, Lee SJ. Delivering care to long-term adult survivors of hematopoietic cell transplantation. J Clin Oncol. 2012;30:3746–51.

Syrjala KL, Jensen MP, Mendoza ME, Yi JC et al. Psychological and behavioral approaches to cancer pain management. J Clin Oncol. 2014; 32 (16): 1703–11.

Tecchio C, Bonetto C, Bertani M, et al. Predictors of anxiety and depression in hematopoietic stem cell transplant patients during protective isolation. Psychooncology. 2013;22:1790–7.

Tichelli A, Labopin M, Rovó A, et al. Increase of suicide and accidental death after hematopoietic stem cell transplantation: a cohort study on behalf of the Late Effects Working Party of the European Group for Blood and Marrow Transplantation (EBMT). Cancer. 2013;119:2012–21.

Tremolada M, Bonichini S, Basso G, et al. Perceived social support and health-related quality of life in AYA cancer survivors and controls. Psychooncology. 2016;25:1408–17.

Clinically Relevant Drug Interactions in HSCT

Tiene Bauters

31.1 Introduction

Patients undergoing HSCT often receive polymedication which carries the potential to result in drug interactions. To avoid unexpected outcomes, attention to drug interactions is crucial especially when drugs with a narrow therapeutic index or inherent toxicity profile are involved (Leather 2004; Glotzbecker et al. 2012; Gholaminezhad et al. 2014).

Drug interactions can be defined as changes in a drug's effect due to recent or concurrent use of another drug, food, or environmental agent. The net effect of the combination can result in enhanced activity of the affected drug, possibly leading to toxicity, or reduced activity leading to therapeutic failure (Thanacoody 2012).

In general, drug interactions can be categorized as being pharmacodynamic, pharmacokinetic, or pharmaceutical in nature.

31.1.1 Pharmacodynamic Interactions

Pharmacodynamic interactions occur when the effect of one drug is changed by the presence of another drug at its site of action. They compete

T. Bauters (✉)
Pharmacy, Pediatric Hemato-Oncology and Stem Cell Transplantation, Ghent University Hospital, Ghent, Belgium
e-mail: Tiene.bauters@uzgent.be

for specific receptor sites or interfere indirectly with physiological systems.

The effect can be additive/synergistic or antagonistic. An example of an additive interac tion is the concurrent use of QT-prolongating drugs (e.g., ciprofloxacin and fluconazole) which substantially increases the risk of torsades dē pointes or other ventricular tachyarrhythmias.

Specific antagonists can be used to reverse the effect of another drug at the receptor site (e.g., naloxone, an opioid receptor antagonist which reverses signs of opioid intoxication) (Lexicomp Drug® Interactions 2018).

31.1.2 Pharmacokinetic Interactions

Pharmacokinetic interactions (PK) occur when one drug alters the rate or extent of absorption, distribution, metabolism, or elimination of another drug resulting in diminished effects or drug potentiation (Palleria et al. 2013). The most frequent and significant drug interactions relate to drug metabolism. These will be further dis cussed here.

31.1.2.1 Cytochrome P450 Enzyme System

Several enzyme families are involved in drug metabolism, cytochrome P450 (CYP450) being the most important one. CYP450 consists of a unique group of isoenzymes grouped into fami lies (1–3) and divided into subfamilies (A–E).

They are primarily found in the liver and are genetically encoded (Ingelman-Sundberg and Rodriguez-Antona 2005; Lynch and Price 2007).

The effect of a CYP450 isoenzyme on a particular substrate can be altered by interaction with other drugs. Drugs can be substrates for a CYP450 isoenzyme and/or may inhibit or induce the isoenzyme (Larson 2018; Glotzbecker et al. 2012; Leather 2004):

Inhibition: Leads to reduced metabolism of the substrate with an increase in the steady-state concentration. It potentiates the effect and might lead to enhanced or toxic effects, especially in drugs with a narrow therapeutic index like cyclosporine and tacrolimus. Its onset occurs within 1–3 days for drugs with a short half-life, while the maximal effect may be delayed for drugs with a long half-life.

Induction: Increases the activity of CYP450 enzymes and usually results in decreased concentration/effect of the affected drug with the risk of therapeutic failure. Since the process of enzyme induction requires new protein synthesis, the effect usually occurs over days to weeks after starting an inducer.

Prodrugs rely on CYP450 enzymes for conversion to their active form(s). The combination of a prodrug (e.g., CFM) with a CYP450 inhibitor may result in therapeutic failure because of little or no production of the active drug. Conversely, an exaggerated therapeutic effect or adverse effect can be expected when a CYP450 inducer is added (Lynch and Price 2007).

In general, any drug metabolized by one of the CYP450 enzymes has the potential for PK- interaction, and concurrent use should be done with caution. As CYP3A4 is responsible for the metabolism of more than 50% of clinically administered drugs (Ingelman-Sundberg and Rodriguez-Antona 2005; Larson 2018), examples of CYP3A4 substrates, inhibitors, and inducers used in HSCT are presented in Table 31.1.

Mutations in CYP genes give rise to four major phenotypes: poor metabolizers, intermediate metabolizers, extensive metabolizers, and ultrarapid metabolizers (Ingelman-Sundberg and Rodriguez-Antona 2005; Ahmed et al. 2016). Polymorphisms in CYP450 are of concern in the study of interindividual altered drug metabolisms and/or adverse drug reactions.

31.1.2.2 Drug Transportation

P-glycoprotein (PgP) is a plasma membrane transporter involved in the excretion of drugs.

Table 31.1 CYP3A4 substrates, inhibitors and inducers commonly used in HSCT (non-limitative list) (Flockhart 2018; Medicines Complete 2018)

Substrates	Inhibitors	Inducers
Benzodiazepines[a]	Amiodarone	**Barbiturates (phenobarbital)**
Budesonide	Aprepitant	**Carbamazepine**
Calcium Channel Blockers[b]	Cimetidine	Corticosteroids
Carbamazepine	Ciprofloxacin	**Phenytoin**
Corticosteroids	**Clarithromycin**	**Rifampicin**
Etoposide	Diltiazem	St John's wort
Immunosuppressives[c]	Erythromycin	
Macrolide antibiotics[d]	Fluconazole	
Statins[e]	Grapefruit juice	
Steroids[f]	**Itraconazole**	
Miscellaneous[g]	**Ketoconazole**	
	Posaconazole	
	Voriconazole	
	Verapamil	

Bold font indicates strong inhibitors/inducers
[a]Alprazolam, diazepam, midazolam
[b]Amlodipine, diltiazem, verapamil
[c]Cyclosporine, tacrolimus, sirolimus
[d]Clarithromycin, erythromycin, NOT azithromycin
[e]Atorvastatin, NOT pravastatin, simvastatin
[f]Estradiol, progesterone, testosterone
[g]Aprepitant, fentanyl, ondansetron, thiotepa, zolpidem

Table 31.2 Drug interactions with busulfan (BU) (non-limitative list)[a]

Interacting drug	Proposed mechanism	Effect	Recommended action
Paracetamol	Competition for glutathione	Increased BU levels	– Avoid paracetamol within 72 h prior to or concurrently with BU – Monitor for increased BU concentrations/toxicity when used concurrently
Metronidazole	CYP3A4 inhibition Competition for glutathione		– Monitor for increased BU concentrations/toxicity when used concurrently
Itraconazole voriconazole	Unclear (probably CYP3A4 inhibition)		
Phenytoin	CYP3A4/glutathione-S-transferase induction	Decreased BU levels	– Use alternative antiepileptic (levetiracetam)

[a]Lexicomp® Drug interactions (2018) and Glotzbecker et al. (2012)

Its activity can be inhibited or induced by other drugs, resulting in increased or decreased bioavailability/clearance of PgP substrates (Ingelman-Sundberg and Rodriguez-Antona 2005; Thanacoody 2012).

Monoclonal Antibodies

Metabolism of monoclonal antibodies (MABs) does not involve CYP450 enzymes or drug transporters; therefore, PK interactions between MABs and conventional drugs are very limited. However, current information in this area is not abundant and more research is needed (Ferri et al. 2016).

31.1.3 Pharmaceutical Interactions

Pharmaceutical interactions manifest when two or more drugs and their diluents are mixed in the same infusion bag/syringe or when infusion lines meet at a Y-site junction. They are the result of incompatibilities as physicochemical reactions (changes in color, turbidimetry, and precipitation). Amphotericin B, for example, should not be diluted or mixed with physiological saline as microprecipitation will occur immediately.

31.2 Drug Interactions in HSCT Practice

Drug interactions can occur as early as during the conditioning regimen. Drugs as etoposide and thiotepa rely on CYP450 enzymes for metabolism, while cyclophosphamide needs to be converted to become functional. A non-limitative list of PK interactions with busulfan and recommendations for management are summarized in Table 31.2.

Many clinically relevant interactions have been reported with calcineurin inhibitors (cyclosporine and tacrolimus) and sirolimus. A non-limitative overview of PK interactions with these drugs is presented in Table 31.3.

31.3 Interactions with Herbal Drugs and Food

31.3.1 Herbal Drugs

The use of herbal drugs is growing worldwide, and a number of serious interactions with conventional drugs have been reported (Enioutina et al. 2017). Patients often do not perceive herbal supplements as drugs and prescribers are not always aware that patients are taking these products. A thorough drug history anamnesis is important and should be performed by asking very specific questions about herbal drug use.

An example of an herbal drug frequently involved in major drug interactions is St John's wort (SJW) (*Hypericum perforatum*). SJW is an over-the-counter product commonly used in HSCT patients for the treatment of mild depression. SJW can reduce the serum concentration of CYP3A4 substrates as cyclosporine and tacrolimus by induction of CYP3A4 or by increasing PgP expression, resulting in lack of response. Concomitant use of SJW with drugs metabolized by CYP3A4 should be avoided or monitored if no

Table 31.3 Pharmacokinetic interactions with cyclosporine (C), tacrolimus (T) and sirolimus (S) (non-limitative list)[a]

Interacting drug	Proposed mechanism	Effect	Recommended action
Anti-epileptics			
Carbamazepine Phenobarbital Phenytoin	CYP3A4 induction	– ▼ C/T/S level	• Monitor C/T/S levels • Increased C/T/S doses will likely be needed • Consider therapy modification (levetiracetam)
Antifungals			
Caspofungin	Unknown	– C: ▲ adverse/toxic effect of caspofungin – ▼ T/S levels	• Monitor liver function/hepatotoxicity in combination with C • Monitor T/S levels and adjust as necessary
Fluconazole Itraconazole Posaconazole Voriconazole	CYP3A4 and/or PgP inhibition	– ▲ C/T/S levels	• Monitor clinical response of C/T/S closely • Monitor C/T/S levels closely • Decreased C/T/S doses will likely be needed • Itraconazole: consider therapy modification (C/T/S) • Posaconazole/voriconazole: consider therapy modification (C/T), avoid combination (S)
Calcium channel blockers			
Diltiazem Verapamil	CYP3A4 inhibition	– ▲ C/T/S levels	• Monitor C/T/S levels • Decreased doses of C/T/S might be needed • Monitor for decreases in blood pressure (C) • Consider therapy modification (C)
Calcineurin inhibitors			
Cyclosporine	CYP3A4 competition	– T: ▲ levels/nephrotoxicity of C/T – S: ▲ levels of S (of specific concern with modified C)	• Discontinue C/T therapy at least 24 h prior to initiating therapy with the other agent • C/T: avoid combination • Monitor for toxic effects of S • S: ▲ risk of C-induced HUS/TTP/TMA • Administer oral doses of S 4 h after doses of C • C/S: consider therapy modification
Tacrolimus		– C: ▲ levels/nephrotoxicity of C/T – S: ▲ adverse/toxic effect of T/S, ▼ level of T	• Avoid combination with C/S (enhanced toxicity of C/T/S)
Corticosteroids	CYP3A4/PgP induction CYP3A4 substrate	– ▲/▼ C/T levels – ▲ corticosteroid levels	• Monitor for changes in C/T levels (likely initial increase, possibly decrease thereafter) and toxic effects of corticosteroids and/or C/T if used concomitantly
Macrolide antibiotics (not azithromycin)			
Clarithromycin Erythromycin	CYP3A4/PgP inhibition	– ▲ C/T/S levels – S: ▲ level of erythromycin	• Monitor C/T/S levels and adjust dose accordingly • Avoid concurrent use
Proton pump inhibitors (PPI, not pantoprazole)			
Omeprazole Lansoprazole	C: unclear T: CYP3A4/ CYP2C19 inhibition	– ▲ C/T level	• Monitor C/T levels closely when starting or stopping therapy with PPI and adjust dosage if necessary (T) • Inconsistent data (omeprazole), rabeprazole or pantoprazole: less likely to significantly interact

Table 31.3 (continued)

Interacting drug	Proposed mechanism	Effect	Recommended action
Statins			
Atorvastatin Simvastatin	CYP3A4 inhibition and inhibition of OATP1B1-mediated hepatic uptake	– C: ▲ level of atorvastatin/ simvastatin – T: limited effect	• Monitor for increased risk for statin-related toxicities (myopathy and rhabdomyolysis) • C: Avoid concurrent use atorvastatin / simvastatin • Consider changing to pravastatin or fluvastatin (less sensitive to this interaction) or alternative therapy • Warn patients to report any unexplained muscle pains or weakness • T: No action needed
Miscellaneous			
Grapefruit juice	CYP3A4 inhibition (intestinal)	– ▲ C/T/S levels (C/T: primarily limited to orally administered C/T)	• Monitor C/T/S levels • Avoid combination with C/S/T
Metronidazole	CYP3A4 inhibition	– ▲ C/T/S levels	• Monitor C/T/S levels
Mycophenolate mofetil (MMF)	Decreased enterohepatic recirculation	– C: ▲ glucuronide metabolite concentrations (associated with mycophenolate adverse effects) – MMF: ▼ C exposure in children – T: does not affect PK of mycophenolic acid (one study suggests ▲ T exposure)	• Monitor MMF dosing and response to therapy particularly closely when adjusting concurrent C (starting, stopping, or changing dose) or if changing from C to T/S
Rifampicin	CYP3A4/PgP induction	– ▼ C/T/S levels	• Monitor levels, increase dose C/T/S accordingly • Avoid combination if possible
St John's wort (SJW)	CYP3A4/PgP induction	– ▼ C/T/S levels	• Consider alternatives to SJW • If it cannot be avoided, monitor C/T/S levels

▼ = decreased; ▲ = increased
[a]Lexicomp® Drug Interactions (2018) and Glotzbecker et al. (2012)

alternative for SJW is available (Enioutina et al. 2017; Lexicomp® Drug Interactions 2018).

31.3.2 Food

Drug interactions with food and drinks are known to occur. Grapefruit juice is a potent inhibitor of intestinal CYP3A4, and many clinically relevant interactions have been reported (e.g., with simvastatin and calcineurin inhibitors). Cruciferous vegetables (Brussels sprouts, cabbage, and broccoli) contain substances that are inducers of CYP1A2 but do not appear to cause clinically important drug interactions (Thanacoody 2012).

31.4 Resources for Drug Interactions

Drug interactions in HSCT can be numerous. Whenever a potential clinically relevant drug interaction is recognized, a management plan should be recommended (modification in drug therapy or closer monitoring of efficacy and adverse reactions) (Tannenbaum and Sheehan 2014). A number of resources are available to help identifying and managing drug interactions (e.g., Lexicomp® Drug Interactions 2018; Clinical Pharmacology® 2018; Medicines Complete® 2018). Interpretation of interactions must be performed carefully to avoid the risk of over-alerting. The patient's clinical status, comorbidities, and severity of the drug interactions presented should always be taken into account.

31.5 Conclusion

Drug interactions can occur at all levels during HSCT. Attention to and management of interactions is crucial to prevent severe clinical consequences. Due to the complexity of the therapy and the risk of drug interactions, an active collaboration in a HSCT multidisciplinary team, including physicians, pharmacists, and nurses, is of paramount importance.

Key Points

- Drug interactions in HSCT are common and can occur at all levels
- Knowledge of mechanisms involved in drug metabolism might help in anticipating interactions
- A multidisciplinary approach is important to reduce the risk of drug interactions

References

Ahmed S, Zhou Z, Zhou J, Chen SQ. Pharmacogenomics of drug metabolizing enzymes and transporters: relevance to precision medicine. Genomics Proteomics Bioinformatics. 2016;14:298–313.

Clinical Pharmacology powered by ClinicalKey. Tampa: Elsevier. http://www.clinicalkey.com. Accessed 16 Jan 2018.

Enioutina EY, Salis ER, Job KM, Gubarev MI, Krepkova LV, Sherwin CM. Herbal Medicines: challenges in the modern world. Part 5. Status and current directions of complementary and alternative herbal medicine worldwide. Expert Rev Clin Pharmacol. 2017;10:327–38.

Ferri N, Bellosta S, Baldessin L, Boccia D, Racagni G, Corsini A. Pharmacokinetics interactions of monoclonal antibodies. Pharmacol Res. 2016;111:592–9.

Flockhart Table P450 Drug Interactions. Indiana University. http://medicine.iupui.edu/clinpharm/ddis/main-table/. Accessed 16 Jan 2018.

Gholaminezhad S, Hadjibabaie M, Gholami K, et al. Pattern and associated factors of potential drug-drug interactions in both pre- and early post-hematopoietic stem cell transplantation stages at a referral center in the Middle East. Ann Hematol. 2014;93:1913–22.

Glotzbecker B, Duncan C, Alyea E, Campbell B, Soiffer R. Important drug interactions in hematopoietic stem cell transplantation: what every physician should know. Biol Blood Marrow Transplant. 2012;18:989–1006.

Ingelman-Sundberg M, Rodriguez-Antona C. Pharmacogenetics of drug-metabolizing enzymes: implications for a safer and more effective drug therapy. Philos Trans R Soc Lond B Biol Sci. 2005;360:1563–70.

Larson AM. Drugs and the liver: metabolism and mechanisms of injury. UpToDate, Post TW (Ed), UpToDate, Waltham, MA. Accessed 16 Jan 2018.

Leather HL. Drug interactions in the hematopoietic stem cell transplant (HSCT) recipient: what every transplanter needs to know. Bone Marrow Transplant. 2004;33:137–52.

Lexicomp Drug Interactions. UpToDate, Post TW (Ed), UpToDate, Waltham, MA. Accessed 16 Jan 2018.

Lynch T, Price A. The effect of cytochrome P450 metabolism on drug response, interactions, and adverse effects. Am Fam Physician. 2007;76:391–6.

MedicinesComplete [online]. London: Pharmaceutical Press. http://www.medicinescomplete.com/. Accessed 16 Jan 2018.

Palleria C, Di Paolo A, Giofrè C, et al. Pharmacokinetic drug-drug interaction and their implication in clinical management. J Res Med Sci. 2013;18:601–10.

Tannenbaum C, Sheehan NL. Understanding and preventing drug-drug and drug-gene interactions. Expert Rev Clin Pharmacol. 2014;7:533–44.

Thanacoody HKR. Drug interactions. In: Walker R, Whittlesea C, editors. Clinical pharmacy and therapeutics. 5th ed. London: Elsevier; 2012.

Role of Nursing in HSCT

Aleksandra Babic and John Murray

32.1 Introduction: HSCT Nursing

With the progress of HSCT in the early 1960s, it became clear that nurses play a crucial role within the multidisciplinary team (MDT) caring for patients and their families undergoing this intense treatment. The distress during the time prior to undergoing HSCT, during isolation, in the recovery phase and the time after (long-term recovery) is not to be underestimated.

The best compliment towards nursing was made by Prof. Edward Donnall Thomas, the 1990 Nobel Prize winner in Medicine who stated that 'nurses and nursing are my secret weapon without whom I could not have achieved my goals' (Appelbaum 2013).

Continuity of care is vital to patient's right from their initial attendance in hospital. Nurses are an advocate throughout the transplant and often act as a motivating force, supporting and advising as well as supplying physical, psychological and emotional care whilst patient's transition from acute care to long-term follow-up clinics. Experienced nurses with high levels of technical competencies offer patients and families excellent care and support in this challenging area.

Patient preparation for HSCT involves the use of chemotherapy and/or radiotherapy to eradicate the underlying disease of the patient. Throughout the transplant procedure, the patient needs special care to overcome the complications associated with treatment. Nurses must be aware of the possible complications in order to play a role in prevention or early detection of alarming signs, such as sepsis, fluid overload and organ dysfunction, taking appropriate measures to minimize adverse effects and restore the clinical balance of the patient. This care is very complex and requires a high level of skill (Wallhut and Quinn 2017).

The field of nursing research in HSCT has evolved from reflecting on symptom management and service development to quality of life and long-term survival topics. The FACT-JACIE International Standards Accreditation requires that the clinical programme has access to personnel who are formally trained, experienced and competent in the management of patients receiving cellular therapy (JACIE 7th edition n.d.). Thus, it is important that training and competency programmes are structured and ongoing, with documented evidence of training topics and dates (Babic 2015).

A. Babic (✉)
IOSI-Istituto Oncologico della Svizzera Italiana, OSG, Bellinzona, Switzerland
e-mail: Aleksandra.Babic@eoc.ch

J. Murray
Haematology and Transplant Unit,
The Christie NHS Foundation Trust, Manchester, UK

32.2 Role of Nursing Throughout HSCT Patient Pathway

HSCT is a standard therapy in a number of malignant and non-malignant conditions.

Pre-transplant assessments must be undertaken, and the results of these along with suitable donor medical clearance and cell availability are essential to ascertain that transplant is a valid option and can proceed safely.

Nurses are pivotal in implementing practices to prevent and manage infections and other serious effects following HSCT (Sureda et al. 2015; Kenyon and Babic 2018) as:

- Bleeding risk caused by thrombocytopenia
- Tiredness and fatigue caused by the decreased haemoglobin levels and lasting effects of chemo-/radiotherapy and associated medications
- Pain due to mucositis
- Sepsis
- Reduced nutrition
- Psychosocial distress
- Isolation

32.2.1 The Role of the Transplant Coordinator (TC)

Many transplant coordinators are nurse specialists who focus their role on the individual needs of the patient and families; however, some centres have medical staff that organize transplants. TC is the person who should:

- Ensure that timely events occur for each patient and their families undergoing HSCT and that the patients are physically and psychologically prepared for the treatment.
- Provide a high level of care and management, inform and educate the patient, have holistic knowledge of the patient, participate in specific or advanced nursing practices (bone marrow sampling, HLA typing, transplant recipient care) and coordinate all the transplant logistics.

- Ensure that a suitable source of cells is available following the high-dose chemotherapy or immunosuppressive treatment that the patient will receive. Make requests to donor search panels, and order cells once the ideal match has been identified by the transplant physician.
- Support the patient with verbal and written information, and educate them about the whole process from typing to transplant. The TC will coordinate all of the care and embodies a clinical nursing function where emphasis is placed on specialization in a clearly defined area of care.
- Actively participate in the JACIE process of accreditation of transplant centres by writing and evaluating SOPs and being a valued member of the MDT and ward team offering teaching and advice.

32.3 Specific Aspects with a Prominent Role for Nurses

32.3.1 Venous Access Device (VAD)

Education and training should not be limited to the care and maintenance after insertion of the VAD but should be focused on well-being and patient safety. An algorithm for choosing the right VAD for the right patient should start with the diagnosis and treatment plan. The best VAD should be chosen based on the pH and osmolarity of the drugs used during the whole treatment period and the vein condition and should include the option for (partial) home infusion treatment.

Within the range of CVAD (central VAD), a peripherally inserted central catheter (PICC) is seen frequently in haematology patients, often as an alternative for a tunnelled CICC (centrally inserted central catheter) such as a Hickman catheter (see Chap. 22).

Nurses are responsible for the safe administration of drugs such as chemotherapy, IS immunosuppressive drugs and blood products as well as parenteral nutrition and symptom control drugs. The accurate handling and taking care of the central venous catheter and infusion pump systems are vital in the process because the catheter is related to the highest risk of infections. The use of an Aseptic Non Touch Technique (ANTT) (Pratt et al. 2007) and its ten principles of care have led to a decrease in catheter-related infections.

GAVeCeLT (*Gli Accessi Venosi Centrali a Lungo Termine*) (Pittiruti and Scoppettuolo 2017) has developed an algorithm for the choice of the most appropriate VAD, based on the best evidence available in the international guidelines, the bundle for the safe implantation of PICCs (see Table 32.1).

Table 32.1 The bundle for the safe implantation of PICCs[a]

The *goals* of the bundle are to minimize
1. Complications related to venipuncture: failure, repeated punctures, nerve injury, arterial injury
2. Malposition
3. Venous thrombosis
4. Dislocation
5. Infection

In order to reach the goal, *the SIP protocol* was developed and needs to be followed
1. Bilateral US scan of all veins at the arm and neck
2. Handwashing, aseptic technique and maximal barrier protection
3. Choice of the appropriate vein at the midarm (vein mm = or >cath Fr)
4. Clear identification of median nerve and brachial artery
5. Ultrasound-guided venipuncture
6. US tip navigation during introduction of the PICC
7. Electrocardiography method for assessing tip position
8. Securing the PICC with cyanoacrylate glue, sutureless devise and transparent dressing

Infections in PICCs to be close to zero if a bundle of *preventive measures* are taken[b]
- Site selection
- Skin disinfection with 2% chlorhexidine in 70% gluconate
- Hand hygiene
- Maximum barrier precautions
- Daily control on indication and on complications

[a]Pittiruti and Scoppettuolo (2017)
[b]Harnage (2012)

32.3.2 Early and Acute Complications

They occur following transplantation when the patient has reduced tolerance due to neutropenia and/or increased intestinal permeability. In neutropenia, the number of white blood cells decreases significantly, resulting in aplasia with an increased risk of infection. An increased permeability of the intestinal wall is caused by intensive chemotherapy damaging the gastrointestinal mucosa. As a result, pathogenic bacteria (bodily bacteria or bacteria from the diet) can enter the bloodstream and cause sepsis.

Early complications generally occur within 100 days post HSCT. In the early phase of HSCT, the main risk factors for infections are neutropenia-barrier breakdown due to mucositis, indwelling catheters, depressed T-cell and B-cell function and aGvHD.

Two of the most common early complications are oral mucositis and sepsis. Some other relatively rare complications are HC, ES, IPS and DAH. TAM and SOS/VOD are analysed in Chaps. 42, 49 and 50. For all complications there are locally agreed recommendations for prevention and principles for nursing care, with monitoring and prompt intervention that may have an influence on patients' morbidity and mortality.

32.3.2.1 Oral Mucositis (OM)

Oral mucositis (OM) has been defined (Rubenstein et al. 2004) as the inflammation of the mucosal membrane, characterized by ulceration, which may result in pain, swallowing difficulties and impairment of the ability to talk. The mucosal injury caused by OM provides an opportunity for infection to flourish and in particular putting the severely immunocompromised patient in the HSCT setting at risk of sepsis and septicaemia.

OM and oral problems in the HSCT setting can be expected to occur in as many as 68% of patients undergoing autologous HSCT and 98% of patients undergoing allogeneic HSCT (EORTC Guidelines). With the increasing use of targeted drug therapies and approaches in the cancer and haematology setting, problems in the oral cavity will increase and become even more of a challenge (Quinn et al. 2015).

All treatment strategies aimed at improving mouth care are dependent on four key principles: accurate assessment of the oral cavity, individualized plan of care, initiating timely preventative measures and correct treatment (Quinn et al. 2008). The assessment process should begin prior to HSCT by identifying all the patient risks most likely to increase oral damage.

The choice of prevention regimens should be guided by evidence based on expert opinion interventions, working with the patient to reduce their potential risk of oral mucositis occurring.

All treatment plans should be based upon the grading of oral damage and patient reports, and these may include the use of topical analgesics and the use of opiates (Elad et al. 2015).

32.3.2.2 Sepsis

Sepsis is a life-threatening condition caused by aberrant and dysregulated host response to infection (Elad et al. 2015). The most important action to prevent infections acquired by exogenous organisms is good hand hygiene performed correctly (Hand Hygiene Guidelines). Appropriate clean work clothes, with short sleeves, no jewellery and no neck tie are the responsibility of all staff. Protective isolation during the neutropenic phase is recommended, and the patient should not be in contact with any staff or visitors with symptoms of infection. For prevention of endogenous infections, oral hygiene and skin care to maintain the mucosal and skin barrier and use of prophylactic antibiotics are the most important actions. Correct handling of any indwelling catheters is also a key nursing responsibility in infection control.

Other areas where infections can be prevented are air and water quality, food hygiene and environmental cleaning. Environmental cleaning includes medical equipment as well.

Early recognition and treatment are vital for a successful outcome of sepsis. Temperature, pulse, blood pressure, respirations and saturation (vital signs) should be frequently monitored.

Signs of infection are not always obvious, but if the patient has a temperature ≥38.0 °C, cultures should be taken, IV antibiotics and IV fluids started or increased and oxygen therapy initiated.

The goal is always to *start antibiotic treatment within 1 h* from detection of fever and is the most critical period in the patient's survival from sepsis. Early recognition and intervention are achieved by frequent monitoring of the patient's vital signs and general condition and paying attention to subtle changes that should be promptly reported, such as mental state alteration or mottled skin.

Alert for immediate action are when a previously well patient only responds to pain or becomes unresponsive, becomes confused and has a systolic blood pressure of <90 mmHg or a fall of >40 mmHg from baseline; an elevated heart rate >130 bpm; a respiratory rate of >25 per min, requiring oxygen to maintain saturations >92%; a non-blanching rash or mottled, ashen or cyanotic skin, not passed urine in the last 18 h; an output of <0.5 ml/kg/h; a lactate of >2 mmol/l; or received recent chemotherapy.

Immediate action is required at the first indication of sepsis. The concept of *the sepsis six and the severe sepsis resuscitation bundle* (Daniels et al. 2011) has been developed as a guide to prioritize interventions in patients where sepsis is suspected:

1. Oxygen therapy aims to keep saturations >94% (88–92% if at risk of CO_2 retention, e.g. COPD).
2. Blood cultures, at least a peripheral set, consider CSF, urine, sputum, chest X-ray and urinalysis.
3. IV antibiotics, according to hospital policy, consider allergies prior to administration.
4. Fluid resuscitation, if hypotensive or lactate >2 mmol/l, 500 ml bolus stat, may be repeated if clinically indicated. Do not exceed 30 ml/kg.
5. Serial serum lactates corroborate high VBG lactate with arterial sample. If lactate >4 mmol/l, call critical care for support. Recheck after each 10 ml/kg challenge.

6. Assess urine output which may require catheterization, and ensure fluid balance chart commenced and completed hourly.

When treatment has been initiated, the patient must be continually monitored to determine the effect of treatment or worsening of the condition. This includes vital signs, fluid balance including weight and assessment of identified and/or potential infection sites (mouth, skin, all indwelling catheters, urine, stools, etc.), mental status, signs of bleeding, pain and general appearance and well-being.

Antibiotics should be delivered with strict adherence to the prescribed time schedule. Antipyretic agents should be avoided since they may mask fever but may under certain circumstances be used to alleviate patient discomfort and pain.

32.3.2.3 Pain

Pain in the HSCT setting is most commonly experienced as a result of mucositis, but patients will also report other pain such as bone pain associated with G-CSF, abdominal pain due to diarrhoea or general discomfort with fluid accumulation. A comprehensive evaluation of the pain, location, characteristics, onset, duration, frequency and severity, exacerbating and relieving factors, should be included. This assessment should be supported by the patient's non-verbal reactions such as facial expression, pallor, tempo of speech, body position, etc. as well as their vital signs.

32.3.2.4 GvHD

GvHD remains a leading cause of non-relapse mortality and is associated with a high morbidity that increasingly affects quality of life (Lee et al. 2003; Dignan 2012). Nursing care of patients with GvHD is highly complex and extremely stressful especially in the acute setting in patients with grades 3–4 skin and GI involvement (Table 32.2). Supportive nursing care to complement medical interventions aims to offer symptomatic comfort and relief.

There are many manifestations of GvHD, and nurses are able to advise patients with respect to many of these including eye, mouth and genital care. Further readings: GvHD chapter in the

Table 32.2 Nursing care of patients with skin and gastrointestinal GvHD

Skin care
1. Maintain integrity of the skin; regular application of cream, ointment or gel; patient choice of vehicle
2. Emollient application, high or low water content to be considered, QV, hydromol or diprobase
3. At least 30-min gap between emollient and steroid cream applications
4. Topical steroids, strength decided by site and length of treatment
5. Menthol cream for painful and pruritic skin, cooling effect
6. Use high-factor sunscreen SPF 50+
7. Always apply creams to make the skin appear shiny; adult body will require 500 g per week
8. Apply in one direction, direction of hair growth, do not scrub on
9. Medical grade silk clothing
10. Good fluid intake and nutrition
11. Organic coconut oil or other natural lipids
12. Aloe vera gels; do not use alone as they will dry the skin

Gastrointestinal
1. Ensure stool samples are taken to exclude infection
2. Adequate oral intake with strict fluid balance
3. Small and frequent high-calorie food and drinks
4. Antiemetics
5. Loperamide, codeine and octreotide may be used to stem diarrhoea
6. Rest bowel and use parenteral feeding
7. Consider the use of radiologically inserted gastrostomy (RIG) feeding
8. Flexi-seal faecal collection device

EBMT Textbook for nurses 2018 (Kenyon and Babic 2018).

32.3.3 Long-Term Complications and Side Effects Post Allo-HCST

Long-term side effects after allo-HSCT include non-malignant organ or tissue dysfunction, changes in quality of life, infections related to abnormal immune reconstitution and secondary cancers. Many of these can be attributed to effects of chronic graft-versus-host disease (Dignan 2012; Bhatia 2011; Mohty and Mohty 2011). With advances achieved in terms of supportive care, it is reasonable to expect outcomes to improve steadily, and consequently increasing numbers of transplant survivors will be facing life after the initial transplant experience. For some survivors the burden of long-term morbidity is substantial, and long-term follow-up of patients who received allo-HSCT is now widely recommended.

Key Points

- Specific technical care activities require nursing knowledge and specific skills in the field of HSCT such as instrument manipulation, knowledge of technologies and the use of special protocols to effectively intervene in complex situations and deal with acute and chronic HSCT complications.
- As patients become more complex, so does the care that they require.
- It is essential that nursing adapts to these challenges and improves in both the quality and expertise that is vital to improve patient survival and overall experience of this life-changing treatment.
- The predominant role for nurses is focused to vascular access device, oral mucositis and other early complications as HC, ES, IPS and DAH. TAM and SOS/VOD, sepsis, pain, GVHD and several late complications.

References

Appelbaum FR. 2013. http://www.hematology.org/Thehematologist/Profiles/1088.aspx.

Babic A. Transplant unit personnel competency maintenance: online testing by sharepoint application. EBMT 2015. Oral presentation N003.

Bhatia S. Long-term health impacts of hematopoietic stem cell transplantation inform recommendations for follow-up. 2011. https://www.ncbi.nlm.nih.gov/pmc/articles/PMC3163085/.

Daniels R, Nutbeam T, McNamara G, Galvin C. The sepsis six and the severe sepsis resuscitation bundle: a prospective observational cohort study. Emerg Med J. 2011;28:507–12.

Dignan FL, Amrolia P, Clark A, Haemato-oncology Task Force of British Committee for Standards in Haematology, British Society for Blood and Marrow Transplantation, et al. Diagnosis and management of chronic graft-versus-host disease. Br J Haematol. 2012;158:46–61.

Elad S, Raber-Durlacher JE, Brennan MT, et al. Basic oral care for hematology-oncology patients and hematopoietic stem cell transplantation recipients: a position paper from the joint task force of the Multinational Association of Supportive Care in Cancer/International Society of Oral Oncology (MASCC/ISOO) and the European Society for Blood and Marrow Transplantation (EBMT). Support Care Cancer. 2015;23:223–36.

Harnage S. Seven years of zero central-line-associated bloodstream infections. Br J Nurs. 2012;21:S6, S8, S10-2.

JACIE 7th Edition Standards. www.Jacie.org.

Kenyon M, Babic A. European blood and marrow transplantation textbook for nurses. Cham: Springer; 2018. isbn:978-3-319-50025-6.

Lee SJ, Vogelsang G, Flowers MED. Chronic graft-versus-host disease. Biol Blood Marrow Transplant. 2003;9:215–33.

Mohty B, Mohty M. Long-term complications and side effects after allogeneic hematopoietic stem cell transplantation: an update. Blood Cancer J. 2011;1:e16.

Pittiruti M, Scoppettuolo G. The GAVeVeLT manual of PICC and midline, indications, insertion, management. St. Paul: Edra; 2017.

Pratt RJ, Pellowe CM, Wilson JA, et al. National evidence-based guidelines for preventing healthcare-associated infections in NHS hospitals in England. J Hosp Infect. 2007;65(Suppl 1):S1–64.

Quinn B, Potting C, Stone R, et al. Guidelines for the assessment of oral mucositis in adult chemotherapy, radiotherapy and haematopoietic stem cell transplant patients. Eur J Cancer. 2008;44:61–72.

Quinn B, Thompson M, Treleaven J, et al. United Kingdom oral care in cancer guidance. 2nd ed. 2015. www.ukomic.co.uk. Accessed 03 Sep 2016.

Rubenstein EB, Peterson DE, Schubert M, Mucositis Study Section of the Multinational Association for Supportive Care in Cancer, International Society for Oral Oncology, et al. Clinical practice guidelines for the prevention and treatment of cancer therapy-induced oral and gastrointestinal mucositis. Cancer. 2004;100(Suppl 9):2026–46.

Sureda A, Bader P, Cesaro S, et al. Indications for allo- and auto-SCT for haematological diseases, solid tumours and immune disorders: current practice in Europe, 2015. Bone Marrow Transplant. 2015;50: 1037–56.

Wallhut E, Quinn B. Early and acute complications and the principles of HSCT nursing care. In: Wallhult E, Quinn B, Kenyon M, Babic A, editors. The European blood and marrow transplantation textbook for nurses. 2017. https://doi.org/10.1007/978-3-319-50026-3_9.

Ethical Issues in HSCT

Khaled El-Ghariani and Jean-Hugues Dalle

33.1 Introduction

Ethics is a branch of philosophy, and, like mathematics, moral philosophy does not give ready-made answers to questions but teaches how one could systematically analyse and resolve a problem. Philosophy's main tool, to achieve this, is logic, where accurate premises are linked together to support a conclusion within a sound and valid ethical argument (West 2009). This chapter aims to explain this process using examples from blood and marrow transplantation practices.

Ethical discourse requires a theory of ethics (Thompson 2005). One requires a landmark to understand their ethical position. One needs to know on what basis one can decide if an action is wrong or right, bad or good; a theory of ethics should help this. It will also allow better understanding of common threats to ethics such as appealing to religion, using relativism to justify accepting different truths to different situations or explaining that ethical stands are unreasonably demanding (Blackburn 2001).

The most known ethical theories are Kant's deontological theory and Bentham and Mill's utilitarianism (Vardy and Grosch 1999). Kant argued for our duty to pursue a set of intrinsically ethical rules that can be universally applied. Ethics is the search for such rules. On the other hand, utilitarianism argues that an action or a rule is moral if their outcomes bring the greatest pleasure and happiness to the greatest numbers of people. No doubt, these theories would ignite an interesting discussion on transplant ethics but may not provide clear enough guidance to health care practitioners to help tackle the dilemmas that they regularly encounter.

During the last four decades, Beauchamp and Childress (2013) defended, and significantly developed, the four principles ethical theory for healthcare profession. These principles include:

1. Respect for autonomy: respecting the decision-making capacity of autonomous persons
2. Non-maleficence: avoiding the causation of harm
3. Beneficence: providing benefits as well as balancing such benefits against risks and cost
4. Justice: distributing benefits, risks and costs fairly.

According to Beauchamp and Childress (2013)

K. El-Ghariani (✉)
Department of Hematology, Sheffield Teaching Hospitals Trust and NHSBT, The University of Sheffield, Sheffield, UK
e-mail: Khaled.el-ghariani@nhsbt.nhs.uk

J.-H. Dalle
Department of Pediatric Hematology-Immunology, Hospital Robert-Debré, Assistance Publique-Hôpitaux de Paris, Paris Diderot University, Paris, France

Beneficence is the primary goal of medicine and healthcare, whereas respect for autonomy, along with non-maleficence and justice, sets the moral limits on the professional's actions in pursuit of this goal.

Ethical obligations towards patients (and sometimes their relatives) are well known to healthcare professionals. In the field of transplantation, management of donors adds another dimension to the ethical complexity. Two more areas of work are morally challenging, and although less well argued for, they are critical and have wide implications: firstly, the moral obligations of professionals to engage with fund holders, commissioners and insurers to ensure fair funding of service and, secondly, the ethical role of experts in the management, reporting and publishing of data and information to ensure accurate practice evidence to inform decision-making. Ethical practice requires one to apply the above four principles to all field of work, every time an ethical issue is raised. Transplantation practice is full with issues that can raise serious and sometimes disturbing ethical concerns. The following is a discussion of some aspects of the ethical implications of high-risk treatment, lack of enough funding for healthcare and issues with donor care.

33.2   Ethical Challenges of High-Risk Treatment

Blood and marrow transplantation is mostly used to treat life-threatening illnesses, but also it carries serious complications that are themselves life threatening. Resistance disease or a recipient with significant comorbidities can make transplant risks too high and brings risks of futility to the equation. Although guidelines and outcomes data are available in the literature, the application of such evidence may require the support of colleagues or other experts within a multidisciplinary team. This should help in striking the desirable balance between expected benefits and possible harm (the beneficence and the non-maleficence principles). Although risks may be too high, one

ought to ask 'is it the best option available for that particular patient with that particular disease?' (Snyder 2016). Moreover, the implications of undertaking a transplant procedure with limited benefits on resources and other patients ought to be considered. The limitation of transplant rooms, for example, may explain how a decision to transplant a particular patient could affect another.

A transplant procedure that carries only 10–20% chance of success can be a source of worry to staff as it brings the beneficence/non-maleficence balance to a critical point. However, the other two ethical principles may help. What the patient wants to do? And will such a transplant jeopardise other patients care or face funding rejection? Obviously for a keen patient and supportive healthcare payers, the decision is less problematic. The balance of forces may be different in another situation with the same clinical ground. This brings uncomfortable variations into practice which can only be minimised by the development of constructive ethical discourse.

An unbiased list of options ought to be discussed with the patient (and possibly with their relatives and even healthcare payers). To obtain an autonomous consent, staff have to ensure that the patient has fully understood all options and has made a choice that is not influenced by any coercive factors. Obtaining such a valid consent requires arrangements and it will take some time and effort. This, however, not only meets our moral obligations but also has practical benefits, as a well-consented patient is likely to cooperate with the demand of treatment and work with staff to fight complications. Respect of autonomy dictates that patients are well informed about decisions that they make, and it also dictates that staff accept such decisions even if decisions sound counterintuitive. A self-funding patient who refuses life-saving transplant to save the money for their young children may pose difficult and very uncomfortable challenges to staff. This patient can be helped through exploring charitable funds for their treatment, but ignoring their autonomous decisions is not an ethical option.

33.3 Engagement with Funding Issues as a Professional Moral Obligation

Establishing funding rules for transplantation treatment has been, on many occasions, considered the job of healthcare payers or insurers. Medical staff are involved in setting up guidelines, publishing data on outcomes and advising in some complex cases. However, an ethical assessment of the issue will put medical staff in the centre of decision-making. After all, healthcare payers and insurers will base all their decisions not only on medical information but also on the interpretation of such information as provided by medical staff. It is prudent to think that it is unethical that medical staff do not engage actively in this process. The same ethical desire that drives staff to treat illness and complications ought to drive their engagement in mending funding practices that do not meet patients' needs, as both issues are detrimental to patients' outcomes.

The respect to autonomy principle dictates involvement of patients' representatives in funding decisions. Most healthcare services have such an arrangement, and the job of the medical staff is to educate representatives to be able to make valid and informed decisions. The principle of beneficent, in this setting, can be applied by gathering, analysing and publishing good data to support funding decisions. Whilst publishing papers may have been considered as an option for academic progression, it seems that it has become an ethical obligation. Nonmaleficence means that delays in introducing new development in the field must be avoided. Transplant field is rapidly changing (for the better), and such delays could devote patients from a helpful treatment modality that could make a difference to them. The principle of justice is in the heart of healthcare funding. However, this ought to not mean 'sticking to the rule'. Most rules have legitimate exceptions and the job of the transplant physician to fight the corner of the patients in this regard. Some healthcare services support cord transplant but not the use of double cord, because of cost implications. This would disadvantage many adult patients with body weight that is too high for a cord blood unit to support. The desire to establish an ethical process of funding may have led the English National Healthcare Service to establish Clinical Reference Groups, including one for transplantation. This group is composed of a medical chair, eight other transplant physicians and three members to represent patient and public voice (NHS England 2018). Medical ethics is mainly seen as a direct issue between a professional and a patient. This discussion showed the ethical obligations of professionals outside the clinic and the hospital ward. This is obviously demanding but also more helpful to patients.

33.4 The Ethical Issues in Donor Management

Transplant donation is a fertile subject for ethical debate as all types of donation carry some moral concerns. These are mainly around respect of donor autonomy, risk of exploitation or possible harm to donor. Unrelated donors are supported by professionals other than staff who look after the recipient, and this is according to national and international guidance. Unrelated donations have some financial and reputational benefits to the donor registries. However, given existing professionalism and code of practice, this has rarely raised concerns. On the other hand, family donors receive less structured protection. The recent success in haploidentical transplantation means that more family donors will be involved, and so ethical grounds of such process needs to be established.

Whilst the balance of risks and benefits of most types of treatment offered to a particular patient can be established, a major dilemma in donor ethics is the fact that assessing harm and inconvenience to one person (the donor) in relation to expected benefits to another (the recipient) is highly problematic. Staff occasionally make the decision themselves and argue that some temporary aches and pains and minimal risks of ruptured spleen (G-CSF side effects) are acceptable risks to justify a life-saving donation, particularly to a family member. Staff position makes 'some sense', but it does not respect donor autonomy, and so it cannot be accepted as a universal rule that could be practiced widely, i.e. it lacks ethical grounds.

Child donors, pregnancies conceived for HCT and donation from a family member who lack capacity have been debated. Minor sibling donors require particular consideration as their autonomy is harder to prove. There is evidence that a child donor is subjected to both physical and psychological implications. This prompted (the) American Academy of Pediatrics Committee on Bioethics to recommend that five conditions are met to ensure morally justified donations from children (AAP 2010). These include lack of suitable adult donor, the expected benefit to recipient is reasonably high, strong relationship between donor and recipient, potential physical and psychological harms to donor must be minimised and, finally, obtaining parents' consent and child assent. Child assent and agreement are hard to confirm, and the availability of independent committee or assessor to look after such donors has been recommended.

Moreover, a family donation from an adult with full capacity can be morally challenging for two reasons. Firstly, not all family members want to donate. Some of them find the process too demanding, and if they were 'given the choice', they will rather not. The story of one such donor was in the news. A newspaper (the Daily Mail, UK) reported the situation using the following headline: 'Sentenced to die by my sister, leukemia victim refused her only chance of transplant' (Oldfield 1997). The sister refused to donate bone marrow because of the phobia of hospitals. The subsequent media debate led the donor to reconsider her position. This is a moral position that is hard to defend. Secondly, the health risks to family donors are not minimum or negligible. They are more likely to encounter significant complications than unrelated donors (Halter et al. 2009). Documented experience from unrelated donations cannot be used to advise family donors, and the comparison between harm to donor and benefit to recipient is even harder in the family donor situation. Many authors (van Walraven et al. 2010; Brand et al. 2011) attempted to raise awareness of these issues, and many argued that a system that is separate to and not influenced by patient care ought to be in place to manage family donors.

Transplantation, like other healthcare practices, requires an accurate balance between expected benefits and possible harm as well as valid patient consent. Given limited resources, the implication of one transplant on another ought to be considered. Given the life-saving and life-threatening nature of this modality of treatment, ethical issues with transplantation are likely to be challenging. Staff are expected to let patients decided for themselves. Moreover, staff ought to escalate complex issues to the legal system or more commonly to the ethics committee within their institution. In the European Union, Directive 2001/20/EC established ethics committees as an independent body to agree complex ethical challenges.

Key Points
- Clinical ethics teaches skills to tackle moral dilemmas but does not provide ready-made answers.
- Clinical ethics now extends, beyond patient clinician relationship, to donor care as well as engagement with fund holders and insurers.
- The four principles ethical theory (autonomy, beneficent, non-maleficence and justices) provides reasonable basis for moral assessment of ethical issues in most fields of practice.
- The donation process requires ethical vigilance. Family donors have high health risks and, given the potential social pressure, are not always autonomous.

References

American Academy of Pediatrics. Policy statement, children as hematopoietic stem cell donors. 2010. http://pediatrics.aappublications.org/content/pediatrics/125/2/392.full.pdf.

Beauchamp TL, Childress JF. Principles of biomedical ethics. 7th ed. Oxford: Oxford University Press; 2013.

Blackburn S. Being good a short introduction to ethics. Oxford: Oxford University Press; 2001.

Brand A, et al. Uniform examination of stem cell donors. ISBT Sci Ser. 2011;6:160–4.

Halter J, Kodera Y, Ispizua AU, et al. Severe events in donors after allogeneic hematopoietic stem cell donation. Haematologica. 2009;94:94–101.

NHS England. NHS commissioning, Specialised, F01. Blood and Marrow Transplantation. 2018. https://www.england.nhs.uk/commissioning/spec-services/npc-crg/blood-and-infection-group-f/f01/.

Oldfield S. Sentenced to die by my sister. Daily Mail. 1997;1:5.

Snyder DS. Ethical issues in haematopoietic cell transplantation. In: Forman SJ, et al., editors. Thomas' hematopoietic cell transplantation. Chichester: Wiley Blackwell; 2016.

Thompson M. Ethical theory. 2nd ed. Coventry: Hodder Murray; 2005.

Vardy P, Grosch P. The puzzle of ethics. London: Fount; 1999.

van Walraven SM, Nicoloso-de Faveri G, Axdorph-Hygell UAI, et al. Family donor care management: principles and recommendations. Bone Marrow Transplant. 2010;45:1269–73.

West AA. Rulebook for arguments. 4th ed. Indianapolis: Hackett Publishing; 2009.

Quality of Life Assessment After HSCT for Pediatric and Adults

Anna Barata and Heather Jim

34.1 Introduction

Methodological advances in the HCT field have increased the population of survivors worldwide. However, HCT is associated with significant morbidity that impairs survivors' recovery and adversely affects their QoL. A significant body of literature has addressed QoL after HCT and highlights significant deficiencies in physical, psychological, social, and role functioning both in adult and pediatric survivors (Pidala et al. 2010). These data are clinically relevant as they help to understand the impact of HCT on patient's lives. Clinically, assessment of QoL can inform patient education and be used to evaluate the benefit of supportive care interventions.

34.2 QoL Assessment

QoL can be considered a patient-reported outcome (PRO). PROs are defined by the US Food

A. Barata (✉)
Department of Hematology, Hospital de la Santa Creu i Sant Pau, Universitat Autònoma de Barcelona, Barcelona, Spain

José Carreras Leukemia Research Institute, Barcelona, Spain
e-mail: ABarata@santpau.cat

H. Jim
Department of Health Outcomes and Behavior, Moffitt Cancer Center, Tampa, FL, USA

and Drug Administration (FDA) as the "measurement of any aspect of a patient's health status that comes directly from the patient, without the interpretation of the patient's response by a clinician or anyone else" (US Food and Drug Administration 2009). Thus, PROs specifically describe the impact that HCT has on patients' lives and provide information unavailable from other sources (Kurosawa et al. 2017; Russell et al. 2006). PROs are also used in pediatric populations, although parents or other proxies might be used as source of information when children are unable to report their own QoL. However, the use of patients' own reports is clearly recommended because significant discrepancies are found when comparing patients' self-reported QoL to reports of physicians, parents, or other proxies (Kurosawa et al. 2017; Russell et al. 2006). In general, measures to assess patient- and proxy-reported QoL are questionnaires.

These instruments can be broadly categorized as general or disease- or procedure-specific. General measures assess QoL of the general population and can also be administered to specific populations, such as HCT recipients. These questionnaires allow comparisons of QoL across populations, such as between HCT survivors and individuals without cancer. In contrast, disease- and procedure-specific instruments examine specific aspects of the health conditions assessed. These measures capture specific PROs that are likely to be important to patients.

34.3 Measures to Assess QoL in Adults and Pediatric Patients Undergoing HCT

There are numerous measures assessing QoL on adults and pediatric HCT recipients. Measures used have been both general and disease-specific. The following sections list some of the most common used questionnaires in the field of HCT.

34.3.1 Adults

Interest in assessing QoL in adult HCT recipients is reflected in the variety of measures used to assess this outcome. However, there is a need for the scientific community to reach consensus about which questionnaires to use in order to facilitate comparison across studies (Shaw et al. 2016). Table 34.1 summarizes alphabetically some of the most common questionnaires to assess QoL in adults.

Table 34.1 QoL questionnaires assessing QoL in adult HCT survivors

(a) General	
European Quality of Life- 5 Dimensions (EQ-5D-5L) (van Reenen and Jansen 2015)	
Aim	Health status
Items	6
Domains/subscales	Mobility, self-care, usual activities, pain, anxiety, depression
Results	Profile of each of the domains assessed, and an index of the health status. Higher scores indicate better health status
Translations	Available in more than 130 languages
Medical Outcomes Study-Short Form (MOS SF-36) (Ware et al. 1994)	
Aim	QoL
Items	36; shorter versions feature 12 items (SF-12) or 8 items (SF-8)
Domains/subscales	General health, physical, role, emotional and social functioning, mental health, pain, vitality
Results	Physical Component Score; Mental Component Score and Global Score. Higher scores indicate better QoL
Translations	Available in more than 170 languages
Patient-Reported Outcomes Measurement Information System (PROMIS) (Cella et al. 2010)	
Aim	Mental, physical, and social health and QoL in healthy populations as well as those with chronic conditions
Items	Multi-item measures varying in length and complexity; for example, PROMIS-29 has 29 items, PROMIS-43 has 43 items, PROMIS-57 has 57 items
Domains/subscales	Each subscale measures a single domain; PROMIS Profile measures assess multiple domain
Results	Higher scores indicate more of the concept being measured. Measures use standardized T-score metric against normative data for the US population
Translations	Available in Spanish and several other languages
(b) Cancer and HCT specific	
European Organization for Research and Treatment of Cancer QoL Questionnaire Core 30 (EORTC QLQ-C30) version 3.0 (Aaronson et al. 1993)	
Aim	QoL in cancer
Items	30 items
Domains/subscales	Functional scales, symptom scale and a QoL scale
Results	Higher scores in functional and QoL scales indicate better wellbeing. Higher scores in the symptom scale indicate worse symptomatology
Translations	Available in more than 100 languages

Table 34.1 (continued)

Functional Assessment of Cancer Therapy—Bone Marrow Transplant (FACT-BMT) (McQuellon et al. 1997)

Aim	QoL in HCT
Items	47
Domains/subscales	Consists of the FACT-G (Cella et al. 1993) and the BMT concerns subscale
Results	Higher scores indicate better QoL
Translations	Available in more than 38 languages

Functional Assessment of Cancer Therapy—General Scale (FACT-G) (Cella et al. 1993)

Aim	QoL in cancer
Items	33
Domains/subscales	Physical, functional, social and emotional well-being
Results	Higher scores indicate better wellbeing and global QoL
Translations	Available in more than 60 languages

34.3.2 Pediatrics

There is less research on QoL on pediatric patients than adult patients. Initial pediatric studies focused on a single aspect of functioning, such as psychosocial and physical limitations. It was not until the early 1990s that pediatric QoL began to be addressed as a multidimensional construct. Most of the measures used in pediatric studies were originally developed to be used in the general population or in children with specific illnesses. Table 34.2 lists alphabetically the most common measures used to assess QoL in pediatric population.

34.4 Challenges when implementing QoL assessment

Improvement in patients' QoL is included among the strategic goals of major cancer organizations such as the American Society of Clinical Oncology and regulatory agencies such as the FDA and the European Medicines Agency. Recognition of the importance of the patient experience is reflected in the increasing incorporation of patient-reported QoL measures in observational research and clinical trials. However,

some aspects should be considered when implementing patient-reported QoL measures.

Historically, studies and clinical trials performed in the USA have often used the FACT instruments, whereas studies performed in Europe have chosen the EORTC. This divergence makes results difficult to compare (Shaw et al. 2016), although efforts are underway to map common QoL measures such as the EORTC QLQ-C30 and FACT-G to one another (Young et al. 2015). Second, the mode of administration should also be considered. PRO measures have traditionally been administered by paper and pencil, but new technologies offer the potential to use electronic measures. Electronic measures administered before or during a clinic visit allow results to be available at the time of consultation and may facilitate symptom monitoring to guide supportive treatment. One example is the PROMIS instrument, which is available using computer adaptive testing or through REDCap software. Computer adaptive testing selects questions based on the previous responses that patients have provided to approximate the construct being measured in the fewest number of questions. The implementation of routine assessment of patients' QoL on clinical care and clinical trials has the potential to improve patients' well-being.

Table 34.2 QoL questionnaires assessing QoL in pediatric HCT survivors

(a) General	
Child Health Questionnaire (CHQ) (Landgraf et al. 1996)	
Aim	QoL
Versions	Parent-reported versions feature 50 items (CHQ-PF50) or 28 items (CHQ-PF28) and are intended for parents of children aged 5–18 years. The child-report version (CHQ-87) has 87 items and is appropriate for children aged 10–18
Domains/subscales	Global health, physical functioning, role/social-physical functioning, bodily pain/discomfort, role/social-emotional functioning, role/social -behavior, parental impact -time, parental impact -emotional, self-esteem, mental health, global behavior, family activities, family cohesion, and changes in health
Results	Higher scores indicate higher physical and psychosocial wellbeing
Translations	The CHQ-PF50 and CHQ-PF28 are available in more than 80 languages, and the CHQ-87 to 34
Patient-Reported Outcomes Measurement Information System (PROMIS) (Hinds et al. 2013)	
Aim	Health and QoL in healthy populations as well as those with chronic conditions
Versions	Multi-item measures varying in length and complexity: PROMIS-25 has 25 items, PROMIS-37 37 items, and PROMIS-49 49 items. PROMIS measures are child- and parent-reported. Child-report measures are intended for children aged 8–17, and parent-report for children 5–17
Domains/subscales	Physical, mental and social health, and a global QoL score
Results	Higher scores indicate more of the concept being measured. PROMIS use standardized T-score metric against normative data for the US population
Translations	Children and proxy measures are available in Spanish and in several other languages
Pediatric Quality of Life Inventory (PedsQL™) 4.0 Generic Score Scales (Varni et al. 2001)	
Aim	QoL in healthy children or those diagnosed with an acute or chronic disease
Versions	Parent-report form for children aged 2–4 has 21 items, and child and parent reports for children aged 5–18 have 23 items
Domains/subscales	Physical, emotional, social, and school functioning
Results	Physical health summary score; Psychosocial health summary score; Total score. Higher scores indicate better QoL
Translations	Available in more than 70 languages
(b) Cancer and HCT specific	
Child Health Rating Inventories (CHRIs)-and Disease-Specific Impairment Inventory-Hematopoietic Stem Cell Transplantation (DSII-HCT) (Parsons 2005)	
Aim	The disease specific (DSII-HCT) module assesses QoL of childhood HCT survivors
Versions	10-item module intended to child-report (aged 5–12), adolescent-report (13–18) and parents-report (5–18)
Domains/subscales	Items are grouped in three domains reported by parents and patients to be most salient to the HCT experience: worry, hassless, and body image
Results	Higher scores indicate better QoL
Translations	The questionnaire is available in English
Peds Quality of Life Cancer Module 3.0 (PedsQL CM™) (Varni et al. 2002)	
Aim	QoL in children with cancer
Versions	Parent-report form for children aged 2–4 has 25 items, child and parent reports for children aged 5–7 has 26 items, and child and parents reports for children more than 8 years has 27 items
Domains/subscales	Pain and hurt, nausea, procedural anxiety, treatment anxiety, worry, cognitive problems, perceived physical appearance and communication
Results	Higher scores indicate better QoL
Translations	Available in more than 100 languages
The Behavioral, Affective and Somatic Experiences Scales (BASES) (Phipps et al. 1994)	
Aim	QoL during the acute phase of HCT
Versions	There are separate versions to be completed by nurses (BASES-N), parents (BASES-P) and children (BASES-C). The BASES-N and BASES-P have 38 items and the BASES-C has 14 items. The questionnaire is intended to be used in child aged 5–17
Domains/subscales	Somatic distress, mood disturbance, compliance, quality of interactions and activities
Results	Higher scores indicate more distress/impairment
Translations	Available in English

Key Points

- Assessing HCT survivors' QoL is essential in order to know the impact that the HCT, its morbidity, its treatments, and related interventions have on survivors' well-being.
- Enhanced efforts should be made to in order to include QoL assessment in routine clinical practice. Engaging clinicians in using QoL assessments, potentially by means of electronic administration, as well as broadening the interpretation of their scores into the clinical field, might facilitate incorporation.
- Further efforts should elucidate to what extent QoL results are incorporated into management decisions, treatment recommendations, and patients' education.
- Additional efforts should also be made to include QoL outcomes in clinical trials.
- The incorporation of QoL assessment into clinical and research practice has the potential to improve HCT outcomes.

References

Aaronson NK, Ahmedzai S, Bergman B, et al. The European Organization for Research and Treatment of Cancer QLQ-C30: a quality-of-life instrument for use in international clinical trials in oncology. J Natl Cancer Inst. 1993;85:365–76.

Cella D, Riley W, Stone A, et al. The Patient-Reported Outcomes Measurement Information System (PROMIS) developed and tested its first wave of adult self-reported health outcome item banks: 2005-2006. J Clin Epidemiol. 2010;63:1179–94.

Cella DF, Tulsky DS, Gray G, et al. The Functional Assessment of Cancer Therapy scale: development and validation of the general measure. J Clin Oncol. 1993;11:570–9.

Hinds PS, Nuss SL, Ruccione KS, et al. PROMIS pediatric measures in pediatric oncology: valid and clinically feasible indicators of patient-reported outcomes. Pediatr Blood Cancer. 2013;60:402–8.

Kurosawa S, Oshima K, Yamaguchi T, et al. Quality of life after allogeneic hematopoietic cell transplantation according to affected organ and severity of chronic graft-versus-host disease. Biol Blood Marrow Transplant. 2017;23:1749–58.

Landgraf JM, Abetz L, Ware JE. Child health questionnaire (CHQ): a user's manual. Boston: Health Institute, New England Medical Center; 1996.

McQuellon RP, Russell GB, Cella DF, et al. Quality of life measurement in bone marrow transplantation: development of the Functional Assessment of Cancer Therapy-Bone Marrow Transplant (FACT-BMT) scale. Bone Marrow Transplant. 1997;19:357–68.

Parsons SK, Shih MC, Mayer DK, Barlow SE, Supran SE, Levy SL, Greenield S, Kaplan SH. Preliminary psychometric evaluation of the Child Health Ratings Inventory (CHRIs) and Disease-Specific Impairment Inventory-Hematopoietic Stem Cell Transplantation (DSII-HSCT) in parents and children. Qual Life Res. 2005;14(86):1613–25.

Phipps S, Hinds PS, Channell S, et al. Measurement of behavioral, affective, and somatic responses to pediatric bone marrow transplantation: development of the BASES scale. J Pediat Oncol Nurs. 1994;11:109–17; discussion 118-119.

Pidala J, Anasetti C, Jim H. Health-related quality of life following haematopoietic cell transplantation: patient education, evaluation and intervention. Br J Haematol. 2010;148:373–85.

van Reenen M, Jansen B. EQ-5D-5L user guide. Basic information on how to use the EQ-5D-5L instrument [Internet]. 2015 [cited 2018 Jan 24]. https://euroqol.org/wp-content/uploads/2016/09/EQ-5D-5L_UserGuide_2015.pdf. Accessed 12 Feb 2018.

Russell KMW, Hudson M, Long A, et al. Assessment of health-related quality of life in children with cancer: consistency and agreement between parent and child reports. Cancer. 2006;106:2267–74.

Shaw BE, Lee SJ, Horowitz MM, et al. Can we agree on patient-reported outcome measures for assessing hematopoietic cell transplantation patients? A study from the CIBMTR and BMT CTN. Bone Marrow Transplant. 2016;51:1173–9.

US Food and Drug Administration. Guidance for industry: patient-reported outcome measures: use in medical product development to support labeling claims. US Department of Health and Human Services. Food and Drug Administration. 2009. https://www.fda.gov/downloads/drugs/guidances/ucm193282.pdf. Accessed 12 Feb 2018.

Varni JW, Burwinkle TM, Katz ER, et al. The PedsQL in pediatric cancer: reliability and validity of the Pediatric Quality of Life Inventory generic core scales, multidimensional fatigue scale, and cancer module. Cancer. 2002;94:2090–106.

Varni JW, Seid M, Kurtin PS. PedsQL 4.0: reliability and validity of the Pediatric Quality of Life Inventory version 4.0 generic core scales in healthy and patient populations. Med Care. 2001;39:800–12.

Ware JE, Kosinski M, Keller S. SF-36 physical and mental health summary scales: a user's manual. Boston: Health Institute; 1994.

Young TA, Mukuria C, Rowen D, et al. Mapping functions in health-related quality of life: mapping from two cancer-specific health-related quality-of-life instruments to EQ-5D-3L. Med Decis Mak. 2015;35:912–26.

Permissions

All chapters in this book were first published in TEBMTH, by Springer; hereby published with permission under the Creative Commons Attribution License or equivalent. Every chapter published in this book has been scrutinized by our experts. Their significance has been extensively debated. The topics covered herein carry significant findings which will fuel the growth of the discipline. They may even be implemented as practical applications or may be referred to as a beginning point for another development.

The contributors of this book come from diverse backgrounds, making this book a truly international effort. This book will bring forth new frontiers with its revolutionizing research information and detailed analysis of the nascent developments around the world.

We would like to thank all the contributing authors for lending their expertise to make the book truly unique. They have played a crucial role in the development of this book. Without their invaluable contributions this book wouldn't have been possible. They have made vital efforts to compile up to date information on the varied aspects of this subject to make this book a valuable addition to the collection of many professionals and students.

This book was conceptualized with the vision of imparting up-to-date information and advanced data in this field. To ensure the same, a matchless editorial board was set up. Every individual on the board went through rigorous rounds of assessment to prove their worth. After which they invested a large part of their time researching and compiling the most relevant data for our readers.

The editorial board has been involved in producing this book since its inception. They have spent rigorous hours researching and exploring the diverse topics which have resulted in the successful publishing of this book. They have passed on their knowledge of decades through this book. To expedite this challenging task, the publisher supported the team at every step. A small team of assistant editors was also appointed to further simplify the editing procedure and attain best results for the readers.

Apart from the editorial board, the designing team has also invested a significant amount of their time in understanding the subject and creating the most relevant covers. They scrutinized every image to scout for the most suitable representation of the subject and create an appropriate cover for the book.

The publishing team has been an ardent support to the editorial, designing and production team. Their endless efforts to recruit the best for this project, has resulted in the accomplishment of this book. They are a veteran in the field of academics and their pool of knowledge is as vast as their experience in printing. Their expertise and guidance has proved useful at every step. Their uncompromising quality standards have made this book an exceptional effort. Their encouragement from time to time has been an inspiration for everyone.

The publisher and the editorial board hope that this book will prove to be a valuable piece of knowledge for researchers, students, practitioners and scholars across the globe.

List of Contributors

Rainer Storb
Clinical Research Division, Fred Hutchinson Cancer Research Center and University of Washington, School of Medicine, Seattle, WA, USA

Alois Gratwohl
Hematology, Medical Faculty, University of Basel, Basel, Switzerland

Mohamad Mohty
Hematology, Hôpital St. Antoine, Sorbonne University, Paris, France

Jane Apperley
Centre for Haematology, Hammersmith Hospital, Imperial College London, London, UK

Irina Evseeva
Anthony Nolan, London, UK

Lydia Foeken
Word Marrow Donor Association (WMDA), Leiden, The Netherlands

Alejandro Madrigal
Anthony Nolan, London, UK UCL Cancer Institute, Royal Free Campus, London, UK

Walid Rasheed and Mahmoud Aljurf
King Faisal Specialist Hospital and Research Centre, Riyadh, Saudi Arabia

Dietger W. Niederwieser
University of Leipzig, Leipzig, Germany

Riccardo Saccardi
Department of Cellular Therapies and Transfusion Medicine, Careggi University Hospital, Florence, Italy

Eoin McGrath
European Society for Blood and Marrow Transplantation (EBMT), Barcelona, Spain

John A. Snowden
Department of Haematology, Sheffield Teaching Hospitals NHS Foundation Trust, University of Sheffield, Sheffield, UK

Simona Iacobelli
Department of Biology, University of Rome Tor Vergata, Rome, Italy EBMT, Leiden, The Netherlands

Liesbeth C. de Wreede
Department of Biomedical Data Sciences, Leiden University Medical Center, Leiden, The Netherlands DKMS Clinical Trials Unit, Dresden, Germany

Alessandro Aiuti
San Raffaele Telethon Institute for Gene Therapy (SR-TIGET)/Pediatric Immunohematology and Bone Marrow Transplantation Unit, IRCCS Ospedale San Raffaele, Vita-Salute San Raffaele University Milan, Italy

Serena Scala
San Raffaele Telethon Institute for Gene Therapy (SR-TIGET), IRCCS Ospedale San Raffaele, Milan, Italy

Christian Chabannon
Institut Paoli-Calmettes, Centre de Lutte Contre le Cancer, Marseille, France Université d'Aix-Marseille, Marseille, France Inserm BCT-1409, Centre d'Investigations Cliniques en Biothérapies, Marseille, France

Attilio Bondanza
Innovative Immunotherapies Unit, Division of Immunology, Transplantation and Infectious Diseases, University Vita-Salute San Raffaele and Ospedale San Raffaele Scientific Institute, Milan, Italy

Ulrike Koehl
University Hospital and Fraunhofer IZI, Leipzig, Germany

Andrea Hoffmann
Department of Orthopaedic Surgery, Laboratory of Biomechanics and Biomaterials, Hannover Medical School, Hannover, Germany

Antoine Toubert
University Paris Diderot and Hopital Saint Louis, Paris, France

Eric Spierings
Laboratory for Translational Immunology, University Medical Center, Utrecht, The Netherlands

Katharina Fleischhauer
Institute for Experimental Cellular Therapy, University Hospital, Essen, Germany

Jürgen Kuball
Department of Hematology, UMC, Utrecht, The Netherlands Laboratory of Translational Immunology, UMC, Utrecht, The Netherlands

Jaap Jan Boelens
Laboratory of Translational Immunology, UMC, Utrecht, The Netherlands Memorial Sloan Kettering Cancer Center, New York, NY, USA

Enric Carreras
Spanish Bone Marrow Donor Registry, Josep Carreras Foundation and Leukemia Research Institute, Barcelona, Catalunya, Spain Hospital Clinic Barcelona, Barcelona University Barcelona, Spain

Alessandro Rambaldi
Department of Hematology-Oncology, Azienda Socio Sanitaria Territoriale Papa Giovanni XXIII, Bergamo, Università Statale di Milano, Milano, Italy

Francis Ayuk
Department of Stem Cell Transplantation, University Medical Center Hamburg-Eppendorf (UKE), Hamburg, Germany

Adriana Balduzzi
Outpatient Hematology and Transplant Department, Clinica Pediatrica, Università degli Studi di Milano Bicocca, Ospedale San Gerardo, Monza, Italy

Arnon Nagler
Department of Medicine, Tel Aviv University, Tel-Hashomer, Israel Hematology Division, BMT and Cord Blood Bank, Chaim Sheba Medical Center, Tel-Hashomer, Israel

Avichai Shimoni
Bone Marrow Transplantation, Chaim Sheba Medical Center, Tel-Aviv University, Tel Hashomer, Israel

Norbert Claude Gorin
Department of Hematology and Cell Therapy, EBMT Paris Office, Hôpital Saint Antoine APHP, Paris, France Paris Sorbonne University, Paris, France

Kai Hübel
University of Cologne, Department of Internal Medicine, Cologne, Germany

Volker Witt
Department of Pediatric Hematology and Oncology St. Anna Kinderspital, Medical University Vienna, Vienna, Austria

Christina Peters
Stem Cell Transplantation Unit, St. Anna Children's Hospital, Vienna, Austria

Patrick Wuchter
Institute of Transfusion Medicine and Immunology, German Red Cross Blood Service Baden-Württemberg – Hessen, Medical Faculty Mannheim, Heidelberg University, Mannheim, Germany

Sergio Querol
Banc Sang i Teixits, Barcelona, Spain

Vanderson Rocha
University of São Paulo, São Paulo, Brazil University of Oxford, Oxford, UK

Michael Schumm, Peter Lang and Rupert Handgretinger
Department of Hematology/Oncology and General Pediatrics, Children's University Hospital, University of Tuebingen, Tuebingen, Germany

Peter Bader
Division for Stem Cell Transplantation and Immunology, University Hospital for Children and Adolescents, Goethe University Frankfurt am Main, Frankfurt, Germany

Montserrat Rovira and Maria Suárez-Lledó
HSCT Unit, Hematology Department, Hospital Clínic de Barcelona, University of Barcelona, Barcelona, Catalunya, Spain

Simone Cesaro
Pediatric Hematology Oncology, Azienda Ospedaliera Universitaria Integrata, Verona, Italy

Federica Minniti
Mother and Child Department, Ospedale della Donna e del Bambino, University of Verona, Verona, Italy

Hubert Schrezenmeier, Sixten Körper, Britta Höchsmann and Christof Weinstock
Institute of Clinical Transfusion Medicine and Immunogenetics Ulm, German Red Cross Blood Transfusion Service Baden-Württemberg-Hessen and University Hospital Ulm, Ulm, Germany Institute of Transfusion Medicine, University of Ulm, Ulm, Germany

Annic Baumgartner
Internal Medicine and Endcrinology/Diabetology/ Clinical Nutrition and Metabolism, Medical University Clinic of Kantonsspital Aarau, University of Basel, Aarau, Switzerland

Philipp Schuetz
Department of Endocrinology, Diabetes and Metabolism and Internal Medicine, Kantonsspital Aarau, University of Basel, Aarau, Switzerland

David Michonneau and Gérard Socié
Hematology/Transplantation, AP/HP Hospital St Louis, Paris, France University Paris VII, Denis Diderot, Paris, France INSERM UMR 1160, Paris, France

Francesca Bonifazi
Institute of Hematology "Seràgnoli", University Hospital S. Orsola-Malpighi, Bologna University, Bologna, Italy

Malgorzata Mikulska
Division of Infectious Diseases, Department of Health Sciences (DISSAL), IRCCS Ospedale Policlinico San Martino, University of Genova, Genova, Italy

Francesca Riccardi
Consultant Hematology Unit, Hemato-Oncology and SCT Pole, Istituto Giannina Gaslini, Genoa, Italy

Elio Castagnola
Infectious Diseases Unit, Department of Pediatrics, Istituto Giannina Gaslini, Genoa, Italy

Rafael de la Cámara
Department of Hematology, Hospital de la Princesa, Madrid, Spain

Alice Polomeni
Service d'Hématologie clinique et thérapie cellulaire, Hôpital Saint Antoine - Assistance Publique- Hôpitaux de Paris, Paris, France

Enrique Moreno
Department of Psychology, Asleuval (ValencianAssociation of Leukemia), Valencia, Spain

Frank Schulz-Kindermann
Pychooncological Outpatient Department, Institute of Medical Psychology, University Cancer Center Hamburg, University of Hamburg, Hamburg, Germany

Tiene Bauters
Pharmacy, Pediatric Hemato-Oncology and Stem Cell Transplantation, Ghent University Hospital, Ghent, Belgium

Aleksandra Babic
IOSI-Istituto Oncologico della Svizzera Italiana, OSG, Bellinzona, Switzerland

John Murray
Haematology and Transplant Unit, The Christie NHS Foundation Trust, Manchester, UK

Khaled El-Ghariani
Department of Hematology, Sheffield Teaching Hospitals Trust and NHSBT, The University of Sheffield, Sheffield, UK

Jean-Hugues Dalle
Department of Pediatric Hematology-Immunology, Hospital Robert-Debré, Assistance Publique-Hôpitaux de Paris, Paris Diderot University, Paris, France

Anna Barata
Department of Hematology, Hospital de la Santa Creu i Sant Pau, Universitat Autònoma de Barcelona, Barcelona, Spain
José Carreras Leukemia Research Institute, Barcelona, Spain

Heather Jim
Department of Health Outcomes and Behavior, Moffitt Cancer Center, Tampa, FL, USA

Index